TECHNOLOGY, DISEASE AND COLONIAL CONQUESTS,
SIXTEENTH TO EIGHTEENTH CENTURIES

HISTORY
OF WARFARE

General Editor

KELLY DEVRIES
Loyola College

Founding Editors

THERESA VANN
PAUL CHEVEDDEN

VOLUME 2

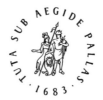

TUTA SUB AEGIDE PALLAS · 1683 ·

TECHNOLOGY, DISEASE AND COLONIAL CONQUESTS, SIXTEENTH TO EIGHTEENTH CENTURIES

Essays Reappraising the Guns and Germs Theories

EDITED BY

GEORGE RAUDZENS

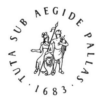

BRILL
LEIDEN · BOSTON · KÖLN
2001

Illustration on the cover: Major Robert Rogers, 1731-1795, led his Rogers' Rangers, American colonial troops and allied Indians, against the French and Indians between 1755 and 1760. He became famous for his long range raiding, scouting, and exploring expeditions, usually taking his frontier fighters further westward into the North American interior than other British forces. Some of his exploits became semi-legendary. Basically he remained an interesting but minor commander during the Anglo-French struggle for North America. But he did typify the use of Native American technologies and skills in warfare. (Illustration taken from *The Story of the Pioneers* by A.L. Mason, p. 177. Courtesy Barry Scott Library, Macquarie University).

This book is printed on acid-free paper.

Die Deutsche Bibliothek – CIP-Einheitsaufnahme

Technology, disease and colonial conquests, sixteenth to eighteenth centuries : essays reappraising the guns and germs theories / ed. by George Raudzens. – Leiden ; Boston ; Köln : Brill, 2001
(History of warfare ; Vol. 2)
ISBN 90–04–11745–8

Library of Congress Cataloging-in-Publication Data

Library of Congress Cataloging-in-Publication Data is also available

ISSN   1385–7827
ISBN   90 04 11745 8

PRINTED IN THE NETHERLANDS

CONTENTS

LIST OF FIGURES

(Figure 8.1–8.6 following page 238)
Figure 8.1. A map of the birchbark country
Figure 8.2. The jade canoe "The Spirit of Haida Gwaii"
Figure 8.3. Dome-shaped lodge and three bark canoes
Figure 8.4. Encampment with conical lodges and canoe
Figure 8.5. Encampment among the islands of Lake Huron
Figure 8.6. Retreat along Lake St. Clair

LIST OF CONTRIBUTORS

Jeremy Black is a Professor of History at the University of Exeter, UK. His recent publications include *War and the World, 1450–2000*, Yale University Press, 1998; *European Warfare 1660–1815*, Yale University Press, 1994; and (as General Editor) *Atlas of World History*, Dorling Kindersley, 1999.

Francis Brooks, PhD, is a retired Senior Lecturer in History at Flinders University, South Australia. His recent publications include "Motecuzoma Xocoyotl, Hernán Cortés, and Bernal Diaz del Castillo: The Construction of an Arrest", *Hispanic American Historical Review* 75(2), 1995, 149–183; and "Revising the Conquest of Mexico: Smallpox, Sources, and Populations", *Journal of Interdisciplinary History* 24(1), 1993, 1–29.

David Cahill, PhD, is a Queen Elizabeth II Research Fellow at the University of New South Wales, Australia, in the Department of Spanish and Latin American Studies. His recent publications include *Hapsburg Peru: Images, Imagination and Memory*, Liverpool University Press, 2000 (jointly with Peter Bradley); and *The Inca and Corpus Christi: The Feast of Santiago in Colonial Cuzco*, CEDLA, Amsterdam, 1999.

Lawrence Clayton is a Professor of History at the University of Alabama, USA. His recent publications include *A History of Modern Latin America*, Harcourt, Brace, 1999 (jointly with Michael Conniff); *Los EE.UU y el Perú: 1800–1995*, Centro Peruano de Estudios Internaciones y Xerox del Peru, 1998; and *Peru and the United States: The Condor and the Eagle*, University of Georgia Press, 1999.

Bruce Hodgins is a Professor Emeritus of Trent University, Canada, and currently Visiting Professor of Canadian Studies at Duke University, USA. He is co-author of *The Temagami Experience*, University of Toronto Press, 1989 (jointly with Jamie Benidickson) and has published extensively on the history of the Canadian North, Aboriginal peoples, Federalism and Canoes.

David McNab, PhD, is a public historian at the Department of Native Studies, Trent University, Canada, and currently a Claims Advisor for Nin.Da.Waab.Jig. Bkejwanong First Nation. His recent publications include *Earth, Water, Air and Fire: Studies in Canadian Ethnohistory*, Wilfrid Laurier University Press, 1998; and *Circles of Time: Aboriginal Land Rights and Resistance in Ontario*, Wilfrid Laurier University Press, 1999.

Linda Newson is a Professor of Geography at King's College London. She specialises in the impact of early Spanish colonial rule on indigenous peoples in Latin America and the Philippines. Her recent publications include *Life and Death in Early Colonial Ecuador*, University of Oklahoma Press, 1995; and she is currently writing a book on the early colonial Philippines.

George Raudzens is a former Associate Professor of Modern History at Macquarie University, Australia, and is currently Honorary Research Fellow there. His publications include *The British Ordnance Department and Canada's Canals*, Wilfrid Laurier University Press, 1979; *Empires, Europe and Globalization, 1492–1788*, Sutton, Stroud, 1999.

Dale Standen is a Professor of History at Trent University, Canada. His recent publications include *Gin Das Winan: Documenting Aboriginal History in Ontario. A Symposium at Bkejwanong, Walpole Island First Nation, September 23, 1994*, The Champlain Society, 1996 (as joint editor with David McNab); and "François Chalet and the French Trade at the Posts of Niagara and Frontenac, 1742–1747," in David Buisseret (ed.), *France in the New World: Proceedings of the Twenty-Second Meeting of the French Colonial Historical Society, Poitiers, 1996*, Michigan State University Press, 1998.

Armstrong Starkey is a Professor of History at Adelphi University, New York. His recent publications include *European and Native American Warfare, 1675–1815*, UCL and University of Oklahoma Presses, 1998. He is particularly interested in the cultural background of eighteenth century warfare and has contributed articles on this subject to the Journal of Military History and War and Society.

INTRODUCTION

George Raudzens

The European colonial conquests in the period between Columbus and industrialization were until the 1960s popularly explained as having been enabled by racial and ethnic superiorities. The expansionists were superior and the native people of the other continents were inferior. Thus it was considered that advanced cultures and improved human beings had replaced backward cultures and undesirable primitive folk. By the 1990s these main explanations had been replaced by much improved alternative scenarios. History students and "general readers" now mostly consider that this "Expansion of Europe", the linking together of all the continents and peoples of the planet which we at the present time call "globalization"—and which is arguably the most important change in the condition of humanity after the introduction of agriculture in pre-history and before industrialization—was caused mainly by two powerful fortuitous factors: Western European combat advantage based on guns; and the impact of epidemic disease on New World populations lacking Eurasian immunities. So it is thought that the colonial conquerors did have two superiorities: the arquebuses, muskets and cannons which gave them unmatched firepower; and the capability of carrying without harm to themselves Old World epidemic diseases, like smallpox, which killed off millions of susceptible potential resistance fighters in the New World.

The historians most responsible for converting this generation to the "guns and germs" theories were led by William H. McNeill, who argued for both things; Carlo Cipolla, who stressed the guns and also added ships; Geoffrey Parker, who popularized the "Military Revolution" theory of superior European combat powers; Alfred Crosby, who best argued the case for epidemic devastations among "virgin soil" populations lacking immunities; and Jared Diamond, the most recent and possibly most widely read synthesisers of the "guns and germs" combination.[1] These "great interpreters" have

---

[1] William H. McNeill, *Plagues and Peoples* (New York: Doubleday, 1977), and *The*

many precursors, supporters, and disciples; and these are noted in the pages of this book. They were "great" because they produced generalizations simple enough yet sufficiently convincing to facilitate effective communication of historical knowledge in ways which maximize consensus. They have expanded our common historical consciousness.

To do this, however, they have also had to oversimplify and distort. The main body of specialist historians over the last two generations have sometimes seemed to be fragmenting historical knowledge so finely as to preclude comments about the main causes of anything; causes too often appear as sum totals of all possible complexities. The quantity of specialist publications expands exponentially despite recent signs of attrition in tertiary history departments. Much of this is beyond the interests or capabilities of non-specialist readers, who cling to broad concepts like "guns and germs". But many of these specialists also bring back insights from their detailed complexities to the wider perspectives of big generalizations. They use their specialities to qualify, modify, and improve the plausibility of older views. The eight essays of this volume, thus, all present different sets of details about key aspects of the colonial conquests which challenge the plausibility of the "guns and germs" theories. None reject the importance of such broad causes, and indeed emphasise the ongoing validity of parts of these generalizations. But all argue that these big theories are oversimplified and that other causes must be added which were from time to time more important than "guns and germs" by themselves. The objective of this work as a whole is to refine and improve the big generalizations historians must make in order to reach the widest possible audience, among themselves and beyond themselves.

Jeremy Black leads off by taking on Michael Roberts' and Geoffrey Parker's "Military Revolution" concepts. He has famously wrestled with the "Revolution" in many other places. Here he updates his arguments, setting the standard of criticism for the other seven con-

---

Pursuit of Power. Technology, Armed Forces and Society Since AD 1000 (Chicago: University of Chicago Press, 1982); Carlo Cipolla, *Guns and Sails in the Early Phase of European Expansion 1400–1700* (London: Collins, 1965); Geoffrey Parker, *The Military Revolution. Military Innovation and the Rise of the West 1500–1800* (Cambridge: Cambridge University Press, 1988); Alfred W. Crosby, *Ecological Imperialism. The Biological Expansion of Europe, 900–1900* (Cambridge: Cambridge University Press, 1986), and Jared Diamond, *Guns, Germs, and Steel. The Fate of Human Societies* (New York: W.W. Norton, 1997).

tributors. First, he accepts that the "Revolution" did have strong effects both in Europe and overseas. Guns, firepower, fortifications, and military and naval efficiencies did indeed help Europeans in combat with non-Europeans. But not always, everywhere, and against everybody. The context of the combats and the character of the opposition often precluded European ascendancy. Only some Europeans, those of the Atlantic regions, deployed successful firepower advantages overseas from time to time; other Europeans did not. Their motives were often as important in producing successful conquests as their war technologies and techniques. So, yes, the "Military Revolution" helped in colonial conquests, but other causes—opposition, time and place, and motivation—were just as important.

I follow these critiques by looking specifically at four colonizing projects: Hispaniola from 1493; Virginia from 1607; New France from 1608; and New England from 1620—which became the most important bases for the subsequent take-overs of the largest New World regions, with the most numerous indigenous populations. Noting in each case that during the critical foundation stages—when the native people had the numbers advantage and best chances of driving the invaders back into the Atlantic—disease outbreaks probably hurt the invaders the most. I go on to show that while there was warfare in every case, with European firepower advantage in evidence, in fact the extent of combat was not large. In each case the continuing flow of invading colonists migrating into the region was more dramatic in effect than battles. Within two decades of each settlement Europeans achieved numerical superiority over native Americans in the areas of continuous contact between the two groups. The logistical efficiency which kept the settlers coming and the motives which drove Europeans to attempt settlement seem at least as important as "Military Revolution" advantages.

Armstrong Starkey continues with an analysis of warfare between English colonists and Amerindians in an effort to compare combat effectiveness. In too many cases, instead of Europeans outfighting Amerindians, things turned out quite the reverse. In the period from 1513 to 1815 there are repeated instances of superior native American combat prowess, often against odds. In terms of endurance, tactics, and individual combat skills Amerindian warriors were generally better than European colonists, and indeed, as is exemplified by the 1755 defeat of Braddock's redcoats, better than Europe's finest professional "Military Revolution" soldiers with their numerical advantages. Not only did the warriors of eastern North America adopt improved flintlock and rifled guns more quickly than the settlers, they learned to shoot them more accurately. They provided the invaders with the tactical models for successful woodland combat using shoulder guns. The Europeans, however, did have long-term numbers and supply advantages that evened the odds, especially at times when successful Amerindian resistance campaigns collapsed for lack of gunpowder. Successful combat in this region was an amalgamation of European material resource superiority with Amerindian skills and methods. When colonists and Amerindians fought as allies they were at their most effective. Certainly the invaders relied on Amerindian militarisms as well as European ones in order to conquer both their Amerindian and rival European opponents. Learning Amerindian war skills was vital to success. Thus invader capacity to adapt to the ways of the natives as well as the advantages of better and more plentiful material resources often outweighed "Military Revolution" factors in the successful colonial conquests.

For David Cahill in his study of the Inca "conquest", "Military Revolution" advantages on the Spanish side—as well as disease impacts—decline in importance close to becoming irrelevant. While popularizers like Jared Diamond focus intensely on the bloody capture of Atahualpa at Cajamarca in 1532 by Pizarro's 168 conquistadors as a prime example of the "guns" thesis, Cahill points out that most of the Inca élite actually welcomed the Spanish invaders as liberators and willingly settled down with them to share rule over Andean farmers and miners. Despite violent episodes, the first three hundred years of Spanish "rule" in the Andes was a partnership with indigenous "kurakas" and caciques who continued to control labour allocations and tax collection. Spanish town-dwellers collected a share and interfered only by promoting Hispanicization and Christianization. The dominant process here was accommodation, or amalgamation, rather than subjugation. The Andean cultures absorbed Hispanic features but the colonists learned to live with Andean ways. Only very gradually, toward the end of the eighteenth century, did the indigenous élites begin to lose their local dominance to mestizo and Creole newcomers of a more Europeanized type. In this long process there was nothing like sudden and forcible subjugation by the "invaders". Perhaps there was only a slow infiltration. But in any case neither guns nor germs help to explain this major episode of European colonial take-over.

Francis Brooks moves on to the effects of disease in the most dramatic of all the colonial conquests, the defeat of the Aztecs by the conquistadors of Cortes. Reiterating earlier criticisms of the credibility of the 1520 smallpox epidemic at Tenochtitlan as a major reason for Spanish victory, he then reviews the whole Western Hemisphere "virgin soil" epidemics historiography and finds much of it flawed or obsolete. It is unlikely that huge epidemics with massive mortalities swept at great speed up and down the two continents just in time to annihilate so many Amerindians that the remnants were too shattered and too few to defend their lands against handfuls of Europeans. The historical demographers of the last generation calculated immense population sizes for the Americas before 1492 on the basis of very little verifiable evidence. Thus epidemics must have killed millions. But so far there is no way to verify such demographic speculation. Indeed, the available evidence supports smaller estimates rather than larger ones. Further, World Health Organization findings about smallpox in 1988 indicate that this disease, nominated by killer disease advocates such as Alfred Crosby as the main destroyer, could not have caused huge fast-moving death rates. So neither population estimates research nor disease research supports the germ theory. Brooks urges a return to the contact details surrounding the invasion—to interactivities which are better explanations for the Aztec subordination process.

Linda Newson extends these approaches chronologically and geographically. Her focus is on the mortality rates of post-conquest indigenous societies under Spanish "rule" in the Mexican and Andean highlands (where both the largest native populations were located and where there was especially intense interaction with Spanish colonizers), and the Philippines (where the people were scattered and contacts were more limited in time and space). In the populous highlands there were large mortality rates early in the "conquest" period, with demographic recovery within some three generations. In the Philippines initial mortality rates were low, but long-term rates tended to continue at higher levels. These rates could not have been caused by "virgin soil" epidemics, where the indigenes, lacking Eurasian immunities, were overwhelmed by new diseases from outside their worlds. The latest research indicates that there are no big differences in immune responses from one group of people—isolated or otherwise—to another. Instead, the incidence of epidemics and their seriousness were more likely to have been caused by the intensity of social, economic and life-style changes generated by contact with the colonizers. Environmental and social factors had bigger impacts on mortality than the types of diseases the Europeans indirectly imported into indigenous societies. Thus things like alterations to agricultural practices and labour demands in the mining regions could have precipitated sharp population reductions in the first post-colonization generation. Again, the context and character of the people who were "conquered" were more important than germs.

Although Lawrence Clayton concedes the importance of artillery as a conquest enabler, he moves away from the "Military Revolution" theory entirely and turns instead to other technologies—superior ships and navigation techniques. Assessing the reasons for the Portuguese and Spanish initiation of maritime expansion and imperialism, he concludes that ship technology and navigation skills were probably the biggest causal factors, but they were important only in a marginal and indirect way. They derived from the Iberian medieval context and the characteristics of Iberian economics, politics, and society. And these means for economic expansion—while sufficiently unique to outclass the maritime transport systems of every other culture that participated actively in sea-faring—were themselves inert without motives. The Iberians were also driven to expand by religious zeal, political and economic ambition, and opportunity. So ships—perhaps even a "maritime revolution"—were important. They were more important than guns or the "Military Revolution". But so were motives and opportunities.

David McNab, Bruce Hodgins and Dale Standen finish this critique by arguing that in some contexts, and specifically north-eastern North America up to the 1820s, European technology and technical skills were more than outbalanced by key native American technologies and skills. In the regions of the birch-tree, which coincided with the cores of both New France first and British Canada second, the people of the birch-bark canoes operated with this unique invention an inland communications system superior to all others until the advent of steam-power and railways. European colonizers controlled communications up to the tidal reaches of Atlantic-coast rivers with their sailing-ships. Beyond these, however, the Amerindians dominated. These native people had a watercraft which Europeans could only borrow and enlarge a bit but with which Amerindians—and a few adopted European allies—could travel the north-eastern North American waterways and forest-lands more efficiently and quickly than anybody else. The canoe dominated inter-Amerindian relations, and relations between Amerindians and Europeans, in cultural exchange, trade, politics, and war. More often than not it gave the Amerindians the advantage over the colonizers. Thus, first the French and then both the French and the British relied on Amerindian trading and war partnerships to make progress in inland expansion or against each other. In some ways it was the Amerindian allies which controlled the French rather than vice versa. Nothing could move very far without canoeists. The main Algonquian and related Ohio tribes survived as independent societies for three centuries because they in fact had the better communications system. European allies were in some ways like naturalised Amerindians because of these transport superiorities. At the least canoes and European sailing ships together were the main factors shaping rates and patterns of colonizer expansion.

All eight contributors seriously qualify aspects of the "guns and germs" generalizations. All stress specific time and place contexts and the characteristics of the opponents of colonial conquerors as key additional influences. Most also emphasize the importance of long-range communication control systems. And most stress motivation as a basic driving force. There are many other criticisms to make and improvements to suggest in this quest for larger but better generalizations. Hopefully this book is a useful start.

1. EUROPEAN OVERSEAS EXPANSION AND THE MILITARY REVOLUTION*

Jeremy Black

Any consideration of the impact of the changes summarized as the Military Revolution on European expansion in the early modern period requires an assessment both of the extent of this expansion and of the nature of the Military Revolution. This essay considers alternative conceptualizations of European expansion in order to offer a critique of the dominant current notion of the global dimension of this Revolution. An approach that, instead, focuses on ideological factors is adopted. This approach, however, is interpreted flexibly. In considering and emphasising the will to deploy resources and to conquer, it is necessary to relate attitudes to means and local opportunities, in order to avoid a misleading assumption that "the West" could conquer whenever it was minded; and that it was all a matter of people making up their minds.

The essay addresses the question of the nature and role of relative military capability in the long early modern period, that from the late fifteenth century to the close of the eighteenth. This question has frequently been discussed in terms of technological determinism, with an emphasis on the role of firepower. Thus, both European conquest and the Military Revolution have been presented as aspects of an early-modern gunpowder revolution, most profitably in the work of Geoffrey Parker. Far from concentrating simply on technology, Parker, like Michael Roberts, argued that weapons (technology) were important as they were marshalled by doctrine and cultural habit of use (technique) and drew connections between military technology and techniques and larger historical consequences.

Especially if the global geographical span of Parker, rather than the narrower European focus of Roberts, is adopted, then European

* I am grateful for the comments of Tom Arnold, Gerry Bryant, Jan Glete, Harald Kleinschmidt, Peter Marshall, Douglas Peers, George Raudzens and Peter Wilson on an earlier draft. I have benefited from the opportunity to present papers at the University of North Carolina-Greensboro, and at the College of William and Mary.

overseas conquest can be seen as *the* Military Revolution, and it is possible to suggest that it was revolutionary in cause, course and consequence, and the aspect of military development that was most important on the global scale. Such an approach classically focuses on the arrival and establishment of Portuguese naval power in the Indian Ocean and the Spanish conquests of Aztec Mexico and Inca Peru, all of which were apparently able to meet these criteria. Their chronological near-congruence, in the period 1500–40, both dates this Military Revolution, or aspect of the Military Revolution, and ensures that arguments of the significance of any one of these events are supported by the presence of the others, the whole contributing to a sense of major change. This approach can be expanded to encompass changes in Christendom's apparent ability to fight the Turks, specifically the contrasts between the Christian failures of 1521–6 (Belgrade, Rhodes and Mohacs) and the successes of 1565–71 (Malta, Lepanto and the length of time Szigetvár held out in 1566).[1]

The standard account of the Military Revolution, however, has been challenged by much of the research produced over the last decade.[2] There has been an emphasis on the variety of factors that contributed to European success, and the nature and extent of this success have also been qualified. The net effect is, first, to ensure that what occurred appears as more complex, and, second, to throw doubt on established patterns of causality. This creates the problem of establishing a new synthesis and of addressing the tension between complexity and the desire for a synthesis, or even simplification, both for its own sake and in order to provide a stage in military history. Unless such a synthesis can be provided by military historians, there is a danger, first, that military history will excessively focus on detail, without the benefit of sufficient contextualization, and, second, that dated and misleading syntheses will be offered. They will be provided either by non-military historians, who have a general tendency both to offer misleadingly structural accounts and to demilitarize military history, or by military scholars who fail to match new conceptualization to fresh empirical research.

---

[1] M. Roberts, *The Military Revolution, 1560–1660* (Belfast, 1956); G. Parker, *The Military Revolution. Military Innovation and the Rise of the West, 1500–1800* (2nd edn., Cambridge, 1996); T. Arnold, "War in sixteenth-century Europe: Revolution and Renaissance", in J.M. Black (ed.), *European Warfare 1450–1815* (London, 1999).

[2] J.M. Black, *War and the World. Military Power and the Fate of Continents 1450–2000* (New Haven, 1998).

The comparative dimension offers a fruitful approach towards a synthesis. It is useful to relate developments in one particular area to those in other regions, to consider land alongside naval warfare, and to provide a global context. Such an approach, of course, faces serious problems.

In particular, there is the danger that a comparative or contextual stance will lead to a hierarchy of military strength, capability and achievement based on the misleading idea that there is a commonality of challenge and an agreed basis that can be established and employed in the judgment of success. In addition, there is a risk that such an approach might lead to a teleology of military progress that is as misleading in its judgment of military success, as it is crude in its understanding of governmental, social and cultural relationships. Instead, there is a need to understand that the plurality of military options and trajectories on the global scale reflect not some hierarchy of success in diffusion and acculturation, but, instead, a complex process of adaptation to a multiplicity of circumstances.

Such a caveat may seem to undermine any process of contextualization, and the very complexity of the task, methodologically and in terms of material, both extent and lacunae, is forbidding. Nevertheless, such a process is still valuable. The practice of comparison is a reminder of military options that forecloses determinism. It adds point to understandings of contemporary debates and, instead, encourages the fruitful modern exercise of counterfactualism. In the last half millennium the shrinking of the world (or looked at differently the expansion of some of its regions), gave particular force to the issue of comparison, not least through the bringing together of hitherto separate military systems and through a greater potential for the diffusion of developments.

Military history is commonly teleological in character, and that helps to account for the popularity of the notion of the early-modern Military Revolution. It takes a role akin to that of the transition from feudalism to capitalism in the Marxist model. If the concept of a Military Revolution did not exist, it would be necessary to devise an alternative in order to explain major shifts that have been discerned, both in terms of state formation within Europe (and, in some theories, elsewhere) and in the world economy. Force explains, and is the *modus operandi* of, what has been seen as a politics and economics of control and expropriation. The Military Revolution apparently fulfils the need for an abrupt and violent close to medievalism and the Middle Ages.

In addition, the Military Revolution is an aspect of the modernity and modernization discerned by many from the late fifteenth century. It is the counterpart of humanism, the Renaissance, printing, European exploration and the Protestant Reformation, the product of a new mental world. As such, it is challenged by arguments that the onset of modernity should be dated later, either to the eighteenth century, with its cult of secular progress, or the nineteenth, with the astonishing transformation in the productive and organizational capability of the Western world that is somewhat misleadingly described as the Industrial Revolution.

Military parallels to such a debate, and, in particular, to the issue of the later onset of modernity, would look not only at the empirical case for the crucial changes as occurring later than the sixteenth century, whether, for example, with flintlock, bayonet, and larger standing armies and navies in 1680–1730, or with the Revolutionary and Napoleonic period of 1792–1815, or with later, nineteenth-century, changes, but, also, at the wider intellectual, cultural, political and social contextualisation of war and armed force. Many of the accounts of conflict in the sixteenth, seventeenth and eighteenth centuries do not readily support the notion of a Military Revolution, understood in terms of a significant increase in European military effectiveness. Major-General John Richards recorded of the British siege of Valencia in May 1705: "our mortars could not be worst served . . . slow . . . they shot as ill as could be . . . the fuses were so ill made that . . . great many of them never burnt at all . . . length of time taking it has delayed us". Moving on to Alburquerque he was affected by the strength of the wall "of a prodigious hard matter, armed with square towers after the ancient manner".[3]

An alternative approach is to argue that many of the changes used to define the Military Revolution, or associated with it, such as larger armies, greater military expenditure, new tactics, and the *trace italienne*, all had medieval precedents.[4] From this perspective, the major

---

[3] Richards Diary, London, British Library, Stowe papers, Vol. 467, fols. 21–3. See also, for example, W. Roth, "L'affaire de Majorque", *Revue d'Histoire Diplomatique*, 96 (1972), 26.

[4] A. Ayton and J.L. Price, "The military revolution from a medieval perspective", in Ayton and Price (eds.), *The Medieval Military Revolution. State, Society and Military Change in Early Modern Europe* (London, 1998), p. 16. I have benefited from reading an unpublished paper by Kelly DeVries, "Was there a renaissance in warfare? Humanism and technological determinism, 1300–1559".

technological innovations in weaponry employed in the sixteenth century occurred earlier, in, or even prior to, the fifteenth century. There was only limited change in firearms technology during the sixteenth century, but an increase in numbers was important. The most sustained and imaginative criticism of the Parker thesis has indeed come from medievalists, although, in response, it can be suggested that their contribution really adds up to a prehistory of the Military Revolution. An analogy can be drawn with the argument that the Renaissance has to be discussed with reference to the achievements of Carolingian, Ottonian and/or twelfth-century Renaissances.

If long-term trends in the later Middle Ages are emphasized, it is unclear that subsequent European territorial and trans-oceanic expansion in any one period of say a half century can either be linked to a unique stage in European military development, or profitably employed in order to focus on a specific period of European military activity. This is even more the case if the evolutionary theories of many historians of technology are employed as models,[5] although Clifford Rogers has recently borrowed the notion of "punctuated equilibrium", an approach that promises to combine both incremental and revolutionary change.[6]

At the length available, this essay cannot hope to be a complete account of a subject that is anyway fast developing. It is important, however, to clarify the linked questions of the putative Military Revolution and the military dimensions of European conquest. First, it is helpful to re-examine the components of the Military Revolution, in particular from the perspective of European overseas conquest. Here, one faces the problem of categorization, namely which of the military changes in the period 1460–1660 are worthiest of note; whether, indeed, there was a staged or episodic early-modern Military Revolution and, if so, when it started and ended; and how far is it appropriate to think of a European military revolution that was different in type from military changes in other parts of the world? This is complicated by the need to consider whether to treat land and sea warfare separately or together.

---

[5] For an emphasis on an "evolutionary" approach to the "gunpowder revolution", B.S. Hall, *Weapons and Warfare in Renaissance Europe* (Baltimore, 1997).

[6] C.J. Rogers, "The military revolutions of the Hundred Years War", in Rogers (ed.), *The Military Revolution Debate. Readings on the Military Transformation of Early Modern Europe* (Boulder, Colorado, 1995), p. 77.

As far as both land and sea are concerned, it is necessary to focus, not on initial "discoveries", but on diffusion, the understanding and regularization of usage, and effective usage at that. From that perspective, it is pertinent to comment on the widespread dissemination of cannon and hand-held firearms in the sixteenth century. The cumulative firepower of European forces thus rose greatly, both on land and at sea, and both in Europe and overseas. A similar emphasis on sixteenth-century diffusion is appropriate for new-style fortifications, employing the *trace italienne*, which were essentially designed to thwart cannon. Whether these changes deserve the designation revolution is unclear. The effectiveness of new geometrical layouts in fortification are open to debate.

It is also unclear how best to evaluate the organizational changes of the period. It is uncertain whether terms such as bureaucratization are appropriate, but the growing role of the European state gradually replaced the semi-independent military entrepreneurs of early days, especially from the mid-seventeenth century. Furthermore, Europeans were well advanced in the field of international finance, enabling states, such as Spain in the sixteenth century, the United Provinces in the seventeenth, and Britain in the eighteenth, to finance their activities, in part, through a well-developed international credit network.

Aside from these questions, there is the issue of the effectiveness of the European military machine overseas, and the applicability there of the linked conceptualization of military change. It can be suggested, first, that there was no Military Revolution and, second, that, even if there was, it did not have a revolutionary effect overseas. This approach can be challenged at once with reference to the Portuguese in the Indian Ocean and the Spanish *conquistadores*. Yet, it is also possible to consider the latter as unique[7] and, in addition, to regard the trajectory and causation of naval success, both in the Indian Ocean and elsewhere, as separate. Alongside these successes, there were numerous European failures, in the New World and the Indian Ocean, as well as Africa.[8] Neither the weaponry nor the orga-

---

    [7] D.H. Peers (ed.), *Warfare and Empires. Contact and Conflict between European and non-European Military and Maritime Forces and Cultures* (Aldershot, 1997), p. xviii.
    [8] P. Powell, *Soldiers, Indians and Silver: The Northward Advance of New Spain, 1550–1600* (Berkeley, 1952); R.C. Padden, "Cultural change and military resistance in Araucanian Chile, 1550–1730", *Southwestern Journal of Anthropology* (1957), 103–21; M. Newitt,

nizational dimension of a European military revolution appeared as apparent a cause or aspect of relative capability in New England or Chile, West Africa or Mozambique, the Swahili coast of East Africa or the Persian Gulf, India or Sri Lanka, Java, Timor or the Amur Valley, as might be implied by the literature on the revolution. It is all too easy to run together a few episodes and create a paradigm that can then be extrapolated.

European failures qualify any account of success, but the fact that it was Europeans pressing against the indigenes of the far continents, and not vice-versa was and is important, while, more generally, it is unclear whether an aggregate measure of achievement is more pertinent than a focus on individual failures, or successes. Such a measure, whether or not used to support the notion of a Military Revolution, fails, however, to address the multifaceted nature of European expansion and military activity. It is dangerous to read from a particular success or failure in order to produce a general account of relative capability.

This is even more the case if the military activity of other expanding global powers outside Europe in this period are concerned. If capability is discussed in terms of particular successes and these successes are then "explained", that cannot, nevertheless, create an explanatory model, because it fails to account for expansion such as that of the Ottomans, the Safavids, the Mughals, the Mongols (in the sixteenth century), Adal, Toungoo, and the Manchus.[9] The great event in sixteenth-century India was the creation of the Mughal empire, not the expansion of Portuguese power. In some cases, it is possible to accommodate such successes to those of the Europeans. Thus, for example, it is possible to incorporate the Ottoman overrunning of Syria, Palestine and Egypt in 1516–17 or the Moroccan conquest of Timbuktu in 1591 or the Satsuma invasion of the Ryuku islands in 1609,[10] into a model that otherwise focuses on

---

Portuguese Settlement on the Zambezi (London, 1973); A. Hess, *The Forgotten Frontier. A History of the Sixteenth-Century Ibero-African Frontier* (Chicago, 1978); R. Law, "'Here is no resisting the country:" The realities of power in Afro-European relations of the West African Slave Coast", *Itinerario*, 18 (1994), 51–2; J. Hemming, *Red Gold: The Conquest of the Brazilian Indians, 1500–1760* (2nd edn., London, 1995), pp. 72–3, 78–9, 90–6.

[9] J.M. Black (ed.), *War in the Early-Modern World 1450–1815* (London, 1999).

[10] D.E. Streusand, *The Formation of the Mughal Empire* (Delhi, 1989); U. Suganuma, "Sino-Liuqiu and Japanese-Liuqiu relations in early modern times", *Journal of Asian History*, 31 (1997), 53.

the *conquistadores*. The "Gunpowder Revolution" may have been important for the early Spanish conquests in the New World (which were achieved with *very* few Spaniards), but they were not in principle very different from other cases, both earlier and contemporaneous, of warriors conquering agricultural societies with much larger populations.

It is unclear how far it is appropriate to distinguish between a European Military Revolution in which new ways of war were invented (around the opportunity presented by firearms), and Ottoman, Mughal, or other non-European use of firearms in accordance with William McNeill's model of gunpowder empires.[11] It can be argued that it was only in Europe that there was a sustained transformation of the culture of war. In contrast, in Ottoman Turkey, and Morocco firearms were adopted as useful force multipliers, as more or differently useful weapons, but the underlying culture of warfare remained the same. Such an approach is important if it is argued that the central issue of the Military Revolution is that of analyzing and comparing European and non-European military institutions and cultures, rather than weapons. The effectiveness of any European transformation of the culture of war in the sixteenth century should not be exaggerated however.

The gunpowder approach to early-modern military history is less commonly employed to focus on non-European powers, not least because, in their case, naval warfare cannot be readily brought in in support of the analysis: the Europeans were more prominent at sea than on land. Seaborne "plunder and trade" empires had existed before the Portuguese intrusion in the Indian Ocean, both there and in the Mediterranean. What was new in the Portuguese achievement was the vast distance from the base to the area of activity. Here guns, new sailing technology and ships built to fight with guns were important, as guns did not require food and water on long expeditions and were not vulnerable to disease. Technological superiority facilitated both attack on and protection of limited objects: ships, forts and islands.[12]

---

[11] W.H. McNeill, *The Age of Gunpowder Empires 1450–1800* (Washington, 1989).

[12] C.M. Cipolla, *Guns and Sails and Empires. Technological Innovation and the Early Phases of European Expansion, 1400–1700* (London, 1965); R.C. Smith, *Vanguard of Empire: Ships of Exploration in the Age of Columbus* (Oxford, 1993).

Furthermore, the use of individual episodes of gunpowder success in order to construct a general theory of military effectiveness, capability, and the rationale for change, is as questionable outside Europe as in the case of the European powers and, anyway, in part, rests on a failure to understand these episodes. Thus, for example, the role of gunpowder firepower in the Ottoman victory over the Safavids at Chaldiran in 1514 is a matter of controversy. The Ottoman cannon were in part important because, once chained together, they formed a barrier to Safavid cavalry charges. It is unclear whether Ottoman firepower or numerical superiority was more important.[13]

An important variable in any discussion is provided by the quality of the firearms. This can be divided into first the refinement of the technology over time during the period 1350–1800, in other words the improvement of the basic models, and of the gunpowder, and, secondly, the age of the firearms in the hands of the soldiers and their maintenance. In the 1750s and 1760s many Indian mercenary troops came into the service of the British East India Company with their own weapons which Company officers considered to be nearly worthless.

It is also necessary to consider how best to incorporate into any thesis of the global impact of firearms conquests by armies that were not infantry-based or the forces of settled societies and "advanced", bureaucratic states. This is true, for example, of Uzbek pressure on Persia in the sixteenth century, the Afghan conquest of Persia in the 1720s, and the successful invasions of India by Nadir Shah of Persia and by the Afghans in 1738–9 and 1757–61 respectively. The continued role and impact of cavalry in Asia, savanna Africa and Eastern Europe has been seriously underrated. Any consideration of such campaigns requires a re-evaluation of comparative global military advantage and capacity and also reopens the question of how best to measure success, whether, in particular, conquest is the best definition.

Successful raiding, indeed, can be seen as a corollary of European coastal positions, both serving as the basis for trade in a situation where trade and tribute were not polar opposites. The slave trades indicated this relationship. They served the requirements of more powerful societies, but were also dependent on a measure of local

---

[13] R. Savory, *Iran under the Safavids* (Cambridge, 1980), pp. 41–4.

support. This was more apparent in the case of the Europeans in Africa[14] than of their Asian and Arab counterparts, but was also true of the latter.

A rebuttal of the concentration on gunpowder conflict, let alone a simple theory of gunpowder triumphalism, does not, however, have to extend to a denial of any role for such weaponry. In particular, it is possible to draw attention to two different, but probably related, developments; first, the increase in aggregate power flowing from the availability of such weaponry and of troops that were trained to use it, and, second, the training, systematization and industrial production that stemmed from the large-scale deployment of such weaponry on land and sea. The second development, in many respects, is the organizational definition of the Military Revolution. Such a definition is a cultural account that avoids some of the critique of technological determinism associated with the emphasis on weapons. Instead, there is a desire to understand the nature and context of weapons systems.

It can be argued that European forces acquired an edge in keeping cohesion and control in battle for longer than their adversaries, and that this permitted more sophisticated tactics in moving and withholding units on the battlefield and more effective fire. These techniques were developed in conflict between European forces. A British participant in Wolfe's victory over the French outside Québec in 1759 recorded,

> About 9 o'clock the French army had drawn up under the walls of the town, and advanced towards us briskly and in good order. We stood to receive them; they began their fire at a distance, we reserved ours, and as they came nearer fired on them by divisions, this did execution and seemed to check them a little, however they still advanced pretty quick, we increased our fire without altering our position, and, when they were within less than an hundred yards, gave them a full fire, fixed our bayonets, and under cover of the smoke the whole line charged.[15]

European forces tended to be able to advance, withdraw and retreat in a disciplined fashion. This ability can be linked to more general issues of administrative and political capability, can be related to the

---

[14] J. Thornton, *Warfare in Atlantic Africa 1450–1800* (London, 1999).

[15] Journal, possibly by Henry Fletcher, Providence, John Carter Brown Library, Codex Eng. 41.

impact of a set of intellectual suppositions centred on Neostoicism,[16] and can be matched by a consideration of the deployment and employment of warships in battle.

This account has many strengths as a discussion of developments within Europe, but is less useful for any consideration of relative capability on the global scale, because it is not clear how to assess organizational effectiveness in a comparative context. In addition, there is a danger that any such assessment will rest on a primitivization of non-European traditions, one that ranges from Siberian tribes to Ottoman armies. Oriental forces appear as "hordes", a Turkish word borrowed by Europeans better to understand the identity of a non-European war-making culture, but one employed to portray undifferentiated masses apparently unable to act in a planned fashion. It would be erroneous to suggest that the deep and real differences observable between European and Ottoman war-making were simply a problem of European perception, an example of "Orientalism". To point out that Ottoman war culture never shrugged off some of the cultural values of the steppe, especially horsemanship and archery, is not to engage in a primitivization of that culture. Yet, too little is known about activities on the battlefield and on campaign to establish the case for any marked lack of organizational effectiveness on their part. It appears, at the very least, to be an exaggeration.[17]

Similarly, it is possible to offer a positive evaluation of the organisation, conduct and effectiveness of African forces. In seventeenth- and eighteenth-century coastal West Africa local forces were perfectly capable of organising their armed forces in ways comparable to those of Europeans. In Angola, in the sixteenth and seventeenth centuries, the Portuguese were successful only when supported by local troops. Tactical and military-administrative developments have been noted in other contexts, for example eighteenth-century Burma.[18]

---

[16] P. Wilson, "European warfare 1450–1815", in J.M. Black (ed.), *War in the Early Modern World*, pp. 193–4.

[17] C. Finkel, *The Administration of Warfare: Ottoman Campaigns in Hungary, 1593–1606* (Vienna, 1988); R. Murphey, *Ottoman Warfare 1500–1700* (London, 1998), especially, pp. 85–129; G. Ágoston, "Habsburgs and Ottomans: Defense, military change and shifts in power", *Turkish Studies Association Bulletin*, 22 (1998), 126–41.

[18] R.A. Kea, "Firearms and warfare on the gold and slave coasts from the sixteenth to the nineteenth centuries", *Journal of African History*, 12 (1971), 185–213, and *Settlements, Trade, and Politics in the Seventeenth-Century Gold Coast* (Baltimore, 1982); R. Law, *The Oyo Empire c.1600–c.1836: A West African Imperialism in the Era of*

Cultural and temperamental differences were important in both strategy and tactics, but there is no satisfactory methodology for the subject. One approach is Darwinian: warfare was such a competitive activity, sometimes a matter of life and death for states, dynasties and communities that a force is arguably always driving to improve performance, even against tradition or fashion. The more continuous war is the more powerful this factor is likely to be, especially with the dissemination of knowledge through the spread of military literature where methods and theories are tested against experience. This approach can be employed to argue that Europe acquired a competitive advantage because of the frequency of war there in the period 1494–1815. Aside, however, from a lack of clarity as to whether the model is appropriate, namely the question whether competitive "evolutionary" pressures are indeed dominant in military culture and development, and, if so, likely to lead to greater comparative capability, it is also unclear that Europe was more violent than, for example, India, Central Asia, or West Africa. Similar socio-political pressures can be seen in these areas. The concept of "social reproduction", an analysis suggesting that African states and warriors fought to sustain their position,[19] can also be applied to European states with the argument that absolutist societies were by their nature war machines.[20]

The political corollary of the military primitivization of the "non-West" is the argument about the frequent importance of disunity, factionalism and treachery among non-European peoples facing European context. This has been seen as particularly important in India and North America, greatly helping European penetration, conquest and subsequent control, and challenging any analysis in terms of "the West versus the Rest"; but the European colonial pow-

---

Atlantic Slave Trade (Oxford, 1977) and "Warfare on the West African slave coast, 1650–1850", in R.B. Ferguson and N.L. Whitehead (eds.), *War in the Tribal Zone: Expanding States and Indigenous Warfare* (Santa Fé, 1992), pp. 103–26; J. Thornton, "The art of war in Angola, 1575–1680", *Comparative Studies in Society and History*, 30 (1988), 360–78; V. Lieberman, "Political consolidation in Burma under the early Konbaung Dynasty 1750–c. 1820", *Journal of Asian History*, 30 (1996), 162, 168.

[19] R.L. Roberts, "production and reproduction of warrior states: Segu Bambara and Segu Tokolor, c. 1712–1890", *International Journal of African Historical Studies*, 13 (1980), 389–419, esp. pp. 400–19.

[20] J. Schümpeter, "Zur Soziologie der Imperialismus", *Archiv für Sozialwissenschaft und Sozialpolitik*, 56 (1918–19); J.M. Black, *Why Wars Happen* (London, 1998), pp. 32, 66–70, 98, 101–2.

ers were themselves divided and willing to arm and support the local opponents of their European rivals. They did so in both West Africa and North America in the seventeenth century, with the Portuguese and French abandoning initial refusals to sell firearms in response to Dutch willingness to do so.[21] In 1741 Etienne de Silhouette, a French agent in Britain, reacted with alarm to the news that the British were arming Negroes in order to use them against Spanish-ruled Cuba. He felt this might be very dangerous for all American Europeans, but argued that the British were too obsessed by their goals to consider the wider implications.[22] Munitions continued to be regularly supplied to non-European forces. In the late eighteenth century Burma obtained cannon and muskets from British, French and Muslim suppliers.

More generally, the "cultural" approach to military difference suffers from the danger of hindsight, from reading back the successes of the West and the westernization of military organization in parts of the world in the nineteenth century. Cultural issues are not therefore less important, nor the cultural approach less relevant, but the emphasis on organization and other dimensions of military activity that can be considered in a cultural light is being asked to bear an excessive explanatory burden, and cannot be employed with adequate precision.

It is unclear how far this analysis should be used even in the case of relations with the Turks, possibly the best studied military "interaction" with Europe and one where a long timeframe for state to state conflict exists.[23] Alongside any emphasis on Turkish organisational obsolescence and its operational consequences, whether located in the wars with Austria of 1593–1606, 1663–4, 1683–99 or 1716–18, comes evidence of Turkish resilience and success, as in 1711–15, 1737–9 or 1788, and recent work emphasizes the continued strengths of the Turkish military machine into the seventeenth and, even, eighteenth centuries.[24] The Turks had not yet been written off. In 1732 the French envoy in Rome wrote to his counterpart in Vienna "La

---

[21] J.P. Puype, "Dutch firearms from seventeenth century Indian sites", in Puype and M. van der Hoeven (eds.), *The Arsenal of the World. The Dutch Arms Trade in the Seventeenth Century* (Amsterdam, 1996), pp. 52–61.

[22] Silhouette to Amelot, French foreign minister, 7 Sept. 1741, London, Public Record Office (hereafter PRO), State Papers 107/49. The letter was intercepted by the British.

[23] G. David and P. Fodor, *Hungarian-Ottoman Military and Diplomatic Relations in the Age of Suleyman the Magnificent* (Budapest, 1994) is an important recent study.

[24] R. Murphey, "The Ottoman resurgence in the seventeenth-century Mediterranean:

grande question est de savoir si les Turcs feront la guerre cette année au Chrestiens ou non".[25] Eight years later, Villeneuve, the experienced French envoy in Constantinople who had mediated the recent Treaty of Belgrade (1739), by which the Austrians returned Belgrade, Western Wallachia and northern Serbia to the victorious Turks, drew attention to Turkish superiority in the recent war, especially the size and logistical capability of their army.[26] The Austrians were greatly helped in their conflicts with other European powers in 1733–5, 1740–8, 1756–63 and 1792–1815 by Turkish passivity in Europe. Austria itself was a conduit for a flow of military ideas that was both from East to West and West to East. Poland occupied a similar position until the early eighteenth century.

It is possible that a similar re-evaluation emphasising the strength and success of the opponents of European states may be pertinent for other military confrontations between European and non-European powers. In this context, it is probably mistaken to read between, and, thus, combine in the same analysis, European landward wars with non-Europeans, and trans-oceanic conflicts between Europeans and non-Europeans. The latter, in particular, have an episodality that reflects the decision whether or not to attempt landward expansion or control from coastal enclaves, and the dominance of essentially commercial roles. The central role of trade ensured that a set of values and relationships that did not focus on control or defence came into play.

This was far less the case with landward frontiers. Issues of defence were often important in the latter case, and they could lead to pressure for expansion. Thus, Tsar Ivan IV of Muscovy's conquest of the Islamic Khanate of Kazan in 1552 can be seen as a defensive response to the Khanate's alliance with the Crimean Khanate: "Muscovy simply took over the frontier area to protect itself".[27] On

---

The gamble and its results", *Mediterranean Historical Review*, 8 (1993), 198–200; G. Agoston, "Ottoman artillery and European military technology in the fifteenth to seventeenth centuries", *Acta Orientalia Academiae Scientiarum Hung.* 47 (1994), 46–78.

[25] Polignac to Bussy, 16 Feb. 1732, Paris, Archives du Ministère des Relations Extérieures, Correspondance Politique (hereafter AE CP) Autriche, supplement 11.

[26] Villeneuve to Amelot, French Secretary of State for Foreign Affairs, 16 Jan. 1740, Paris, Bibliothèque Nationale, Manuscrits Français 7191, fol. 5; Frederick William I of Prussia to Charles of Brunswick-Bevern, 24 Aug. 1737, Wolfenbüttel, Staatsarchiv, 1 Alt 22 Nr. 609, fol. 164.

[27] D. Ostrowski, *Muscovy and the Mongols. Cross-Cultural Influences on the Steppe Frontier, 1304–1589* (Cambridge, 1998), pp. 187–8.

landward frontiers, the Europeans did not offer the "protection" that they could provide in South Asia. Naval and military skills were the major skills in which Europeans had an edge over South Asians up to the eighteenth century, and this made them useful allies. South and East Asia sold various high-quality manufactured goods that Europe could not produce. The trade was made up by European exports of (American) silver and "protection".[28]

Partial parallels between different relationships may still be drawn or considered. As far as both land and sea are concerned, it is striking how, after the initial period of European impact and expansion, which can be variously dated, but may be centred on the period 1492–c. 1560, there was a long stage during which expansion slowed or halted, or, in some cases, was reversed. This can be seen with the Portuguese in Angola, Mozambique and Morocco, particularly the last,[29] although expansion continued in Brazil. The Portuguese defeat at Azalquivir in 1578 was not like the Italian disaster at Adua in 1898, a simple exception to the rule of European expansion. Within forty years of 1898 the Italians had conquered first Libya and then Ethiopia. There was no comparable Portuguese expansion after Azalquivir. On Europe's land frontier, Ivan IV's conquests of Kazan and Astrakhan in the 1550s were not followed by any over-running of the Ukraine or war with the Crimean Tatars. The Crimea was not conquered until 1783.

With both Spain and the Dutch the slowing down came later than with the Portuguese. In the first case, there was a burst of continuing activity, especially in the 1560s and 1570s, as in the Philippines, and in the Mediterranean against the Turks, but, thereafter, this diminished. It might be attractive to suggest that this was due to a concentration of resources upon warfare within Christian Europe, an argument made for the second case by Fernand Braudel.[30] Yet, such a concentration had also been true of the early decades of the century, when Spain had been heavily committed in the Italian Wars. Furthermore, the energy for expansion, in large part, came from

---

[28] S. Subrahmanyam, *The Portuguese Empire in Asia 1500–1700* (Harlow, 1993), pp. 77–8; O. Prakash, *European Commercial Enterprise in Pre-Colonial India* (Cambridge, 1998), pp. 139–43.

[29] W. Cook, *The Hundred Years War for Morocco. Gunpowder and the Military Revolution in the Early Modern Muslim World* (Boulder, 1994).

[30] F. Braudel, *The Mediterranean and the Mediterranean World in the Age of Philip II* (2nd edn., London, 1981).

within the existing Spanish colonial possessions, Mexico leading to
the Philippines[31] and the latter to Taiwan. Instead, it is more pertinent to draw attention both to a slackening in expansion and to
the strength of resistance, as in Chile, and to the north of Mexico,
and on Mindanao.

In the case of the Dutch, later entrants on the colonial scene,
expansion, and attempted expansion, in 1590–1670, was largely at
the expense of other European powers, especially the Portuguese,[32]
and initial gains elsewhere, as at Cape Town and on Java, did not
lead to widespread expansion.[33] Again, this, in part, reflected a limited interest in territorialisation. Dutch merchants did not seek to
create *latifundia* across the world. The Dutch expedition sent in 1696–7
to explore the West Coast of Australia reported that the "Southland"
offered little for the East India Company. The Dutch had been driven from Taiwan by Coxinga in 1662. They never re-established
their position there.

Similar limits could be seen elsewhere, for example with the English
on Sumatra. The French established bases on Madagascar in the
1660s and the 1740s, but did not conquer the island until 1894–5.
In 1793 Captain John Hayes hoisted the British flag on the north-west
coast of New Guinea, and on behalf of George III took possession
of what he called "New Albion", but the British Governor-General
of India, Sir John Shore, and his council refused to support this private initiative, and in 1795 Fort Coronation and the colony were
abandoned.[34] This was a matter of political will as well as military
capability. Both were important to conquest and resistance. They
can be noted in the relatively small European forces sent to North
America, Africa and South Asia. The first centuries of the European
presence in Asia were limited to seaborne activity, fortress building
and control of certain important islands; the Philippines, an extension of the Spanish empire in America, was, in part, a different case.

---

[31] G.D. Winius, *The Fatal History of Portuguese Ceylon: Transition to Dutch Rule*
(Cambridge, Mass., 1971).

[32] J.L. Phelan, *The Hispanization of the Philippines: Spanish Aims and Filipino Responses,
1565–1700* (Madison, Wisconsin, 1967).

[33] M. Ricklefs, "Balance and military innovation in seventeenth-century Java",
History Today, 40 (1990), 40–6.

[34] A. Griffin, "London, Bengal, the China trade and the unfrequented extremi-
ties of Asia: The East India Company's settlement in New Guinea, 1793–95", *British
Library Journal*, 16 (1990), 151–73.

There were no vast territories, huge agricultural populations or long land borders to defend.

With superior technology, ships could defend themselves and help defend European island and littoral bases. The fortresses and their guns also represented a superior technology, but were seldom built in areas where they confronted major Asian rulers. When attacked, these fortresses were vulnerable. Parker devotes attention to Portuguese-held Malacca's success in fending off repeated attacks by the Sumitran Sultanate of Aceh, but, as he also notes, Muscat fell to the Omanis in 1650, Fort Zeelandia to Coxinga in 1662 and Mombasa to the Omanis in 1698. In 1686 when the Mughals vigorously pursued a dispute with the East India Company the English evacuated their Bengal base of Hooghly and surrendered that of Bombay. They were only able to continue trading after apologising and paying an indemnity.[35] Until the mid-eighteenth century, Europeans mainly defended themselves and their trade and, if they acted aggressively, did so, in part like nomadic raiders, against Asian mainland territories and Asian maritime trade which were taken under European protection.

Limited interest in conquest may, in part, be traced to the military factors discouraging expansion in the period c. 1560 to 1748.[36] Furthermore, it is necessary to consider the problems of conquest understood as the creation of new authority. This was less difficult where, as in Europe, there were existing political structures to take over or with which to reach an accommodation. It *could* be easier to force the more sophisticated, "civilized" peoples into accepting new structures, just as it *could* be easier to defeat them.

In contrast, Amerindian resistance to the Europeans was at its most effective when it was "primitive", especially if aided by difficult terrain or eco-systems, as in Amazonia and with the Araucanians of Chile.[37] Many such peoples practised dispersed warfare, not possibly as a consequence of deep reasoning, but because it was a transition from hunting and a result of low population density. Such warfare could frustrate more sophisticated, cohesive, concentrated European formations, as the Russians discovered in north eastern Siberia in

---

[35] B.P. Lenman, "The East India Company and the Emperor Aurangazeb", *History Today*, 33 (1982), 36–42.

[36] P.J. Marshall, "Western arms in maritime Asia in the early phases of expansion", *Modern Asian Studies*, 1 (1980), 13–28.

[37] D. Sweet, "Native resistance in eighteenth-century Amazonia: The 'Abominable

the eighteenth century. Less urban, market-based cultures could be harder to conquer. If peoples were nomadic, or with scattered or remote settlements, they presented the Europeans with fewer or poorer fixed assets to threaten. The British in India found this a fundamental problem in "pacification" operations.

In such areas there were also fewer political structures that could be acknowledged or with which to reach an accommodation. As a consequence, a European presence could more readily lead to conquest, while, in the absence of recognition, let alone mutuality, it was easier to justify the seizure and settlement of land.[38] This contrast could also be related to differences in the demographic relationship. In India it was easier, more profitable, and more necessary, to create a European presence short of conquest than was the case in North America, South Africa and Australia.

There was a major difference between the establishment of a "plunder and trade" presence, or even empire, and conquering and establishing authority over far-flung but lightly-populated territories. Agricultural societies with many fixed assets were vulnerable to nomads and raiding warriors, such as Vikings, Mongols and Manchus, and could be conquered by determined warrior groups able to guarantee protection against such enemies. The ability to protect created authority, and the Vikings, Mongols and Manchus understood this process. This mechanism also worked in the Spanish conquest of America. The Aztec and Inca empires rapidly fell and the Spaniards took the role of rulers and protectors. The conquest of extensive lightly-populated territories with nomads and "primitive" people, such as North America, Australia, and Kazakhstan, on the other hand, was a long-term project largely achieved by emigration by a large number of Europeans.

In suggesting that a re-evaluation of the Military Revolution is necessary, it is appropriate not to go too far. A margin of European

---

Muras' in war and peace", *Radical History Review*, 50 (1970), 467–81. For the difficulties that the European environment posed for invaders see, for example, D. Sinor, "Horse and pasture in inner Asian history", *Oriens Extremus*, 19 (1972), 181–2; R.P. Lindner, "Nomadism, horses and Huns", *Past and Present*, no. 92 (1981), 14–15; J. Gommans, "The Eurasian frontier after the first millennium A.D.: Reflections along the fringe of time and space", *Medieval History Journal*, 1 (1998), 132.

[38] W.E. Washburn, "The moral and legal justifications for dispossessing the Indians", in J.M. Smith (ed.), *Seventeenth-Century America: Essays in Colonial History* (Chapel Hill, 1959), pp. 24–32; A. Frost, "New South Wales as *terra nullius*: The British denial of Aboriginal land rights", *Historical Studies*, 19 (1981), 513–23.

superiority in naval capability was maintained, and this was also true of amphibious ability, especially the combination of ships, fortresses and garrisons. Non-Europeans were less successful in this sphere, although there were exceptions, such as the Turks in Cyprus in 1570–1. It is difficult to erode this European superiority by talk of germs. Yet, even there, it is possible to draw attention both to the limited inshore effectiveness of European warships and to the success of non-European navies, particularly those of the Turks and the Omani Arabs.[39] Furthermore, the unwillingness of the Chinese, Japanese and Koreans to maintain their powerful naval forces directs attention to the role of volitional factors, and thus to culture, identity, ideology, and politics.

Discussion of an early-modern European Military Revolution has to note that the transformation in naval capability in the period 1820–1920 or 1855–1955 was greater than in any previous century. Scientific developments had been utilised earlier. In 1788 Dr Charles Blagden visited the harbour works at Cherbourg which he described as "a new experiment in mechanics".[40] However, such experiments were more successful a century later.

From the seventeenth century, substantial navies were deployed by only a handful of non-European powers, principally in the East Indies, for example Aceh, the Mediterranean—the Barbary States of North Africa and the Ottoman empire—, and in the western basin of the Indian Ocean—Persia, the Omani Arabs based on Muscat, and the Maratha Angria family on the Konkan coast of India. Their ships were longer range than the war canoes of Madagascar, Oceania and West Africa, and more closely approximated to European warships, but they lacked the destructive power of the latter and the organisational sophistication of the European navies. The Barbary, Omani and Angria ships were essentially commerce raiders, rather than the more regimented and standardized fleets of the European navies with their heavy, slow ships designed for battering power. The latter were also increasingly able to operate effectively in sizeable

[39] A. Deshpande, "Limitations of military technology. Naval warfare on the West Coast, 1650–1800", *Economic and Political Weekly* [Bombay], 25 Ap. 1992, 902–3.

[40] Blagden to Lord Palmerston, 9 July 1788, New Haven, Beinecke Library, Osborn Shelves C114. For the deficiencies in attempts to improve techniques of fortification construction, I. Coutenceau, "Neuf-Brisach (1698–1705): La Construction d'une place forte au début du XVIIIe siècle", *Revue Historique des Armées*, No. 171 (1988), 20.

numbers at a considerable distance from Europe. This owed much to the provision of local bases and these were seen as important to European naval effectiveness. Thus in 1788 the French Foreign Minister wanted to know if the British were constructing warships in Bombay.[41]

Furthermore, despite qualification of the concept of an early modern Military Revolution, there were important European land gains in the seventeenth and early eighteenth centuries. This was especially the case in Siberia, North America and Brazil. Such conquests were different to those made earlier at the expense of the Aztecs, Incas and, later, from the 1750s, at the expense of Indian powers, because the demographic balance in Siberia, North America and Brazil favoured the Europeans, especially at the point of contact, or was less unfavourable than it was before and after. That does not, however, minimise the importance of advances into areas such as Siberia, Canada, British North America, and Louisiana.

In addition, European projectors were eager to propose schemes for gains in many areas. Thus, in the early 1730s, a London merchant of Portuguese origin, John Da Costa, persuaded first a group of British merchants and nobles, then the Russian envoy, Prince Kantemir, and then an influential Russian minister, to support his scheme for a colony on a section of the Atlantic coast of South America allegedly unclaimed by any Atlantic European power. Da Costa proposed to gain the region with two warships and 500 troops.[42]

British and Spanish diplomatic representations led to the end of the scheme, but, in the same period, the British established a colony in Georgia, and they were followed by Russian expansion across the Bering Sea into the Aleutian Islands and, then, Alaska. However, Portuguese projectors were less successful in 1635 and 1677 when they sought to advance up the Zambezi to gain the mines of Monomotapa.

The period c. 1560 to 1748 can also be considered by contrasting it with the subsequent period, by assessing how far there was a "tipping point" into the latter, and how far this was due to a case of more of the same or how far to a new set of circumstances. In North

[41] Montmorin to Luzerne, envoy in London, 6 Ap. 1788, AE. CP. Angleterre 565, fol. 53.
[42] L.A. Tambs, "Anglo-Russian enterprise against Hispanic South America, 1732–1737", *Slavonic and East European Review*, 48 (1970), 357–73.

America from 1748 there was no dramatic change, whether revolution or not, in terms of weaponry, but there was a new energy in European activity that essentially arises from competition between Britain and France. The same was also the case in India.[43] There was no particular increase in the quality gap, if any, in favour of European military methods, but more troops were deployed. Governor William Bull of South Carolina reported in 1761 that Anglo-American prisoners released by the Cherokees claimed that

> their young men from their past observations express no very respectable opinion of our manner of fighting them, as, by our close order, we present a large object to their fire, and our platoons do little execution as the Indians are thinly scattered, and concealed behind bushes or trees; though they acknowledged our troops thereby show they are not afraid, and that our numbers would be formidable in open ground, where they will never give us an opportunity of engaging them.[44]

Nevertheless, there was no common "tipping point" in the mid-eighteenth century. In the case of the eastern Mediterranean for example, although interest in the conquest of Egypt was expressed in 1739,[45] and then, again, from 1784, no attempt was mounted until 1798. The French were successful that year, their rifles "like a boiling pot on a fierce fire", but the British were far less so in 1807 and Egypt was not conquered and held until the British invasion of 1882. Further west, a Spanish attack on Algiers in 1775 was unsuccessful, and when in 1786 Algiers signed a treaty promising to end piracy against Spanish shipping and to return Spanish captives, Spain had to pay 2.2 million pesos, including 1/2 million for redeeming the captives and 1 million as indemnification for the attack of 1775 and the bombardments of 1783–4.[46]

---

[43] The Indian National Trust for Art and Cultural Heritage, *Reminiscences. The French in India* (Delhi, 1997).

[44] Bull to General Amherst, 15 Ap. 1761, PRO CO/5/61, fol. 277. Cited in S. Brumwell, *The British Soldier in the Americas, 1755–1763* (unpublished PhD thesis, Leeds, 1998), p. 203.

[45] F. Charles-Roux, *France, Egypte et Mer Rouge, de 1715 à 1798* (Cairo, 1951), pp. 1–2.

[46] R.L. Tignor (ed.), *Napoleon in Egypt. Al-Jabarti's Chronicle of the French Occupation, 1798* (Princeton, 1993), p. 37; G. Douin and E.C. Fawtier-Jones, *L'Angleterre et L'Egypte. La campagne de 1807* (Cairo, 1928); J. Dunn, "All Raschid al-Kebir. Analysis of the British defeats at Rosetta", paper read at the conference of the Consortium on Revolutionary Europe, Baton Rouge, 1997; J. Sabater Galindo, "El Tratado de

In Burma and South-East Asia there was no major deployment of European force until the following century. French influence in Burma collapsed in 1757 when Pegu was occupied by Alaugpaya. It is also worth noting the difficulties that Europeans encountered in the period of expansion from the late eighteenth century. Aside from issues of conquest, there were grave problems in creating adequate political, organisational, commercial and financial rationales and patterns for control or influence.[47] In addition, subduing and controlling far-flung territories involved ideological, as well as operational, issues.

Interest in such conquests rose during the period 1792–1815. The French Revolutionary and Napoleonic wars led to another age of political "projectors". Although the conflict of that period was concentrated in Europe, the French devoting a greater share of their military resources to conflict there than had been the case during the Seven Years' War (1756–63), competition between the great powers led to interest in the non-European world. In 1812 Major General Charles Stevenson sent the Earl of Liverpool, Secretary for War and the Colonies, a memorandum urging the need to gain control of Timbuktu, a town only recently explored by Mungo Park:

> Africa presents a new country and new channels for your industry and commerce, its soils favourable for your West India productions, it produces gums, drugs, cotton, indigo . . . gold . . . iron . . . this to England is infinitely of more consequence than the emancipation of South America . . . the teak wood so famous for ship building might be cultivated with success in some of its various soils . . . the possession of Thombuctoo [sic] would secure you the commerce of this quarter of the world and give you a strong check upon the Moorish powers of the Mediterranean by being able to intercept all their caravans and refusing them the commerce of the interior. It would likewise give you a complete knowledge of Africa to the borders of the Red Sea and to Ethiopia . . . at the same time you could raise black armies for your East Indies and save your white troops for other service . . . [Napoleon knows] he can from the Niger pass his battalions in echellons to Cairo . . . not all the power of Great Britain can dislodge him if he first adopts the plan of establishing a chain of posts from the Upper

Paz Hispano-Argelino de 1786", *Cuadernos de Historia Moderna y Contemporánea*, 5 (1984), 57–82.

[47] For a recent example, A. Webster, "British expansion in South-East Asia and the role of Robert Farquhar, Lieutenant-Governor of Penang", *Journal of Imperial and Commonwealth History*, 23 (1995), 1–25.

Senegal to the Niger ... I was not destined to conquer Africa, but bridle it, in order to have a check upon its Kings to protect British commerce as well as the African in its transit through the different kingdoms, by which means we should hold the country in check without the expense of defending it and by good management make the greater part of its sovereigns our friends, by supporting some, protecting others and augmenting their powers, and, as Allies, drawing from them whatever black battalions we may want.[48]

An emphasis on ideological issues offers an approach to global military history that displaces attention from the technological interpretation with its world conceived of as some type of isotropic surface. Politics was not simply a question of the mobilisation of resources, but also one of the nature of a political society. This was crucial, both in terms of internal strength and of foreign policy. The ability of polities to incorporate insiders and outsiders varied (and varies), and was a crucial aspect of military strength. This was an aspect both of politics and of armies, the two not being separate in this context.

The Manchu state demonstrates the point. The successful integration of the Chinese and the Mongols in the Manchu state and army in the seventeenth century was crucial both to their conquest and to the subsequent success of the Manchu in conquering Tibet, Xianjiang and eastern Turkestan.[49] This paralleled the British conquest of India, which was dependent on the integration of large numbers of Indians into the British military system. Such a mixed military was crucial to the imperial systems of the last millennium, especially before the dynamic nexus of the nineteenth century: demographic expansion, nationalism and conscription. The process of acquiring crucial political and military allies was most apparent with European imperial states operating across the oceans. It was also a factor, however, with powers operating against contiguous territories, such as the Russians in Kazan, Siberia, Central Asia and the Caucasus, the Mughals, and the Chinese. Local allies could offer crucial military skills. Thus in the 1740s the British used Mohawks against pro-French Micmacs on Nova Scotia, while in 1742 Creeks helped the British block a Spanish advance on Savannah.

---

[48] Stevenson to Liverpool, 1 Feb. 1812, Exeter, Devon County Record Office 152M/C1812/OF27.

[49] F. Wakeman, *The Great Enterprise. The Manchu Reconstruction of Imperial Order in Seventeenth-Century China* (2 vols., Berkeley, 1985).

The ability to win and retain allies was not simply a matter of diplomatic success in specific conjunctures. It was also a product of a cultural flexibility that can be regarded as a crucial politico-military resource. The Manchu dynasty can, in many respects, be seen less as the government of China than as an imperial authority ruling China, Manchuria, Mongolia, Tibet, Korea and Xinjiang. The rulers consciously addressed themselves to different racial groups. Documents written in Chinese and Manchu, and originally thought to be simply translations, proved to say different things in the two languages. There was also an explicit use of Buddhism to control both the Tibetans and the Mongolians. In Kashgar and Tibet, although not Xinjiang, the Chinese left government in the hands of the indigenous elite.

Organisational capability and operational method were also important in the projection of power and the winning of distant allies. The creation of effective long-range logistical systems, such as those employed by the Turks to supply their forces and by the Chinese in supporting their armies in Mongolia, Dsungaria and Tibet, served to create and sustain patterns of conquest, incorporation and alliance-creation that were very different to those of long distance cavalry raiders. Indeed, it would be wrong to contrast the former with the European oceanic systems in order to suggest that the Europeans were necessarily more organised, even bureaucratic.

Effective logistics was not simply a matter of supplying forces. It was also important in winning the backing of local societies. Thus, the Turks rented, rather than seized, pack animals and wagons. Local support in frontier areas was also instrumental in the provision of accurate intelligence.

Characterising the conquest of Xinjiang in the 1750s as a Chinese conquest of Turkic people is, therefore, problematic, and Ross Hassig and John Thornton have made similar points about the Spanish conquest of the Aztecs and Portuguese campaigns in Angola.[50] Much of the Chinese army was composed of Manchu and Mongol banner-men. The banner system enabled Mongols, Chinese and Manchus to work as part of a single military machine. As already suggested, it might be argued that the Manchu use of Chinese troops was much

---

[50] R. Hassig, *Aztec Warfare, Mexico and the Spanish Conquest* (Harlow, 1994); J. Thornton, "The art of war in Angola, 1575–1680", *Comparative Studies in Society and History*, 30 (1988), 360–78.

like the British use of *sepoys* in India. However, the degree of acculturation and assimilation of the Manchus into Chinese culture was greater, and, therefore, it is more appropriate to use the term China. The contrast with the situation in India indicates the value of comparison. The strength of Manchu China owed a lot to the extent to which much of the territory that formed the initial Manchu homeland and acquisitions had been the source of intractable problems for the previous Ming dynasty.

The overcoming of the frontier as a challenge to China was as much, therefore, a matter of political reconfiguration and reconceptualisation as of specific military achievements.[51] There is, however, a danger that the notion of militarily advanced and backward currently defined in technological terms will be replaced by a similarly simplistic use of political concepts. Thus, there will be an emphasis on the ability of different state structures and political societies to mobilise military resources and to sustain struggles, a form of political economy that has direct military consequences. Such an interpretation could be used to explain the success of expansionist states, for example Manchu China or Russia, at the expense of other political cultures, such as those, respectively, of Dsungaria, and of Kazan, Siberia, the Caucasus and Central Asia.

This approach is not without its serious problems, both empirical and methodological, as any consideration of the variety of powers defeated by French Revolutionary and Napoleonic France would suggest, but it does open the possibility of discussing the domestic background of war in a fashion that is at once systematic and theoretical. However, it is also based on the creation of a deficient "other" whose defeat in some way justifies its victim status. This is problematic from the moral perspective, but also entails a failure to understand the particular nature of military challenges. Powers such as the Khanate of Kazan in 1552 or the Dsungars in 1755–7 might be destroyed, but that does not mean that they were bound to be so. The notion of political determinism in military history is as misleading as those of technological and economic determinism have been.

This can be seen if a counterfactual perspective is adopted. Counterfactualism can be employed by looking for alternative trajectories, such as demographic disaster for the European colonists in

---

[51] T.J. Barfield, *The Perilous Frontier: Nomadic Empires and China 221 BC to AD 1757* (Oxford, 1989).

Latin America, East Asian naval development and expansion, or the defeat of the British in India by the local rulers, especially Mysore and the Marathas. Counterfactualism can also be employed by applying a more complex critique to the cultural politics of conquest. The notion of an early-modern European world as a prelude to the modern Western world is an artificial and misleading contract that exaggerates aspects of modernity in Europe, gives them a false causal power and underrates conservative social, cultural and intellectual patterns in the sixteenth and seventeenth centuries, presenting a false antithesis to the rest of the world.

Conservatism in the European world was disrupted in the eighteenth century by the "Enlightenment", but it was far from inevitable that the new ideas and governmental practices of the period would do more than shore up existing structures, as in Turkey. Indeed, the interactions of change, novelty, reform and revolution in the eighteenth century were far from fixed, and this remained the case until the utilitarian hegemony of the mid-nineteenth century.

Counterfactualism needs to be directed to this cultural politics. Prior to the mid-nineteenth century a desire as well as a practice of global dominance had only a limited purchase in Europe. It is necessary to understand the cultural and racial ideas of the Europeans and other societies in order to apply counterfactual perspectives to the notion of drive for ascendancy and the trajectory towards an appropriating psyche. The mercantile/utilitarian conception of territorialisation—of land that could and should be profitably seized even if not then settled—developed late and was not inevitable.

In short, European dominance did not have to take the forms it did. In many respects a distinctive form did not arise until quite late, and this is more apparent if the cultures of European descent in the New World are omitted. A further perspective can be provided by disaggregating Europe and comparing and contrasting the Atlantic West and the Continental powers. Without primitivizing the latter, it is possible to suggest that expansion by Austria and, especially, Russia,[52] once the mercantile (Cossack) phase of Siberian conquest was over, was not too different to expansion by non-European

---

[52] A.S. Donnelly, *The Russian Conquest of Bashkiria, 1552–1740* (New Haven, 1968); M. Khodarkovsky, *Where Two Worlds Met: The Russian State and the Kalmyk Nomads 1600–1771* (Ithaca, 1992).

empires; in short that Euro-Asian conquest is not an easy parallel to the maritime theme of Western Europe.

It is possible that different political developments within Europe would have affected the character of maritime and Continental expansion and the balance between them. The suppression of the Dutch Revolt, the Jacobite success in Britain,[53] and the Napoleonic victory over Britain and Russia were all possible. It is also necessary to consider whether domestic developments within individual European states would have made a major difference. These would have included the triumph of the Huguenots in France in 1560–1600 and of radicalism in Britain in 1780–1800. These domestic suppositions would have affected the cultural suppositions that moulded the use and choices of power. Thus, an understanding of Europe as fluid in its development can be seen as crucial to any counterfactual analysis of her expansion.

The greater pace of European activity in the second half of the eighteenth century had an organisational dimension, conflating political, cultural and military factors, in the shape of a greater deployment of regular forces in North America and the development of *sepoy* forces in India. The latter was more important in the long term, because it led to a major and permanent increase in the armies available to the Europeans in South Asia, and reduced the extent of the need for multiple capability on the part of their armed forces.

Furthermore, the degree of incorporation into Western models was an important organisational shift. It is unclear whether it would necessarily have been less efficient to retain Indian priorities, especially in light cavalry. The British (and French) were largely dependent on allied forces for these and this limited them gravely. The role of such contingents has been minimised, because of the emphasis on *sepoys*, but that may have led to a misguided emphasis on "westernisation" in organisational capability. The role of political choice emerges in the failure of the British to create an Indian cavalry army. There were other factors, including the difficulty of obtaining horses on the east coast, the cost, approximately twice that of infantry man for man, and the intractability of Muslim horsemen, but an unwillingness to train Indians in better cavalry tendencies was also important, as was the preference of London for a defensive stance, rather than the aggressive possibilities offered by cavalry.

---

[53] J.M. Black, *Culloden and the '45* (Stroud, 1990).

As far as the impact of the *sepoys* was concerned, it may be that the demographic dimension was more significant than the organisational. *Sepoys* may be more remarkable, not in terms of an organisational capability gap, but as providers of the numbers without which the Europeans would have been overwhelmingly dependent on warships, artillery fortresses and allies, as they were in West Africa, Angola and Mozambique. This issue was more serious in South Asia than in North America, because of the nature both of the demographic balance with the native population and of the local environment. Disease was far more of a killer in India. As Colonel Gordon wrote in 1808 about the possibility of a campaign elsewhere in the Tropics: "My fears on that subject are the climate, the climate, the climate!!".[54] Demographic factors put far more pressure on European organisational capability. Thanks to small numbers, the Europeans had to worry about how many of their men deserted or died of starvation. Logistics and the reliability of payment were both important.

An absence of a military multiplier in a part of the world where the Europeans were under pressure could have serious consequences for their territorial impact. This was the case on the Swahili coast of East African whence the Portuguese were driven by the Omani Arabs and, for long, on that of West India.

Such an emphasis can be countered by suggesting that the European powers in this period were not primarily concerned with territorial gain, and that it is, therefore, inappropriate as a measure of relative capability. This is also pertinent in the case of transoceanic conflict between European powers. The British were helped in their conquest of Canada in 1758–61 by the presence of more units than the French. This permitted recovery from defeat and enabled the pursuit of more objectives. However, this imbalance in regular forces in North America was a product of choice, as much as resources. In 1755 the French had chosen to send a relatively small force to North America, whereas in 1756 they successfully invaded Minorca, in 1757 sent substantial forces into Germany and in 1759 prepared to invade Britain.

---

[54] Gordon to General Craig, 7 May 1808, London, British Library, Dept. of Western Manuscripts, Additional Manuscripts 49512, fol. 17. He was referring to "the Caraccas".

Differences in resource availability owed much to political and military choices in expenditure, allocation and use,[55] and it is necessary to employ this perspective when considering relations, confrontations and conflicts between European and non-European powers, or, indeed, between the latter. Thus, for example, perceptions of Turkish military effectiveness in the late eighteenth century, not least vis-à-vis the Europeans, might have been affected had there been a major conflict with Persia that Turkey had won. That, however, might also have provoked a process of military adaptation in which the Turks focused on the Persian challenge,[56] rather than on that from European powers.

To the list of major struggles that did not occur, for example that of China and Portugal in the sixteenth century, may be added much of the transoceanic European presence, especially in the Old World in the period 1650–1750. This situation did not completely cease in 1750, as can be seen by comparing the policies of British Governors General of India. Under Sir John Shore, who was in India in 1793–8, there was an emphasis on trade, not territorial expansion. Shore used the army under the Commander-in-Chief, Sir Alured Clarke, to depose and replace the ruler of Oudh, but he, otherwise, adopted a cautious approach. The Maratha leaders and the Nizam of Hyderabad were able to develop their military power, and Shore did not take vigorous steps against Tipu Sultan of Mysore. The situation was to be very different under Shore's aggressive successor, Richard Wellesley. Such changes in policy were not restricted to European expansion. The death in 1723 of the Kangxi emperor was followed by a more limited Chinese policy towards both Tibet and Xianjiang under his less bellicose successor the Yongzheng emperor (1723–36).

When European overseas bases were not used to support major and sustained programmes of conquest, this can be explained functionally in terms of limited population growth and major conflict within Europe. However, such functional and global explanations are of limited value. It is necessary to consider motivation and purpose.

---

[55] J.M. Black, *Britain as a Military Power 1688–1815* (London, 1999).

[56] R.W. Olson, *The Siege of Mosul and Ottoman-Persian Relations 1718–1743* (Bloomington, Indiana, 1975). For the different Safavid system, see R. Matthee, "Unwalled cities and restless nomads: Firearms and artillery in Safavid Iran", *Pembroke Papers*, 4 (1996), 389–416.

One of the strongest arguments against the general concept of the Military Revolution is that it enforces a uniform perception of the world as a single global entity, an approach that invites a presentation in systemic terms. This was a tenable perception for Europe since the late eighteenth century, but systemic perceptions of the world by Europeans over the previous three centuries sharply distinguished between overseas expansion in the Old World and the New. European warfare in Africa and South Asia was largely private and conducted under the supervision of chartered trading companies. This helped ensure a different deployment for European regular forces than was the case in the New World. Issues of cost were much more important in Africa and Asia, as was seen with debates inside the English and Dutch East India Companies on the question of the building and maintenance of fortresses during the later seventeenth and the early eighteenth centuries. We have been too focused on the quality (and quantity) of the means applied to major developments in European expansion, and military history, and not sufficiently focused on motives.

To close on such a note might appear unhelpful. There is no intention of offering a demilitarization of military history, or of ignoring the contingent, the conjunctural and the operational dimension. Nevertheless, a cultural interpretation that focuses on reasons for conquest or for the avoidance of aggressive warfare and conquest, rather than on technological or organisational enablers, directs attention to moods as well as moments. Such an interpretation also focuses on the methodological difficulties of devising a general theory of military capability and change in the early-modern world. An awareness of attitudes, diversity and difficulties is more appropriate than any simplistic and deterministic model that may be helpful to systems theorists of state formation and the global economy, but inappropriate for scholars trying to understand the nature of military power.

2. OUTFIGHTING OR OUTPOPULATING?
MAIN REASONS FOR EARLY COLONIAL CONQUESTS,
1493-1788

George Raudzens

The notion that handfuls of European invaders colonized the New World by defeating one great horde of indigenous defenders after another is still with us. Historical generalizers keep stressing either the superior combat powers of the invaders, or their disease infliction capabilities, or both. For the preceding generation of such writers, these greater killing powers brought victories over heathen primitives and expanded the domain of a higher and better civilization. For many current writers, such powers were the unfair advantages of land-stealing and genocidal imperialist aggressors. But whether the colonial conquests are judged good or evil, too often the central acts of conquest are seen almost entirely as armed assaults and/or forms of inadvertent germ warfare. There is surprisingly little detailed evidence offered up in support of these perceptions, and it seems timely to re-examine the linkages between generalizations and evidence.

With the exception of the Spanish invasion of Mexico under Hernan Cortes between 1519 and 1521, there are few details supporting concepts of major invasion wars and battles in the other early colonies in the Americas or Australia. What the sources instead show is that fighting between colonizers and defenders was the exception more than the rule, and that invasion "battles" were small fights even by contemporary European standards. In most of the foundation colonies which became permanent bases for subsequent European expansion over the continents behind them—notably Hispaniola, Virginia, New England, and New France—invasions "succeeded" not when some or other group of indigenes was outfought in some type of combat, but rather when the influx of settlers grew large and continuous enough to numerically overwhelm the native populations in the colonial target areas. Direct disease impacts were exceptional and debatable. As often as not the fighting was a consequence of territorial outnumbering rather than a cause, as multiplying settlers sought to clear native communities off lands for European living-space needs.

The Cajamarca Paradigm

Probably the biggest single source for the belief in amazing victories against huge odds is the story of Pizarro's capture of the Inca Atahualpa at Cajamarca in Peru on November 16, 1532. Amazingly, less than 200 Conquistadors overthrew some tens of thousands of armed Incas in something like one hour, seizing the Inca emperor and his entire empire.[1] The Aztec conquest is the second most dramatic example of the handfuls versus hordes theme. It is a perennial in general histories of European expansion, and it is supported by some specialists. Geoffrey Parker states that European overseas expansion rested, more than anything else, on ". . . the absolute or relative superiority of Western weaponry and Western military organization over most others", especially in the cases of the Aztec and Inca conquests where the invaders were so few and the defenders so many.[2] The latest expression of this amazing theme is in Jared Diamond's important anthropological study of the rise and fall of world cultures. He starts his book with Cajamarca. In *Guns, Germs and Steel* he entitles Part One "From Eden to Cajamarca", and his chapter 3 is "Collision at Cajamarca".[3] For him, a ". . . ragtag group of 168 Spanish soldiers . . .", surrounded by an Inca army of 80,000,[4] ". . . crushed a Native American army 500 times more numerous, killing thousands of natives while not losing a single Spaniard".[5] They probably killed 7000 Incas.[6] They did this because they had the massive advantages of guns, steel armour and cutting and thrusting weapons, horses, and the benefit of Eurasian diseases which had pre-

---

[1] Garcileso de la Vega. *The Incas* (New York: Avon, 1961), pp. 400–401. De la Vega writes that there were 160 Spaniards in the massacre, and that they killed 5000 Incas, including 1500 women, children, and other non-combatants. F.A. Kirkpatrick, in *the Spanish Conquistadores* (London: Adam and Charles Black, 1967), pp. 156–160, states that Pizarro led 106 infantry and 62 horsemen at Cajamarca, against a possible 30,000 fighting Incas, of which the Spanish probably killed 4000. According to Edward Hyams and George Ordish in *The Last of the Incas* (New York: Dorset, 1963), Pizarro started his march to Cajamarca with 213 men and 64 horses (p. 142) and killed 3,000 to 4,000 Incas in less than one hour, at a rate of 10 to 30 Incas per conquistador (p. 225).

[2] Geoffrey Parker, *The Military Revolution* (C.U.P., 1988). The quotation is on p. 115. See also p. 119.

[3] Jared Diamond, *Guns, Germs and Steel. The Fates of Human Societies* (New York: W.W. Norton, 1997).

[4] Ibid., p. 68.

[5] Ibid., p. 75.

[6] Ibid., p. 73.

viously devastated the Inca empire. If we accept the figure of 168 Spaniards and 7000 Inca casualties as real, each conquistador on average must have killed 41.7 Incas, in about an hour. This could be an all-time face-to-face killing record. If Cajamarca is then listed among the other great European imperialist invasion victories, it clearly stands out as the greatest. It outshines the greatest of Portugal's Asian victories, Malacca in 1511, where the great Affonso da Albuquerque led 900 Portuguese men at arms and 200 Indian mercenaries in a successful one-day assault against some thousands of the war-elephant equipped defenders, at the cost of only 28 Portuguese battle deaths.[7] It is also greater than the Aztec conquest battles of Cortes and the Conquistadors, perhaps the best known of such amazing invasion triumphs. With never more than 1500 men at arms, Cortes overthrew an Aztec empire with a population of no less than 12 million people, and possibly even 25 million.[8] But this conquest took 30 months, from February 1519 to August 1521, and so Cajamarca stays as the victory over the biggest odds, and the strongest example of a technologically and biologically determined triumph over mind-numbing odds. There are, of course, a long series of lesser examples, both in scholarly writing and in popular culture. The settlers usually beat off the various swarms of hostile natives throughout the literature, and the films.

But while Cajamarca is accepted as a victorious battle against odds, to what extent is such acceptance justified? Diamond calls it a battle. Others are less specific, with good reason. The slaughter central to the story was in fact much more a *coup d'etat* than any sort of military contest. The best evidence suggests the Incas offered no serious or sustained military resistance. According to chronicler Garcileso de la Vega, Atahualpa ordered his people not to resist, and they did not fight.[9] The so-called battle was a diplomatic conference in which the guest negotiators turned suddenly against their unsuspecting hosts while the latter were most vulnerable and massacred a large number of them. It can be argued that this bloodbath proved nothing much about military power but plenty about the greater nastiness of the Spanish over the Incas. Whatever the

---

[7] B.W. Diffie and G.D. Winius, *Foundations of the Portuguese Empire, 1415–1580* (Minneapolis, MN: University of Minnesota Press, 1977), pp. 256–7, 258–9.

[8] The best recent studies of the Aztec conquest are those of Ross Hassig. See his *Mexico and the Spanish Conquest* (New York: Longman, 1994).

[9] Garcileso de la Vega, op. cit.

possible range of interpretations allowed by sources which are both one-sided and incomplete, to call Cajamarca a battle seems doubtful.

But battle or not, what about the huge disparity of odds? It is, however, already obvious from the vagueness and contradictions about numbers in the traditional accounts that hard and fast conclusions about the odds are not possible. To exaggerate opponent numbers expanded conquistador achievements. The Incas left no specific information about their version of events, or their own numbers. And the 1530s were not yet a statistically minded age even in Europe. When it came to emotive experiences such as battles and massacres, Europeans back home, recording their own bigger and more frequent battles, could not manage accurate statistical details much of the time. For the period 1503 to 1670, when large formal battles at home coincided with aggressive New World colonization, and when the incidence of such battles was higher than ever before and in any other continent, the participation and casualty numbers were collected with increasing care by state bureaucracies. Nevertheless, for 54 of these battles, as they are reported by our most respected military historians, the discrepancy rates in 18 of them are so great that the standard deviations for the basic numbers in various sources are 30% and over. Only in 18 other cases do all the authorities agree on all the figures.[10] Where quantifications were made by one side only, as in the Mexican and Peruvian conquests and where conditions for accurate counting were marginal due to after-combat stresses and continuing tensions, the likelihood that historians can agree about even the most basic comparative numbers seems small. In any case, Diamond's statement that Pizarro's men overcame odds of 500 to one seems entirely too confident.[11] If the so-called "battle" then lasted an hour, as Diamond and other sources agree, and if the Atahualpa estimate of 7000 Inca casualties is accepted, then each conquistador must have averaged 41 or 42 Inca killings.[12] Edward Hyam and George Ordish reduce this to 10 to 30 Incas per conquistador in less than an hour,[13] but even so the killing rate seems fast even by World War II death-camp standards.

---

[10] George Raudzens, "In search of better quantifications of war history. Numerical superiority and casualty rates in early modern Europe", *War and Society*, Vol. 15, No. 1 (May 1997), 1–3. See especially p. 30.

[11] Diamond, op. cit., p. 75.

[12] Ibid., p. 73.

[13] Hyman and Ordish, op. cit., p. 225.

The explanation for this amazing rate has so far been largely technological, given that disease did not directly impinge on the "battle" itself. As Pizarro himself, Garcileso de la Vega, and other chroniclers describe the Cajamarca violence, it was initiated by Spanish cannon and arquebus fire, followed up with a charge by 62 armoured cavalry, and completed by armoured men at arms on foot with swords. Firearms were present and apparently exercised a strong shock effect on the Incas. Horses, too, had a powerful shock effect. But the guns were few, and probably fired only once. The slaughter zone was in an urban built-up area, with little room to deploy or manoeuvre cavalry effectively. Incas too had body armour, though not as good as Spanish steel. But most of the chroniclers and experts also agree that most of the Spanish killing was done with swords.[14] If this was a technological edge over stone and copper-tipped Inca thrusting and slashing arms, it was marginal rather than monumental. And, in any case, it seems the Incas did not offer serious armed resistance, or perhaps any sort of resistance. If we take only the 10 to 1 killing rate above, it remains an isolated incident rather than any kind of credible suggestion that Spanish men at arms had the capability of overcoming 10 to 1 Inca odds on any sort of regular basis.

Evidence for a massive overall combat superiority based on technological advantage—or anything else—is also missing for the Aztec conquest. Implications about the odds disparity range from 500 to 1500 conquistadors versus from 12 to 25 million subjects of the Aztec empire in the Valley of Mexico. Even extended over a series of battles during 30 months, this was an odds ratio ranging from 8,000 to one (for 12 million Amerindians and 1,500 conquistadors) to 50,000 to one (for 25 million Amerindians and 500 conquistadors). These are clearly fantasy figures. As Ross Hassig has argued, the effective fighting force of Tenochtitlan, with which the Aztecs controlled the entire Valley of Mexico with its possible 12 to 25 million people, numbered no more than 8,000 men.[15] The soldiers of many of the other cities in the Valley in fact joined the Spanish side, in rebellion against their sacrifice-levying Aztec dominators. Thus, the biggest odds were more like 1,500 conquistadors versus 8000 Aztec warriors, about 1 to 5, similar to the claimed kill ratio

---

[14] See the accounts listed in Note 1 above.
[15] Hassig, op. cit., p. 24.

odds of the German forces against Soviet combatants between 1941 and 1944. In virtually every important battle the conquistadors were supported by numerous Amerindian allies. The conquest was more like an internal revolution against Aztec rule than a European invasion of an Amerindian state.[16] These battles were the biggest and most frequent large-scale set-piece combats in the entire Americas invasion experience to the nineteenth century, but by contemporary European standards they were still small-scale affairs.[17] The odds were probably much more even than the types of conjectural figures which require large technological and biological factors to make them plausible seem to suggest.

Defeated Invasions

In the other main colonizing invasions of the Americas the European handfuls versus Amerindian hordes interpretation is even less relevant. In fact, where the odds did favour the defenders, they repelled the Europeans. The first and possibly biggest example of such a successful Amerindian defence was in Vinland around the year 1010. The Viking invaders, armed with steel swords and helmets, and steel-reinforced shields not very different from the basic equipment of Pizarro's men-at-arms at Cajamarca, were driven out of Newfoundland by superior numbers of Skraelings armed with wood, stone and bone weaponry. At least this is as strong a conclusion of the Norse Sagas and recent archaeology suggest.[18]

The total number of colonists under Thorfinn Karlsefni and Freydis Eriksdotter probably came in one ship and totalled 60, mostly men. Freydis then started an internal blood feud and organized the killing of some of her fellow Vikings. Meanwhile, the initial friendly relations with the Skraelings began to break down as individuals from the two groups got into a variety of disputes, in a pattern that was to be repeated in later invasions. Soon hostilities became general and the Skraelings mounted a concerted attack on the settlement.

---

[16] George Raudzens, "So why were the Aztecs conquered, and what were the wider implications? Testing military superiority as a cause of Europe's pre-industrial colonial conquests", *War in History*, Vol. 2, No. 1 (1995), 87–104.

[17] Ibid., p. 101.

[18] See Else Roesdahl, *The Vikings* (Harmondsworth: Penguin, 1991), and F. Donald Logan, *The Vikings in History* (London: Routledge, 1991).

Freydis tried to rally the Vikings, and her individual sword-play is said to have intimidated her attackers. As the Vinland Saga states

> Karlsefni and his men came over to her and praised her courage. Two of their men had been killed and four of the Skraelings, even though Karlsefni and his men had been fighting against heavy odds ...

> Karlsefni and his men had realized by now that although the land was excellent they could never live there in safety or freedom from fear, because of the native inhabitants.[19]

Whatever the actual events were, the Vikings departed and attempted no subsequent settlements.

Their Iceland settlements from about 870 and the Greenland settlement led by Erik Raudsen from 985 were made in uninhabited lands. The most westerly Greenland settlement prospered modestly for about three centuries, though the population stayed small. In 1345, however, Inuit people, driven southward out of the Arctic by the colder climatic conditions after about 1300, wiped out the Norse settlements of western Greenland. By 1410 there was no more regular contact between Greenland and Europe.[20] Thus, where European settlers were few, it seems even the unwarlike Inuit could drive the Europeans out of lands they desired.

There were a number of other repelled invasions. In 1492, Columbus left 39 of his men, with a year's provisions, at Navidad on Hispaniola as he headed for Spain to announce his discovery. There seemed no threat from the Amerindians. When he returned, however, the 39 were gone and Navidad was a ruin. It appears the local Tainos had contributed considerably to their demise.[21] They did not wipe out the much more numerous Hispaniola settlers of 1493, and Spanish colonization by the early years of the next century became irreversible. But not in places where they sent only small groups of invaders. From 1513 to 1542 the Florida Amerindians consistently repelled well-armed Spanish exploring and colonizing expeditions, often after winning pitched battles. In 1513 three ship-loads of Ponce de Leon's men were driven back into the sea by Calusa archers. In 1521 he invaded again with 200 men at arms, and was again repelled

---

[19] Quoted in M. Magnusson and H. Palsson, trans. and intro., *The Vinland Sagas. The Norse Discovery of America* (Harmondsworth: Penguin, 1985), p. 100.

[20] See G.J. Marcus, *The Conquest of the North Atlantic* (New York: O.U.P., 1981). See especially pp. 5–15, 24, 39, 76.

[21] C.O. Sauer, *The Early Spanish Main* (Berkeley: University of California Press, 1981), pp. 31, 72.

and himself killed. In 1526 500 Spanish men at arms attempted another settlement but were effectively starved out by blockading Creek Amerindians. In 1527 Panfilio Narvaez, a hero of the Aztec conquest, led another 500 men into Florida only to be defeated in sustained combat by the Apalachee people. In 1539 Hernando de Soto landed at Tampa Bay with 330 infantry and 270 cavalry. After a series of battles with various groups of Amerindian warriors the expedition reached the lower Mississippi River, but de Soto died and his men were a shattered remnant. In 1565 Spanish colonists finally set up a lasting base at St Augustine, but only after a sustained effort fully funded by the home government. In his analysis of these failed invasions Ian K. Steele concludes that European guns and steel weaponry were not sufficient to overcome the deadliness of Amerindian archery, and that diseases and climatic conditions hurt the Spanish invaders much more than imported Eurasian diseases hurt the Florida Amerindians, at least at that time.[22]

Some of the early invasion efforts of the other European colonizers were also wiped out. The biggest disaster was suffered by the French colonizers of 1541 to 1543 under Jacques Cartier and Jean François de la Roche, seigneur de Roberval, near the site of the Iroquois town of Stadacona on the St Lawrence River. This was supposed to be the start of a New France. There were 1500 original settlers, about the same number as in the 1493 Hispaniola invasion, and like the Spanish colonizers the French too had armour and guns. But the local Iroquois almost immediately identified the French as enemies, and after killing 43 of them, drove the rest to abandon the colony by 1543. Unlike the Spanish on Hispaniola, the French had no prospect of reinforcements from home, and faced hostile Amerindians from the start. There were more Iroquois than settlers, and the Iroquois won.[23] The English also had an early failure, on a smaller scale, the disappearance of the Roanoke Island colonists of 1584–1587. According to Helen C. Rountree this small expedition might have been either wiped out or scattered or assimilated by the Chesapeake Amerindians. The small invader numbers enabled the original landowners to hold on to their territories.[24]

---

[22] Ian K. Steele, *Warpaths. Invasions of North America* (O.U.P., 1994), pp. 7–19.

[23] Ibid., p. 61.

[24] Helen C. Rountree, *Pocahontas's People. The Powhatan Indians of Virginia Through Four Centuries* (London: University of Oklahoma Press, 1990), pp. 20–21.

In all the rest of the serious colonizing invasions, the defenders always lost. For present purposes four foundation colonies are suggested as the main examples of invasion successes. Mexico and Peru are exceptions to the patterns in Hispaniola, Virginia, New England, and New France, each of which became vital staging areas and bases for further major invasions. Even such large ventures as the colonization of Brazil were in many ways reactions to Hispaniola and other Spanish initiatives. In any case Aztec and Inca conquests were take-overs of Native American governments and their populations as much as anything else; the sudden injections of foreign minorities into the ruling elites of politically disrupted Amerindian socioeconomic structures. These involved sustained large-scale military operations only in the Aztec case, and even here with most of the combat between Amerindians on the Aztec side against Amerindians on the Spanish side.[25] By contrast, in Hispaniola, Virginia, New England and New France large-scale military operations in the first generation of settlement were uncommon. The term infiltration may be more appropriate here than invasion. In the more derivative settlements of Brazil, the Greater Antilles, New Holland and the French and English West Indies, large-scale combat against Amerindians was even less frequent, and population displacement—by the injection of African slaves as well as European migrants—even more pronounced.

Hispaniola, 1493–1514

After the Vikings the first serious effort to colonize the Americas was the 1493 Hispaniola venture led by Columbus. It was a project fully supported by Queen Isabella's Castillian government and state funding. When it became clear that it was not in Asia, royal enthusiasm weakened, but it was still enough to keep the colony going and then

---

[25] Douglas M. Peers, ed., *Warfare and Empire. Contact and conflict between European and non-European military and maritime forces and cultures* (Ashgate: Variorum, 1997), p. xviii. Peers in his introduction argues the urgent need for more detailed studies of Europe's military and naval conquests in the "wider world" after c. 1450; among his criticisms of superficial historiography in this area is his statement that ". . . Spain's spectacular gains over the Aztecs and Incas in the sixteenth century are arguably unique. We must recognize the exceptional character of this encounter and that it did not establish a precedent for Europe's later military encounters with non-European peoples." Eurasian diseases and Aztec and Inca political weaknesses, he states, gave the conquistadors unique advantages.

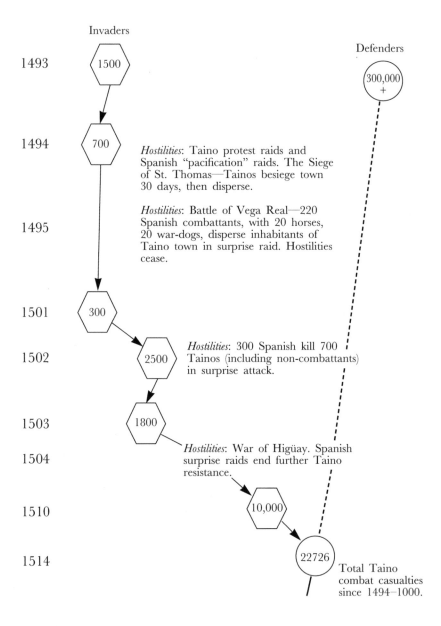

Figure 2.1. Hispaniola 1493–1514.

send the big 1502 settler reinforcement. Initially Hispaniola held out the same types of promises as the Moorish regions of Iberia and the Canary Islands to adventurous colonists, lands and workers with which to build agricultural estates. In addition, there was gold. But between 1493 and 1502 the first 1,500 or so settlers dwindled to 300 males. Death from diseases caused most of the decline, though some colonists returned to Spain. In 1502 the government sent 2,500 reinforcements. These also suffered a disease death rate of more than 50%, but were now continuously replaced by additional settlers so that the Spanish population began to grow steadily. By 1510 there were about 10,000 permanent Spanish residents on Hispaniola. The remaining indigenous Tainos were by this time well on the way to being fully Hispanicized.[26]

Serious Taino resistance to this influx was probably over as early as 1495. In that year they still greatly outnumbered the newcomers. At the start of colonization Bartolome de las Casas estimated there were a million Tainos, or Arawaks, on Hispaniola. Modern scholars suggest 300,000 as more likely. They were fairly evenly spread over the island, in towns surrounded by cassava gardens. But the overall odds were perhaps 300,000 Tainos, counting their non-combatants, versus 1,500 interlopers in 1493, and 700 only in 1494. These 700 were equipped with 100 "hacabuche" hand cannons, 100 "espingarde" guns, and the usual armour and steel equipment of European men at arms. In fact they seem to have had a rather higher proportion of advanced technology guns than was common in European armies in the 1490s.[27] In addition they had horses and war dogs, both armoured, and both a big shock to the Tainos. But these obvious advantages were seldom deployed in large or even medium-scale combat against more poorly equipped Taino warrior forces.

One explanation for the low frequency of combat has been that Eurasian diseases were already slaughtering Tainos on a massive scale. William H. McNeill, Alfred Crosby, and now Jared Diamond, all argue that Tainos were devastated by imported pathogens to which they had no immunities. But there is little evidence of serious

---

[26] D.J.R. Walker, *Columbus and the Golden World of the Island Arawaks* (Kingston, Jamaica: Ian Randle, 1992), p. 309.

[27] M.L. Brown, *Firearms in Colonial America, 1492–1792* (Washington, D.C.: Smithsonian Institution Press, 1980), pp. 35–6.

epidemic disease among the Tainos until about 1510. Meanwhile it was the invaders who were sickening and dying at rates exceeding 50%.

Neither technology nor disease seem to have been central in this first conquest of Amerindian territory. The local Tainos did not contest the initial Spanish landings, and did not identify the newcomers as a threat. They traded, and supplied food to the sick and struggling Europeans. They allowed the invaders to build a total of four fortified towns by 1494, from which the invaders began to make more and more demands on adjoining Taino towns for food and also for labour services. Only when these demands exhausted their small food surpluses and imposed culturally intolerable work ethics did the local towns unite under Caonabo in an organized resistance movement. Only those in close contact with the invaders joined. Individual disputes grew into exchanges of violence and into small-scale raids. Columbus interpreted these as acts of rebellion and launched "pacification" counter-raids against those Taino towns assumed to be hostile. As the violence reached its peak, Caonabo led possibly 10,000 warriors against part of the surviving 700 invaders in the new town of St Thomas, besieging the inhabitants for 30 days, but filing to wipe them out. He had to call off operations for logistical reasons, to let his warriors return to their towns for food. In 1495, after more fighting in smaller engagements, the Spanish settlers struck back against one of the Taino towns containing allegedly 100,000 Amerindians. In a surprise attack with 200 armoured infantry, 20 armoured cavalry, and 20 armoured war dogs they dispersed the defenders and put many to the sword. This they called the Battle of Vega Real. It was probably the biggest organized military operation of the conquest; by European standards it was a small raid and a massacre of mostly non-combatants. Caonabo and his followers sued for peace and submitted to Spanish rule. Other Taino towns in the areas further from the Spanish settlements continued low-level hostilities after this. Murders, raids and counter-raids went on, but to call these "wars" and "battles" of a European kind is inappropriate. The closest the Tainos came to wearing the invaders down in this disorganized fashion was in 1501, when only 300 Spanish settlers remained on the island. The next year, after the great reinforcement, the invaders escalated their anti-Taino raids. In 1502 the biggest of these was one attack by 300 Spanish men at arms which inflicted up to 700 casualties counting non-combatants. In 1503, having expanded their fortified towns to a total of 14, the invaders finished off the last pockets of Taino resistance in what they called "The War of Higüay". Afterwards there was no more serious combat between settlers and Tainos of any sort. Since 1493 Taino combat deaths were probably not much over 1,000. Spanish casualties from disease alone exceeded 2,000. From 1510 Spanish numbers rose above 10,000 In the first official census of surviving Tainos in 1514, the total was 22,726, or a bit more than two Tainos to one invader. By 1540 the remaining Tainos had merged with the settlers, culturally assimilated, and annihilated as a distinct people.[28] The military side of this process boiled down to two serious but small fights, the siege at St Thomas in 1494 and the "Battle of Vega Real" in 1495, with hardly a defender horde anywhere to confront the invader handfuls, technology and disease to the contrary notwithstanding.

Virginia, 1607–1622

The English invasion of Powhatan lands from 1607 was different in many ways but similar in other ways to the Hispaniola conquest. The colonists were not as well supported by government, but the business interests and migration urges driving the flow of settlers were persistent, continuous and spontaneous. About 1,700 settlers invaded the Jamestown area between 1606 and 1616. As in the Hispaniola case between 1493 and 1502, most of these also died soon after landing, from disease and acclimatisation problems. The death rates were 60% in 1607; 45% in 1608 and 1609, and over 50% in 1610. By 1616 there were only 351 survivors.[29] Until they began to grow tobacco for export in the latter year, they were constantly short of food, struggled with the unaccustomed extremes of heat and cold, and often lacked adequate fresh water in their locations on the brackish and tidal James River. While they made no moves to convert the local Powhatan and Pashpahegh people into

---

[28] For details of the Hispaniola invasion, see Sauer, op. cit., Walker, op. cit., and George Raudzens, "Why did Amerindian defences fail? Parallels in the European invasions of Hispaniola, Virginia and beyond", *War In History*, Vol. 3, No. 3 (1996).

[29] J.J. McCusker and R.R. Menard, *The Economy of British America, 1607–1789* (Chapel Hill: University of North Carolina Press, 1985), p. 118.

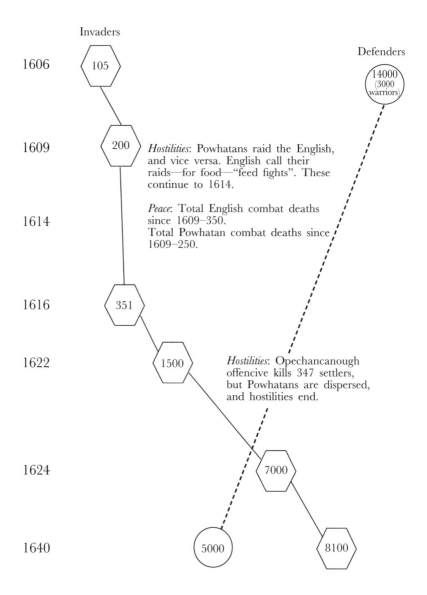

Figure 2.2. Virginia 1606–1624.

their labourers, as the Hispaniola invaders had done with the Tainos, they instead relied on Amerindian surplus corn production to keep them alive for much of the time. It was not an impressive conquering presence.

Opposite Jamestown and its modest outworks were as many as 14,000 Algonkin-speaking Amerindians in the 6,000 square miles of coastal Virginia accessible to the invaders by small boat. Many of these Amerindians were loosely united under the influence of Powhatan, their most powerful politician.[30] Between 1,470[31] and 3,200[32] of them were warriors of fighting age. Powhatan population density was probably no more than two per square mile, by contrast with England's density of 88.[33] Among other things these Algonkin people therefore needed something like 16 to 20 times as much land for sustenance, to produce corn, fish and game, than did European agriculturalists.[34] In terms of contact with the English at Jamestown, therefore, only a minority of the 14,000 indigenes—and perhaps 3,000 warriors— were within trading or fighting range of the invaders. The bulk of the latter, unlike the Amerindians, were men of fighting age, mostly well equipped with armour, pikes, and swords, and some with matchlock arquebuses or muskets. In relative combat strength, therefore, the Powhatans clearly outnumbered the English, but not by hordes versus better-armed handfuls. Nothing like a horde of Powhatans struck the invader beachheads when invader numbers were smallest. The first possible horde, rather dispersed, rose up only in 1622, when it was too late to win.

As on Hispaniola but longer, first contacts in 1606, 1607 and 1608 were amicable. In each of these years about 300 English settlers arrived, but about half died. The Powhatan odds against them were at their highest level, but instead of attacking them the Amerindians fed them. Only after slowly escalating individual disputes and steadily expanding food demands did the good feelings dissipate. When in 1609 the Powhatans ran out of corn for themselves and refused to keep supplying the English, the invaders assumed deliberate malice,

---

[30] Rountree, op. cit., p. 3.
[31] Raudzens, "Why did Amerindian defences fail?", p. 335.
[32] Steele, op. cit., p. 37.
[33] See M. Livi-Bacci, *A Concise History of World Population* (Oxford: Blackwell, 1992), pp. 31, 69, and elsewhere.
[34] Russell, Bourne, *The Red King's Rebellion. Racial Politics in New England 1675–1678* (New York: Atheneum, 1990), pp. 88–90.

and after some individual killings on both sides, began to mount organized small raids against nearby towns and Amerindian cornfields. Those became the typical forms of settler-Amerindian combat, "feed fights" as the invaders called them. They went on, with Amerindian retaliation raids, until 1616. There were no large or even medium set-piece combats between fully-armed and prepared warriors and fully organized armoured musketeers. Mostly each side tried to ambush the other's unsuspecting non-combatants. There were more non-combatants among the Powhatans, and in this sense they were more vulnerable than the invaders. Also, Jamestown fortifications were much stronger than Amerindian palisades, and stayed unchallenged. The Powhatans chose to ambush individuals outside the walls; as some colonists complained, it was not safe to relieve oneself in the bushes. In 1611 the English added a second fort at Henrico, which also proved invulnerable to Powhatan attacks.

Among the biggest fights up to 1616 was the English raid of August 9, 1610, when 70 armoured musketeers attacked a Pashpahegh town, killing 40 warriors and 25 non-combatants.[35] There were nasty casualties in the smaller fights. In 1609 the Powhatans killed a total of 253 settlers, in 1610 they killed 18, in 1611 59, and up to 1614 a grand total of 350. They, in turn, lost about 250 warriors in direct combat.[36] Towards the end the Powhatans relied more and more on food denial in an effort to starve out the invaders, as Tainos had done between 1495 and 1502. But by 1614 they gave up the fight and made peace on invader terms, by giving up big pieces of territory.

After 1616 the English population began to rise. By 1624 there were 7,000 invaders in Virginia. Two years earlier, Powhatan leader Opechancanough for the first time organized a mass attack to drive the English out. In a series of co-ordinated raids against the most exposed English farms—but not their fortified towns—his warriors killed 347 settlers, a third of all the invaders in Virginia. In the English counter-attacks there was only one fight which looked like a battle. In July 1624 on the York River 60 armoured musketeers attacked another Amerindian town. For a change the defenders stood to fight it out for two days, but in the end were driven off.[37]

---

[35] Rountree, op. cit., pp. 54–5.
[36] Raudzens, "Why did Amerindian defences fail?", p. 346.
[37] Ibid., p. 351 and Steele, op. cit., p. 47.

In 1644 Opechancanough tried one more mass attack, with much less success. There were now 8,000 English people in Virginia, but only 5,000 Powhatans, being driven off their lands westward or to cultural extinction within a European society. There was only one more "Indian War" in Virginia, during Bacon's Rebellion in 1675–6, against small Amerindian refugee groups from wars with other European invader communities, now moving into the colony's frontier regions. The settler forces were decisively victorious. Their campaigns were mostly nasty massacres.[38]

New England, 1620–1676

The first invaders of New England were very different from both those of Hispaniola and Virginia. They were politically alienated Pilgrim Fathers and Puritans who came as a more or less complete social slice, with their own rich elite and workers, their own funding, and all their wives and children. North America was their biblical promised land. Since they came as fully articulated societies with self-sufficient logistics they created stable communities faster than the early Virginians. They were very few to start, 102 landing at Cape Cod and settling at Plymouth in Massachusetts between July 22 and November 9, 1620. But on landing they already outnumbered the local Amerindians and, while about half died during the first winter, much as in the early days of Hispaniola and Virginia, they were steadily reinforced. In 1630 came the first of their more numerous Puritan associates, in the largest self-supported migration flow across the Atlantic to that time. By 1640 20,000 people had come to New England, of whom, with surviving Pilgrims, 13,700 were alive in that year. By 1650 there were 22,900 English residents in New England, by 1660 there were 33,200, and the growth was accelerating both from migration and natural increase.[39]

As with other Amerindian population figures there is uncertainty about how many lived in the New England area in 1620. Neal Salisbury cautiously suggests between 114,000 and 126,000 in 1600, 90% of whom were dead from waves of Eurasian epidemic diseases

---

[38] Steele, op. cit., pp. 55–6.
[39] McCusker and Menard, op. cit., p. 103 and elsewhere.

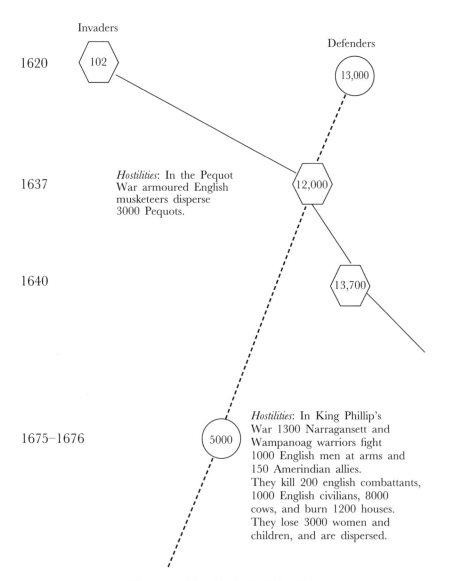

Figure 2.3. New England 1620–1676.

by the time the Pilgrim Fathers landed.[40] At best this translates into 11,400 survivors. The Pilgrims found deserted villages and cleared but unplanted cornfields. They found only very few Amerindians, established peaceful interactivities, and persuaded some of these original inhabitants to teach them how to grow corn on their former fields. There was no serious violence between invaders and defenders for over a decade. In this sense the term "invasion" seems inappropriate. The violent part of this colonization was the disease onslaught, the only clear case of disease as a big factor in helping European colonizers among the main foundation colonies. And those who brought the pathogens did not benefit from the Pilgrim and Puritan land seizures.

As the English settlements expanded in the early 1630s they began to encounter pockets of surviving Amerindian communities. Among the largest of these were the Pequots. In 1633 there may have been 13,000 of them. Smallpox struck later in the year and reduced them to about 3,000. But this was still too many for the expanding settlers. After the usual low-level violence deriving from European encroachments, in May 1637 the Boston authorities organized a force of 90 English armoured musketeers from the colonial militia, recruited 70 Mohegan (or Mohecan) Amerindian allies, and launched a dawn attack on the sleeping inhabitants of the main Pequot town. They were met by 150 surprised warriors, who failed to stop the assault. The Pequot women and children were massacred and the warriors dispersed. This was the only "battle" in the "conquest" of New England, more of an early example of ethnic cleansing than a military operation.[41] By this time there were already many more English settlers in the colony than Amerindians, and it was English hordes versus Pequot handfuls. No greater forces were needed to deal with the Native Americans. The first English troops committed to North American combat by London authorities were 300 soldiers sent against the Dutch at New Amsterdam in 1664.

The bloodiest warfare between New Englanders and Amerindians came in 1675 and 1676, as part of the same type of ethnic cleansing and land-grabbing process as the Pequot War. In 1675 the Boston authorities declared King Philip of the Wampanoags and his 300

---

[40] Neal Salisbury, *Manitou and Providence. Indians, Europeans, and the Making of New England, 1500–1643* (OUP, 1984), pp. 26–7, 22–30.

[41] Ibid., pp. 221–2 and Steele, op. cit., p. 92.

warriors to be in breach of the peace, but sent a militia force to attack the unsuspecting Narragansetts instead. With 1,000 armoured musketeers and 150 Mohegan and Pequot allies they struck at down launching "The Great Swamp Fight". But the surprised Amerindians also had muskets, killing 70 attackers and wounding 150 for a loss of 97 dead, 48 wounded, and up to 1,000 women and children slaughtered. About 1,000 surviving warriors joined King Philip's Wampanoags. In 1676 these 1,300 warriors killed 200 English combatants, 1,000 English civilians, 8,000 English cows, and burned 1,200 houses. In return they lost 3,000 men, women and children before giving up the fight because they ran out of food and gunpowder supplies. Most of them were driven inland or culturally, if not physically, annihilated if they stayed among the Europeans.[42]

So while disease played a part, the Amerindians never had a big numerical advantage and the invaders never had much of a technological edge in weaponry. Instead, European settlers infiltrated into what they saw as unowned land, surrounded surviving Amerindians by population growth and, in 1637 and 1675–6, dispersed the remnants by force of arms. There were three years of "war" in this 56-year process.

New France, 1541–1665

The founding colonizers of the St Lawrence Valley had initial interactions with local Amerindians which were again different from the other main invasion experiences. In both Hispaniola and Virginia, to start with the Amerindians vastly outnumbered the European newcomers, but within the first two decades were themselves outnumbered. In New England the invaders in the contact zones always outnumbered the Amerindians. In the St Lawrence Valley, the Amerindians outnumbered the Europeans for the entire time it took the French to create an irreversible occupation. In some ways the French during their entire North American empire period lived as a minority group among Amerindian societies, some of whom, such as the Iroquois, were hostile, but most of whom were friendly. Despite their trade networks, missions and farms they were more like naturalized Amerindians than conquering invaders.

---

[42] Steele, op. cit., pp. 102–8, and Salisbury, op. cit., pp. 103–120.

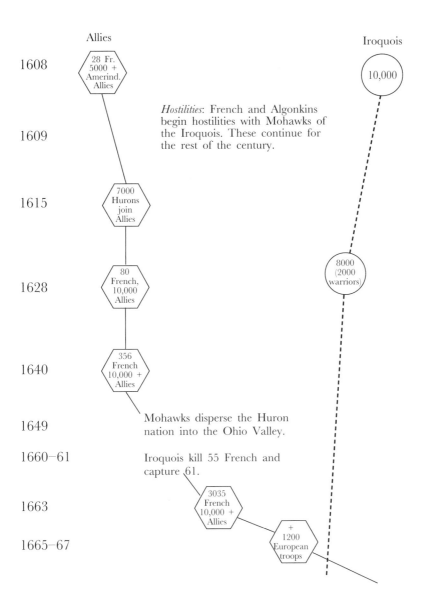

Figure 2.4. New France 1608–1667. (1541–43: Iroquois drive 1500 French out of St Lawrence Valley, killing 35.)

In 1608 Samuel Champlain followed up earlier fur trading ventures by building an outpost at Quebec with 28 men.[43] The site he
chose was the one from which Cartier's and Roberval's colonists had
been driven by the resident Iroquois in 1543. It was now unoccu-
pied. There were several thousand Algonkin-speaking people elsewhere in the St Lawrence Valley but not close enough to feel
threatened by the European newcomers. Twenty of Champlain's men
died the first winter, but others came, and a steady fur trade—
exchange of beaver pelts for manufactured and other European
goods—developed and expanded with the Algonkins and the Hurons
further inland. The Algonkins were hunter-gatherers with birchbark
canoes which gave them an unrivalled inland mobility.[44] The trade
was just profitable enough to keep the Champlain settlement going.
To the Amerindians it was something of a materialist bonanza.
European steel, for example, gave them unprecedented hunting capabilities, and thus more wealth and power. Those closest to the French
gained the most and sought to keep the newcomers as their special
clients, friends, and even relatives. Algonkin canoes were light enough
to carry over gaps in the great inland river and lake networks but
big enough for bulk transport, and so, while the French controlled
the sea transport, their new hunter-gatherer allies monopolized the
interior water ways. The French trade, missions and farms became
dependent on the canoe infrastructure.[45] The agricultural Hurons
were integrated as corn producers, to feed part of this trade. With
perhaps 7,000 warriors, these Iroquois relatives became the friends
and partners of both the Algonkin canoe people and the French.

---

[43] For the basic details and most scholarly interpretations of early French colo-
nization, see W.L. Eccles, *Essays on New France* (Toronto: OUP, 1987), and his *The
Canadian Frontier, 1534–1760* (New York: Holt, Rinehart and Winston, 1969). On
Canada's Amerindians, see Bruce G. Trigger, *Natives and Newcomers. Canada's "Heroic
Age" Reconsidered* (Kingston and Montreal: McGill-Queens University Press, 1985).
On the Iroquois, George Hunt's *The Wars of the Iroquois* (Madison: University of
Wisconsin Press, 1967) is still a worthy starting point. Richard White, in *The Middle
Ground. Indians, Empires, and Republics in the Great Lakes Region, 1650–1815* (CUP, 1991)
does an excellent study of the consequences of early colonization on the Ohio
Amerindians. Steele, op. cit., is a standard reference for combat between Amerindians
and Europeans throughout.

[44] Trigger, op. cit. In Trigger's opinion definite figures for the number of Algonkins
in the Quebec area in 1607 are not possible, but there were some thousands of
them. See pp. 231–242.

[45] See the essay by David McNab, Bruce Hodgins and Dale Standen in this
volume.

On the other hand, the Iroquois corn growers south of the St Lawrence Valley were off the main Algonkin canoe and fur routes and were excluded from the trade. Almost from the start of the Champlain settlement, therefore, they became the implacable enemies of the fur alliance. Thus the gradual Europeanization of the St Lawrence Valley took place in the context of a dominant Amerindian alliance in which the French were a minority, more or less permanently at war with a numerically smaller but more cohesive nation of the Iroquois or Five Nations. The French operated on Amerindian terms, and at the limits of Iroquois war-making powers.

Both the Algonkin alliance and Iroquois wars began with Champlain's "battle" with the Mohawks on Lake Champlain on July 29, 1609. A Montagnais and Huron war party of 60 warriors took Champlain and two other Frenchmen with them on a raid against the Mohawks. They encountered 200 of the latter, probably on their way to do something similar to them. Champlain killed three Mohawks with the first triple-shotted blast of his matchlock musket. His two companions also fired. The Iroquois had no previous experience of firearms. They broke in shock, fled, and lost several more warriors, some killed and 12 captured.[46] Here at last was a genuine example of a small group beating a large one with advanced war technology. But most of the small group were also Amerindians, and once the shock among the Iroquois wore off, they not only withstood gunfire as well as European soldiers but also became as well armed with guns as the Europeans were. In 1628, when six Dutch musketeers went with a Mohegan war party on a raid against Mohawks similar in many ways to the 1609 Champlain "battle", Dutch firepower was entirely ineffective; four of the Dutch musketeers were killed by Mohawk arrows, and a fifth was roasted and eaten.[47] Subsequently the Dutch became the principal suppliers of guns to the Iroquois.

Meanwhile, as the Iroquois began to attack Algonkin canoe fleets in and out of Quebec, by 1615 Champlain was leading his Algonkin and Huron warriors against the nearest Iroquois villages. Casualties were small. In 1624 a brief peace was made. By 1628 there were about 80 permanent French residents in the colony. By 1640, with the support of Cardinal Richelieu's government, the French numbers rose to 356. But as population rose, Iroquois hostility increased.

---

[46] Steele, op. cit., pp. 64–5.
[47] Ibid., p. 115.

By 1635 the French were arming their allies with guns, but the Dutch were arming the Iroquois from New Amsterdam. Hostilities between the Algonkin-Huron allies and the Iroquois escalated steadily until 1648, when the Mohawks began to attack the main Huron towns in southern Ontario. In 1649 Seneca and Mohawk Iroquois organized probably the most formidable Amerindian offensive since Opechancanough's attack on the Virginia settlers in 1622 or the Aztec defence of Tenochtitlan in 1520 and 1521. With 1,000 warriors they struck the Huron towns of St Ignace and Saint Louis, overran the defenders, and scattered 6,000 Hurons westward and southward into cultural annihilation among Algonkins, where their remnants became generally known as the Ottawas of the Ohio Country.[48] This stunning victory over the vital allies of the French was by Amerindians over Amerindians, both sides armed with European guns.

Only in 1660, however, did the Iroquois begin to kill serious numbers of French settlers. That year 800 of them annihilated Dollard des Ormeaux, 17 French musketeers, 40 Hurons, and 4 Algonkins at the Long Sault rapids, at a cost of 20 of their own warriors killed. In 1661 the Iroquois raiders killed 38 settlers and captured 61. But the European population was now rising, to 3,035 in 1663. The new colonial minister of King Louis XIV, Jean Colbert, began to allocate large amounts of funding in order to consolidate the French hold on North America. He sent thousands of new state-assisted migrants. In 1665 he committed the first fully articulated professional regiment of European veterans against the Iroquois; these were 12 companies, 1,200 men, of the Carignan-Salières Regiment, among the first unit to be fully equipped with new flintlock muskets. Other government soldiers were sent later. These troops had modest military success against the Iroquois, but the latter were impressed enough by their potential power to sue for peace, temporarily. The biggest Iroquois blow against the French settlers was in 1689, when they annihilated the entire town of Lachine, but by then there was no serious hope of winning against the colonists. By 1685 there were well over 10,000 Europeans in New France while the Iroquois could seldom muster 1,000 warriors. The Amerindian allies of the French outnumbered the Iroquois, and European professional troops out-

---

[48] White, op. cit., pp. 1–3, and elsewhere.

gunned them. So the Iroquois allied themselves to the expanding English colonists to balance out the odds, until the end of the French empire. Of all the Amerindians they stayed unconquered the longest, and held their territory from 1609 until the American Revolution. But they never had a real prospect of driving out the French. It was they who constantly battled against odds, armed with European guns. They owed their territorial integrity more to geography, their location between the main areas of European expansion, than to other factors.

Thus no Amerindians directly resisted the European colonization of New France in a serious way. The Amerindians actually assimilated the French more than they opposed them. Some regretted the end of the French empire. During Pontiac's Rebellion of 1763–1765, when the Ohio tribes finally mounted a united defence against further European expansion, many kept up their morale by circulating rumours that the French king was about to lead his soldiers back to North America to save them.[49] He did not come, and they too were dispersed.

Conclusion

There was one other big continental invasion which overran indigenous defenders, Australia in 1788. Here too there were no battles. From the first landings the British military and the convicts outnumbered the local Aboriginal residents of Port Jackson. Perhaps this was because of an imported small-pox epidemic. But the other killings were a consequence of conquest, not a means to it.[50] In any case, none of the four main North American invasion stories fit the

---

[49] Gregory Evans Dowd, "The French king wakes up in Detroit: Pontiac's war in rumour and history", pp. 254–271 in Douglas M. Peers, op. cit.

[50] As in the foundation invasions of North America, initial contacts between the concentrated Europeans of the First Fleet and the more thinly spaced local Port Jackson Aborigines were amicable. Hostility developed as Aborigines began to perceive a threat to their food supplies. See Keith Willey, *When the Sky Fell Down. The Destruction of the Tribes of the Sydney Region 1788–1850s* (Sydney: Collins, 1979), pp. 42–55. Noel Butlin suggests that the most widely cited estimate for total Aborigines in the Cumberland Plain is 4,000 in 1788. The First Fleet landed about 1,000 Europeans at Port Jackson, probably inhabited by only a portion of the estimated 4,000 defender people. See N.G. Butlin, *Economics and the Dreamtime. A Hypothetical History* (Melbourne: Cambridge UP, 1993). See especially pp. 137 and 142.

Cajamarca format either. Except in New England, the Amerindians outnumbered the first waves of Europeans substantially or even greatly, but did not concentrate numerical superiorities against the newcomers in the invasion zones. Almost all the sources and histories probably exaggerate Amerindian numbers, and perhaps the odds were not so great. But the odds were not exploited, whatever they were.

In the cases of Hispaniola, Virginia and New France the defenders failed to identify the Europeans as invaders. Both the Spanish and English newcomers were initially pathetically weak, struck down by diseases and dependent on Amerindian food. In the French case, the settlers seemed desirable allies. When hostilities developed in the first two cases, they came from disputes among individuals and from too much pressure on Amerindian food supplies. The Amerindians began to fight seriously only to avoid starvation. There was little sustained combat all the same. Serious fighting came after the Amerindians were already outnumbered, as in Virginia in 1622. The most formidable counter-invasion alliance north of Mexico was probably Pontiac's effort of 1763–1765, much too late.

As for disease and technology, disease helped the invaders only in New England, and technology was a marginal influence. In the rare cases of serious combat, cannon, arquebuses, muskets, armour, pikes and swords were clearly better than Amerindian arms. Europeans also generally built fortifications which Amerindians could not penetrate, and sometimes used cavalry as well. But none of the main invasions was decided by military operations and, in any case, Amerindians became remarkably well equipped with European guns very early.

If failed invasions are contrasted with successful ones, perhaps the critical difference was the strength and continuity of the European migrant flows in the several cases. In the failures small unreinforced invader groups were defeated and driven away. In the successes, migrant flows were continuous, and relative to local Aboriginal population densities—as far as these can be estimated—substantial. In Hispaniola and from the 1660s in New France European governments funded the migrations. In Virginia private capitalists paid the bills and in New England the migrants brought all their own capital with them. But whoever provided the means—for its time and place a big effort—it was the dynamism of the settlers themselves which probably made the main difference. Those average migrants who were driven to risk a frightening ocean voyage, deadly diseases, and perceptions of Amerindian hostility, in order to try to build new homes for themselves on a new and scary continent, were the critical difference. For many reasons, Europe from the 1490s already had enough people willing and able to colonize overseas and keep colonizing. Despite much scholarly effort, the expansionist forces driving ordinary Europeans to new lands still need further illumination.[51]

---

[51] What drove the critical migrant flows has been studied as a whole in works such as Nicholas Canny's *Europeans on the Move Studies on European Migration, 1500–1800* (Oxford: Clarendon Press, 1994), and for North American migrants by specialists such as David Cressy, in *Coming Over. Migration and Communication Between England and New England in the Seventeenth Century* (CUP, 1987). But more research and analysis is probably needed. The "push" and "pull" factors needed to overcome the physical and psychological challenges of crossing the Atlantic and pioneering in a strange environment are too often neglected by historians who at least in an earlier generation were educated on assumptions about the self-evident benefits of colonization.

3. CONFLICT AND SYNTHESIS: FRONTIER WARFARE IN NORTH AMERICA, 1513–1815

Armstrong Starkey

During the sixteenth and seventeenth centuries, North American Indians confronted a series of European invaders who appeared to possess decided military advantages. These invaders were seldom professional soldiers, but they were beneficiaries of European "military revolutions". The timing and nature of such revolutions remain matters of historical debate, but during the sixteenth century the war-making powers of European societies were transformed relative to the capacities of American Indians.[1] Central to this change was naval power in the form of long distance sailing ships, floating castles which could support the establishment and maintenance of settlements on the North American seaboard and which in many cases could penetrate its bays and rivers. Second was the new European reliance on gunpowder weapons in preference to bows and catapults. The introduction of infantry firearms occurred slowly and at an uneven pace over the sixteenth century: the English trained bands, the élite units of the militia, completed the exchange of bows for muskets only by the end of the century and it is debatable whether the musketeers of the day, equipped with slow and cumbersome matchlock weapons, were superior to trained archers. English conversion to firearms may have been more the consequence of the decline in English archery standards than a commitment to modernization. However, whatever the limitations of sixteenth century European military power in hindsight, when weighed in the balance against the resources available to Indian peoples, it seems formidable indeed. This power increased in the seventeenth and eighteenth centuries, particularly with the professionalization of European armies in the

---

[1] Michael Roberts, *The Military Revolution 1560–1660. An Inaugural Lecture delivered before the Queen's University of Belfast* (Belfast, 1956); Geoffrey Parker, *The Military Revolution: Military Innovation and the Rise of the West* (Cambridge: Cambridge University Press, 1988); Jeremy Black, *A Military Revolution? Military Change and European Society 1550–1800* (Atlantic Highlands, N.J.: Humanities Press International, 1991).

eighteenth. Demographics, initially often in favor of Native Americans, had shifted against them by the end of the seventeenth century.

Nevertheless, as the balance of power weighed against them, Indian forces throughout the period inflicted numerous defeats upon well equipped European armies and wars between the two peoples were often fought to a standstill. Indian resistance to European invasion, which may be said to have begun with the 1513 Florida expedition of Juan Ponce de Leon in 1513, was overcome east of the Mississippi only by 1815. Considering clear imbalance of power between the two societies, why was the final defeat so long in coming? The story of Native American resistance serves as a reminder that victory in war is not simply a question of resources.

Richard Overy's recent book on World War II, *Why the Allies Won*, demonstrates that allied advantages in men and material could not always be applied at the point of conflict. Often the margin of victory was very narrow indeed. In some cases, such as at Midway, the balance of resources favored the enemy. Similar conditions prevailed in the first three centuries of conflict between Euopeans and Indians in eastern North America. The continent's vast wilderness and poor communications served to neutralize European material advantages. European invading forces, hampered by poor logistics, seldom reached the size of contemporary armies in Europe. Thus European-Native American warfare was usually small in scale, a factor that worked to the advantage of Indian warriors. Furthermore, whatever numerical superiority Europeans may have enjoyed was often offlset by the quality of their opponents. Battlefield performance counts in the end; leadership, training, skill, and motivation play a critical role in the outcome of war. In the Indians the Europeans encountered martial peoples whose mastery of forest warfare provided them with tactical advantages which frequently reversed strategic imbalances. Given the vast size and remoteness of the territory relative to the settler population, this tactical skill was sufficient to delay European conquest for centuries. Indeed, not until Europeans could adapt to the Indian way of war could they achieve the military conquest of eastern North America.

European soldiers who fought alongside Indian warriors often complained of their lack of discipline and their inconstancy in battle. However, James Smith, an eighteenth century veteran of frontier war and a former Indian captive, scoffed at "the British officers" who "call the Indians undisciplined savages, which is a capital mis-

take—as they have all the essentials of discipline . . . Could it be supposed that undisciplined troops could defeat Generals Braddock,
Grant [generals defeated by Indians in attempts to capture the French
Fort Duquesne at the forks of the Ohio River] . . .?"[2] Smith's description of Indian military discipline stands in sharp contrast to that of
British armies which might lead to victory on the fields of Flanders,
but was useless in the woodland terrain of North America. Ironically,
Indian discipline manifested the qualities advocated by eighteenth
century British military reformers, particularly those interested in the
development of light infantry. "Is it not the best discipline that has
the greatest tendency to annoy the enemy and save their own men?"[3]
In keeping with the reformers views, Indian discipline was founded
on individual honor rather than corporal punishment; leaders were
chosen according to merit based upon courage and experience instead
of privilege or purchase. According to Smith, commanders were concerned to save their men's lives and believed that victory did not
justify unnecessary sacrifice. There was no disgrace in retreating to
await a more favorable occasion for battle. Indian leaders taught
their men to move in scattered order to take advantage of the ground,
to surround the enemy, and to avoid being surrounded. They practiced running and marksmanship and were accustomed to endure
hunger, inclement weather, and hardship with patience and forti-
tude. Although they avoided unnecessary casualties, they were prepared to sell their lives dearly in defense of their homes. Smith
believed that these were moral qualities which provided the Indians
with the ability to oppose enemies possessing seemingly overwhelming advantages in numbers, material, and state power.[4]

The Indian warrior's moral advantage was enhanced by physical
endurance which only the hardiest Europeans could equal. Captives
who survived Indian raids often perished on the brutal marches to
Indian villages. They were expected to maintain the pace of Indian

---

[2] *Scoouwa: James Smith's Captivity Narrative* (Columbus, Ohio: Ohio Historical Society, 1978), p. 161.

[3] Ibid., p. 167.

[4] Smith's account of the Indian way of war is supported by many informed observers including the ranger commander Robert Rogers. See his *A Concise Narrative of North America* (London, 1753), pp. 229–235. Also the comments of the experienced frontier diplomat Conrad Weiser in Paul A.W. Wallace, *Conrad Weiser 1696–1760, Friend of Colonist and Mohawk* (Philadelphia: University of Pennsylvania Press, 1945), p. 201.

warriors who could march 30–50 miles in a day, frequently without food. Mrs. Mary Rowlandson, taken in a raid on Lancaster, Mass. on February 16, 1676, was forced to carry a wounded child through the snow. An Indian threatened to kill the child if she did not keep pace with the party. The only food available on this march was broth made from a horse's leg. She found that Indians could exist on diets at least as demanding as those of modern military survival courses: acorns, ground nuts, horse guts and ears, skunks, tree bark, rattle snakes, and extracts from old bones. Her comment on her captivity experience says at least as much about Indian values as it does about her own religion: *"It is good for me that I have been afflicted. The Lord has shown me the vanity of these outward things."*[5]

Robert Rogers, the famous frontier commander of the Seven Years War, observed that the Indians "have no stated rules of discipline, or fixed methods of prosecuting a war; they make attacks in as many different ways as there are occasions on which they make them, but generally in a very secret skulking, underhand manner, in flying parties that are equipped for the purpose, with thin light dress, generally consisting of nothing more than a shirt, stockings and mogasins, and sometimes almost naked."[6]

Indian rules were not stated in military manuals, but they were clear enough to veteran frontier opponents. "The principles of their military action are rational, and therefore often successful. . . .", wrote one such commander. "In vain may we expect success without taking a few lessons from them."[7] The ability to exploit particular situations was a hallmark of experienced Indian warriors trained in the Indian way of war from the age of twelve. The rigid and inflexible discipline of European armies was a means by which inexperienced and unmartial peasants might be transformed into soldiers. This was unnecessary for Indian warriors possessing the skills and self-discipline of modern commandos or special forces and capable of adapting to unique circumstances. They were masters of the "secret, skulking" way of war: the raid, the ambush and the retreat. Their clothing is indicative of their practicality. Many whites came to pre-

---

[5] *Narratives of the Indian Wars 1675–1695*, ed. Charles Henry Lincoln (New York: Scribner's, 1913), p. 167.

[6] Rogers, *Concise Narrative*, p. 229.

[7] General John Armstrong to President Washington, December 23, 1791, in *The St. Clair Papers*, ed. W.H. Smith, 2 vols. (Cincinnati: Robert Clarke, 1882), II, p. 277.

fer Indian dress to European uniforms and shoes. Frontier rangers such as Rogers, George Rogers Clark, and Daniel Boone clothed themselves in Indian fashion. General John Forbes, leader of the successful British march on Fort Duquesne in 1758, ordered many of his men to adopt Indian dress: "I must confess in this country, wee must comply and learn the Art of Warr, from Ennemy Indians or anyone else who have seen the Country and Warr carried on in it."[8]

In addition to clothing, Europeans adopted many native crafts for use in frontier warfare. Light birchbark canoes were excellent vessels for men moving quickly on inland waterways interrupted by frequent portages. The seventeenth century Massachusetts Indian superintendent Daniel Gookin observed that one man could carry a five passenger canoe on his back for several miles.[9] Snowshoes made possible long distance wintertime raids; easily portable maize rations helped sustain them.[10] Indians seem to have been able to apply any material to practical use in an emergency. Mary Rowlandson's captors eluded their English pursuers by crossing a river on rafts made from brush. Her would-be rescuers were forced to give up the chase. On the other hand, Indians prized the products of European iron working industries. These trade goods which transformed the Indian way of life included tools such as knives, chisels, drills, and hammers. Iron hatchets were valued both as tools and weapons. In addition, woolen blankets provided warmth unmatched by any Indian materials. But it was the introduction of firearms which fundamentally transformed the Indian way of war.

Samuel de Champlain is generally credited with being one of the first to introduce the Indians of northeastern North America to the use of firearms in a battle against the Mohawks in 1609. By the end of the seventeenth century, the Indians of the region were well supplied with muskets. The Indian preference for the musket over the bow and arrow requires some explanation.[11] Early seventeenth

---

[8] *Writings of General John Forbes Pertaining to his Service in North America*, ed. Alfred Proctor James (Menosha, Wisc.: Collegiate Press, 1938), p. 125.

[9] Daniel Gookin, "Historical collections of the Indians in New England", *Massachusetts Historical Society Collections*, 1st Series, I (1792), p. 153.

[10] My discussion of Indian technology is based primarily upon Patrick Malone, *The Skulking Way of War: Technology and Tactics Among the New England Indians* (Lanham, MD.: Madison Books, 1991).

[11] In addition to Malone on this point, see also Thomas B. Abler, "European technology and the art of war in Iroquoia", *Cultures in Conflict: Current Archeological Perspectives*, eds. Diana Claire Tkaczuk and Brian C. Vivian, Proceedings of the

century matchlock guns, fired when the powder was ignited by a
slow burning fuse or match, were unreliable, inaccurate, cumbersome and slow. In wet weather they were useless. Indeed, sixteenth
century Spanish troops continued to rely upon crossbowmen and
swordsmen in battles with Indian opponents. Indians preferred the
self-igniting flintlock musket introduced during the seventeenth century. However, one modern expert who has tested the flintlock against
the bow has found the latter to be superior in almost every respect.[12]
Flintlock muskets were also inaccurate single shot weapons which
were difficult to load in any position other than standing. While the
musket's discharge produced a frightening noise, the sound and the
smoke emitted by black gunpowder was inconsistent with a skulking
way of war. Europeans may have converted from bows to early
firearms because it was easier to train new recruits to become musketeers rather than archers. But Indian boys were accustomed to
bows from an early age. Patrick Malone, the expert on seventeenth
century New England Indian technology, believes that the Indians
saw that bullets travelled faster than arrows and took a more direct
route to the target, thus making a musket easier to aim. Bullets were
less likely to be deflected by brush and were more damaging on
impact. Indians were skilled at dodging arrows, almost impossible in
the case of bullets. Muskets could be loaded to fire several small bullets with one shot making it easier to strike targets.[13]

During the eighteenth century lighter and more practical weapons
became available for hunting and woodland warfare. European officers
noted the Indian preference for the short barreled and light weight
fusil. In the latter half of the century rifled barrel muskets with
increased accuracy and range became common on the frontier.
European soldiers often scorned rifles because they were slower to
fire and more fragile than the standard issue smooth bore muskets
which could also support a bayonet. But rifles were marksmen's

---

Twentieth Annual Conference of the Archaeological Association of the University
of Calgary (1989), pp. 273–282; and Brian Given, "The Iroquois and native firearms",
Native Peoples, Native Lands Canadian Indians, Inuit and Metis, Carleton Library Series
No. 142, ed. Bruce Alden Cox (Ottawa: Carleton University Press, 1987), pp. 3–13.
The standard work on firearms for the period is M.L. Brown, *Firearms in Colonial
America: The Impact on History and Technology 1492–1792* (Washington: Smithsonian
Institution Press, 1980).

[12] Abler, p. 10.

[13] Malone, p. 31. Both Malone and Abler reached their conclusions by comparative tests of the musket against the bow.

weapons suitable for hunting and Indian military tactics. One officer present at General Edward Braddock's defeat in 1755 attributed the slaughter of the British troops to the Indians' effective use of rifles. By the mid-1760's, the veteran frontier commander Colonel James Bradstreet became so concerned about the large number of rifles acquired by Ohio and Great Lakes Indians that he "submitted if it would not be a public benefit to stop making and vending of any more of them in the colonies, nor suffer any to be imported."[14] Indians did not entirely abandon bows. They had value as stealth weapons and could be resorted to in ammunition shortages, but by the end of the seventeenth century firearms were the principal weapons of the Indians of eastern North America.

Indians soon demonstrated skill in the use of firearms superior to their European opponents. Since they made no distinction between hunting and warfare, they trained to achieve accurate marksmanship in both. From an early age Indian men spent their lives acquiring these skills and they became second nature. In contrast, the peasantry were disarmed by law in most European countries. When recruited as soldiers they were trained to fire rapid but unaimed volleys rather than to aim at marks. Destructive enough at close quarters on European battlefields, this method of fire was ineffective in the woods. European settlers in North America brought their military training with them. While they possessed firearms for self defense, they remained for the most part an agrarian people with no special skill in hunting or marksmanship. As Malone observes, "Unfortunately, our popular image of the sharp-shooting frontiersman is questionable even for the early nineteenth-century settlers of Kentucky and is far removed from the reality of the seventeenth-century colonists of New England."[15]

Ironically, the North American Indians not only adapted firearms to their own use, but became among the most formidable marksmen of the seventeenth and eighteenth century world. The challenge that this skill presented to European soldiers cannot be overestimated. The Indian commitment to firepower is even more striking when placed in the context of the eighteenth century European theoretical

---

[14] See numerous references to fusils in the *Writings of General John Forbes*. Also to military affairs: "Colonel Bradstreet's thoughts on Indian affairs", *Documents Relative to the Colonial History of New York*, ed. E.B. O'Callaghan, VII (1856), p. 692.

[15] Malone, p. 60.

debate over shock versus fire. Many European officers believed that
infantry firearms did relatively little damage and expressed a preference for attacks with cold steel. Generals such as Maurice de Saxe
and, early in his career, Frederick the Great advocated advancing
on the enemy with shouldered muskets. The Sieur de Folard urged
the reintroduction of the pike and the revival of something resem-
bling the Macedonian phalanx. Folard had many disciples; his advo-
cacy of the column in preference to the line (the natural formation
for volley fire) would influence French military thought through the
Napoleonic wars and beyond. There were examples of shock prevailing over fire in the eighteenth century, but it appears in hindsight that Indian tactics based on aimed fire represented an advance
over much of the best in contemporary European military thought
and practice.[16]

Indian conversion to firepower meant a dependence on European
suppliers for arms and ammunition. If Indian-European warfare had
been a simple conflict between two monolithic blocks, this would
have been a fatal dependency. Colonial governments often sought
to prevent arms sales to Indians, but such regulations were seldom
effective. Not only did French, Dutch, and English governments pursue different arms sale policies, the English colonies themselves often
failed to cooperate. Arms were an economic as well as a security
issue and an important commodity of exchange in the fur trade.
Furthermore, while it was clearly desirable to deprive hostile Indians
of firearms, it was equally desirable to equip one's allies. Indeed,
failure to provide arms and ammunition could drive an Indian ally
into the hands of the enemy. These complex economic and political conditions assured that the Indians of eastern North America
were equipped with firearms by the end of the seventeenth century.[17]

Firearms required extensive maintenance and repair thus presenting
the Indians with new technological challenges. On the whole, native
artisans adapted well. During the seventeenth century, New England
Indians acquired the art of casting bullets and making gunflints.

---

[16] Maurice de Saxe, *Reveries on the Art of War*, trans. Thomas R. Phillips (Harrisburg,
1944), p. 32; Frederick the Great, *Instructions for His Generals*, trans. Thomas R.
Phillips (Harrisburg, 1960), p. 92; Sieur de Folard, *Nouvelles découvertes sur la guerre*
(Paris, 1726), pp. 83, 253–274. The best discussion of eighteenth century military
thought is Azar Gat, *The Origins of Military Thought from the Enlightenment to Clausewitz*
(Oxford, 1989).
[17] Malone, pp. 42–51.

There is evidence that Indian blacksmiths became proficient in the repair of muskets and in assembling them from parts. Gunpowder manufacture, however, required concentrations of capital and technological expertise beyond the capacity of Indian societies. While weapons could be repaired and reused, gunpowder was an expendable commodity which only Europeans could supply. Ammunition shortages could contribute to the sudden collapse of promising Indian military efforts such as King Philip's War in New England in 1676 and the Pontiac uprising in the mid-west in 1764.[18]

Artillery remained a virtual European monopoly although the Swedes provided the Susquehannock Indians of the Delaware Valley with cannon in the 1660's. They used them to beat off an attack by an army of Five Nations Indians and later to defend a fort against a siege by Virginia and Maryland militia.[19] Palisaded Indian villages were rendered defenseless against European troops equipped with cannon. Indians learned that their forts could easily turn into death traps and often abandoned their towns on the approach of a European army. European commanders had to content themselves with burning the towns and the crops. Slender food reserves might force the Indians to make peace, but such hardships usually did not impair their ability to retaliate by ambushes and raids against white settlements. Indians were seldom prepared to risk casualties in assaults on fortified positions. Settlers fortunate to gain the security of a blockhouse or stockade were relatively safe from attack by Indian raiders. However, it was difficult for settlers to watch their homes and fields go up in smoke and often, as in the case of the celebrated Wyoming Valley "massacre" in Pennsylvania in 1778, they sallied forth into disastrous ambushes. Without cannon the Indians could seldom overcome forts. Often they employed fire arrows, carts loaded with combustibles, and sometimes mining against fortifications. They were skilled at seizing posts by ruses as at Michilimackinac in 1763 when they gained entrance to the fort in pursuit of a lacrosse ball.

Firearms seem to have transformed inter-Indian warfare in the seventeenth century. Pre-European contact warfare was often characterized by hand to hand encounters between large forces which resulted in relatively few casualties. Indians were able to dodge arrows

---

[18] Ibid., pp. 71–72; Jenny West, *Gunpowder, Government and War in the Mid-Eighteenth Century* (The Royal Historical Society: The Boydell Press, 1991).

[19] Steele, *Warpaths*, p. 53.

and sometimes wore wooden or leather armor which provided a
measure of protection. Indian success in war was frequently measured by captives taken rather than deaths inflicted. The seventeenth
century Iroquois, their population levels under stress from epidemic
disease and the rising level of violence associated with the fur trade
wars, placed a high value on captives whom they adopted in order
to sustain their numbers. Despite their fearsome reputation, Iroquois
warriors did not take unnecessary risks and were prepared to yield
an apparent victory on the field if the cost in life was too high.
Some Indians appear to have been shocked by the level of violence
introduced by European soldiers. During the New England Pequot
War of 1637, Connecticut troops and their Indian allies surrounded
a palisaded Pequot village on the Mystic River. The Connecticut
men overwhelmed the defenders by musket fire, burned the houses,
and killed all of the inhabitants including women and children. Many
of the English Narragansett Indian allies departed rather than par-
ticipate in such an atrocity and those who remained denounced the
unnecessary slaughter. European arms and methods altered Indian
styles of warfare. They could ill afford to compete in the open field
against the murderous volley fire of European musketeers. During
the seventeenth and eighteenth centuries Indian warriors discarded
armor useless against musket balls and avoided hand to hand combat unless the enemy was in disarray. The skulking way of war was
a logical response to new conditions and was employed by parties
of warriors whose numbers might range from a handful to several
hundred.[20]

Indian warfare is often portrayed as being marked with special
cruelty or savagery. Indian warriors were not constrained by European
military codes and did not draw the same distinctions between com-
batant and non-combatant or between war and murder. Their style
of war was equivalent to that of the modern commando or guerilla

---

[20] James Axtell, *Beyond 1492: Encounters in Colonial North America* (New York and
Oxford: Oxford University Press, 1992), pp. 141–142; Ian Steele, *Warpaths: Invasions
of North America* (New York Oxford University Press, 1994), pp. 92–93; Adam Hirsch,
"The Collision of Military Cultures in Seventeenth-Century New England", *The
Journal of American History*, Vol. 74 (1987–1988), 1187–1212; Neal Salisbury, *Manitou
and Providence: Indians, Europeans, and the Making of New England, 1500–1643*, (New
York: Oxford University Press, 1982), pp. 221–225; Daniel Richter, "War and
Culture: The Iroquois Experience", *The William and Mary Quarterly*, Series 3, Vol.
40 (1983), 528–559.

fighter, one which even today cannot be easily waged according to the principles of international law and military codes. For example, commandos may find themselves in possession of prisoners whom they cannot safeguard and whose liberty would endanger them. Would they be justified in killing the prisoners in such circumstances? While military lawyers generally answer in the negative, some officers believe that necessity must prevail.[21] The eighteenth century ranger Robert Rogers killed prisoners in such circumstances and it would be surprising if Indians showed greater scruples. In fact Indians probably had greater motivation for keeping prisoners alive than did Rogers.[22] The Indian "skulking" way of war included many practices that Europeans regarded as unfair or inhumane: ambushes, surprises, attacks on civilians, and cruel treatment of prisoners. Aimed fire was a controversial issue in itself. Indian sharpshooters had no reservations about firing at sentries and officers, a practice which many European regulars regarded as tantamount to murder.

The Indian way of war paralleled the male Indian's life as a hunter. One European observer concluded that the Indian warrior "uses the same stratagems and cruelty as against the wild beasts. . . ."[23] Some aspects of Indian cruelty towards captives including torture, scalping, beheading, and cannibalism may be explained by the close relationship between warfare and hunting. Indian cosmologies did not award humans a position superior to other creatures. Hunters believed that animals deserved respect; they could be killed for food, but possessed a spiritual nature that required ritual attention. Similarly, many Indians do not seem to have regarded as fully human non-members of their tribal group. Many captives could expect no better than death nor torture, but others passed through adoption rituals which gave them full membership in the tribal family. Thomas Gist was captured near Fort Duquesne in 1758 and was fortunate to be adopted into an Indian family as a replacement for a dead member. He recalled that: "I was led into the house where I was to live,

---

[21] Telford Taylor, *The Anatomy of the Nuremberg Trials: A Personal Memoir* (New York: A. Knopf, 1992), p. 253.

[22] Robert Rogers, *Journals of Major Robert Rogers* (Readex Microprint, 1966), pp. 128, 145; Rogers, "Journal of a Scout" Jan. 25, 1757, Huntington Library, San Marino, Ca., Loudon Papers, LO 2704 A&B.

[23] William Smith, *An Historical Account of the Expedition Against the Ohio Indians in the Year MDCCLXIV under the Command of Henry Bouquet. . . .* (Philadelphia, 1766), p. 38. Smith based this account on information provided by Bouquet.

there strip'd by a female relation and then led to a river. There she wash'd me from head to foot. . . . As soon as this ceremony was over I was clad from head to foot; then there was an interpreter brought to tell me which of my kin was the nearest to me. I think they re[k]onded from brother to seventh cousin."[24]

The purposes of the brutal torture and cannibalism are not clear. In some cases torture seems to have been rooted in tribal rituals. In others the motive was revenge for an injury suffered at the hands of the enemy. For example, the brutal torture of Colonel William Crawford after his defeat by the Delawares at Sandusky, Ohio, in 1782 was a response to the massacre earlier in the year of a peaceful village of Moravian mission Indians by undisciplined frontiersmen. Not all Indians engaged in cannibalism and some rejected torture. The Delawares were never cannibals and expressed contempt for Mohawk "man-eaters". By the mid-eighteenth century eastern tribes had generally abandoned the practice. The Ottawa resistance leader Pontiac was criticized by his Indian allies for cannibalism and later became known for his "lenity and gentleness" with prisoners. The great Shawnee chief Tecumseh was well known for his antitorture views.[25]

Scalping was the most notorious Indian rite of war. However, it paled in comparison to beheading and other cruelties and some scalping victims survived to tell of their experience. While there have been allegations that scalping was introduced by Europeans, it now seems firmly established that it was a pre-Columbian custom widely spread among North American Indians.[26] In the seventeenth century European frontier fighters also began to scalp their opponents and the practice continued throughout the period. European authorities

---

[24] Howard Peckham, "Thomas Gist's Indian captivity narrative 1756–1759", *The Pennsylvania Magazine of History and Biography*, Vol. 80, No. 3 (July, 1956), 299. For the Indian "Rites of War" see Gregory Evans Dowd, *A Spirited Resistance: The North American Struggle for Indian Unity 1745–1815* (Baltimore: Johns Hopkins University Press, 1992), pp. 9–22.

[25] Jennings, *The Invasion of America*, pp. 160–163; White, *The Middle Ground*; Great Britain, Scottish Record Office, Edinburgh, "Journal of a detachment of the 42nd Regiment going from Fort Pitt down the Ohio to the country of the 'Illenoise'. . . .", Hunter, Harvey, Webster and Will Collection, G.D. 296\196, pp. 144–145; R. David Edmunds, *Tecumseh and the Quest for Indian Leadership* (Boston: Little Brown, 1984), p. 44.

[26] James Axtell and William C. Sturtevant, "The unkindest cut, or Who invented scalping?", *The William and Mary Quarterly*, 3rd Series, Vol. 37, No. 3 (July, 1980), 451–472.

began to offer bounties for scalps which transformed the practice into a financial transaction and encouraged its spread. Experienced frontier diplomats warned that bounties prompted indiscriminate killings which only inflamed the frontier. By the mid-eighteenth century some white leaders worried about the moral or at least the public relations consequences of scalp bounties, but that did not stop the practice. Scalp bounties created a kind of war by body count which played havoc with attempts to establish good Indian relations.[27]

These good relations were crucial to successful frontier military efforts. European commanders found Indian allies to be indispensable in the wilderness. Successful ranger leaders such as Benjamin Church and Robert Rogers included a large number of Indians in their commands while generals such as Edward Braddock and John Forbes lamented their absence. Few Europeans could equal the Indians' wood craft, scouting ability, and marksmanship. At the very least, it was best to seek them as allies rather than to confront them as enemies. Indians allied themselves with Europeans for a variety of reasons. Some sought advantages against rival Indian nations. Christian Indians were prepared to ally with Europeans as a means of accommodation. The mission Indians of Canada supported the French partly as the result of the influence of Jesuits who sometimes accompanied their raids. Christian or "praying" Indians sided with the New England settlers during King Philip's War. In the late seventeenth century, New England authorities recruited Indian mercenaries whose pay was an important source of income at a time when they were losing their lands.[28] Economic decisions sometimes dictated alliances. During the seventeenth century, the French allied with the Hurons against the Iroquois because of the former's strategic position in the fur trade. This ignited a period of prolonged war which devastated the Hurons. The Iroquois continued to contest the control of the fur trade with western Indian tribes and the French in the latter part of the seventeenth century. Although the small Quebec colony suffered heavily in these conflicts, the Iroquois were defeated by an alliance of French and Great Lakes Indians who now matched the Iroquois in firearms. The failure of New York to honor

---

[27] Wallace, *Conrad Weiser*, p. 434; *Frontier Advance on the Upper Ohio, 1778–1779*, ed. Louise Phelps Kellogg (Madison, 1916), p. 385; *Frontier Retreat on the Upper Ohio, 1779–1781*, ed. Louise Phelps Kellogg (Madison, 1917), pp. 183–184.

[28] Richard C. Johnson, "The search for a usable Indian: An aspect of the defense of colonial New England", *The Journal of American History*, Vol. 64 (1977), 623–651.

commitments to support the Iroquois in these wars caused the latter to retreat into a policy of neutrality during the first half of the eighteenth century. Indian economic dependence on European trade goods including arms and ammunition often formed the basis of political alliances. During the American War of Independence, the inability of impoverished Revolutionary authorities to supply friendly Indians undermined the efforts of American diplomats to secure frontier alliances.

The cardinal mistake made by some white authorities was the assumption that Indians could be forced into alliances or dependent roles against their interests. Indian tribes did not regard themselves as subject peoples and often rejected commitments made by their own chiefs which they believed ran counter to their well being. Richard White has demonstrated that French influence in the Great Lakes region during the eighteenth century rested upon diplomacy and commerce rather than force. The Indians of the region referred to the Governor of Quebec as Onontio, the great mountain, the keeper of peace and harmony. When the French sent an expedition into the Ohio country in 1747 to claim formally the area for the French king it was met with hostility. Subsequent construction of French forts led the Indians to explore an alliance with British authorities. Only when British leaders proved unwilling or incapable of protecting Indian lands from English settlers, did the Indians reluctantly ally with the French.[29] British General Jeffrey Amherst, who led the Anglo-Americans to victory over France in North America, developed an Indian policy that was a prescription for disaster. He scorned the ability of Indian warriors and was determined to secure by force the Great Lakes region, ceded by France in 1763, without consulting its Indian inhabitants. On the one hand, he severely reduced expenditures for presents to the Indians which they considered to be the tangible sign of good will; on the other, he spread a number of inadequately garrisoned forts across the region which provoked Indian hostility without overawing them. The result was the 1763 uprising known as Pontiac's rebellion which shook Britain's grip on the region. In two years of war the Indians fought the British Empire to a draw.[30]

---

[29] Richard White, *The Middle Ground: Indians, Empires, and Republics in the Great Lakes Region, 1650–1815* (Cambridge: Cambridge University Press, 1991), pp. 199–232; Michael N. McConnell, *A Country Between: The Upper Ohio Valley and its Peoples, 1724–1774* (Lincoln: University of Nebraska Press, 1992), pp. 61–120.

[30] Steele, *Warpaths*, pp. 234–237; White, *The Middle Ground*, pp. 256–261; McConnell, *A Country Between*, pp. 147–181.

Some eighteenth century military commanders such as John Burgoyne and Barry St. Leger unfairly blamed their Indian allies for their lack of success. Some modern historians have also disparaged the Indians as unreliable allies and useless fighters. Often these writers fail to appreciate the qualities of Indian warriors who had no interest in fighting in the European style or for European objectives. These critics also assume that the Indians were passive clay who could be "used".[31] Although Indians were sometimes recruited by colonial authorities to serve as rangers, relatively few American Indians served as mercenaries; they were not Sepoys. Instead they fought for motives of their own and in their own way. They had to be convinced that their ally's cause justified their participation. The Western Abenakis of Vermont were thus prepared to fight English settlers during the Seven Years War whether or not the French Governor wanted them to. But they were not enthusiastic about participating in the American War of Independence. A few hundred were coerced into joining General John Burgoyne's march from Canada to New York in 1777, but deserted him as his prospects dimmed.[32] On the other hand, the Shawnees of Ohio, determined to protect their lands from American settlement and to drive settlers from their Kentucky hunting grounds, were at the forefront of a British-Indian alliance that retained the military initiative in the mid-west until the conclusion of peace between Britain and the United States.[33] The Indians were thunderstruck when they learned that Britain had ceded the region to the new American government. Not until 1815, after suffering a series of military humiliations, were the Americans able to impose their claims upon the Indian peoples.

---

[31] Those who fail to appreciate the abilities of Indian warriors and thus the value of Indian allies include Robert L. Yaple, "Braddock's defeat: The theories and a reconsideration", *Journal of the Society for Army Historical Research*, 46 (1968), 194–201; and Howard Swiggett, *War out of Niagara: Walter Butler and the Tory Rangers* (New York: Columbia University Press, 1933; repr. Port Washington, N.Y.: Ira J. Friedman). Those who conclude that the British did not properly "use" the Indians in the American War of Independence include Jack M. Soison, *The Revolutionary Frontier 1763–1783* (New York: Holt, Rinehart and Winston, 1967), p. 105; and Henry Steele Commager and Richard B. Morris, eds., *The Spirit of "Seventy-Six: The American Revolution as told by Participants"* (Indianapolis and New York, 1958), 2 Vols., II, p. 999.

[32] Colin G. Calloway, *The American Revolution in Indian Country: Crisis and Diversity in Native American Communities* (Cambridge: Cambridge University Press, 1995), p. 72.

[33] Ibid., p. 39.

Although they were expected to see to their own defense, few of the Spanish, English, French and Dutch who came into conflict with North American Indians during the sixteenth and seventeenth centuries were "professional" soldiers. Sixteenth century Spanish soldiers were warlike military volunteers and adventurers. They came from the strong martial tradition of the *Reconquista* but are not to be confused with the professionals of the *tercios* which projected Spanish power in Europe. English settlers brought with them their native militia institutions and methods of warfare. The Iroquois war prompted the French government to send professional troops to Canada in 1665, but the regulars achieved limited success. The Quebec militia, many of whom gained experience of the Indians way of life by participating in the fur trade to the interior, proved to be more effective in frontier warfare than any of the regulars dispatched from home. The latter were usually best assigned to garrison duty.[34] British regulars did not make a significant appearance in North American warfare until the 1750's. Their first campaign, Braddock's march to the Monongahela, was an unmitigated disaster. Some British regular officers such as Forbes and Bouquet adapted well to frontier warfare. Others, such as Amherst, never bothered to learn.

English colonists arriving in Virginia based their defense on an ancient institution: the militia which had its roots in the Anglo-Saxon fyrd. As feudalism became militarily obsolete and politically suspect during the Tudor period, the militia gained renewed significance for the defense of the realm. Elizabeth I's government gave increased attention to the training and equipment of the militia and established élite trained bands to provide a well trained and well armed core. By the end of the reign the trained bands had exchanged bows for firearms and began to be trained in the volley fire techniques common to European battlefields. This militia organization and the adoption of firearms were the two important elements of English military life that the first settlers brought to Jamestown. They were crucial to the salvation of the colony when war erupted with the Powhatan Indian confederacy in 1609. Even so the colony was almost abandoned before a new governor arrived with reinforcements including experienced soldiers and introduced a strict military discipline upon the inhabitants. The new commanders included men who had

---

[34] W.J. Eccles, *The Canadian Frontier 1534–1760* (New York: Holt, Rinehart, and Winston, 1969), pp. 122–124.

served in Elizabethan wars in the Netherlands and in Ireland. One expert concludes that "at present there is little evidence to permit an evaluation of the tenuous but indisputable relationship between English military experiences in Ireland and developments in Virginia."[35] The parallels are certainly clear. The Irish successfully used guerilla tactics against the English, winning most of their victories by ambush. They were also better shots. The English responded with a strategy that was to be the staple of their wars against North American Indians: to seek out and destroy the enemy in open battle; to seek aid from the Irish themselves; to hem in the enemy with fortifications; and, in the last resort to devastate the countryside so that the hostile force could not live upon it.[36] The English defeated the Powhatan confederacy by a similar strategy. The Powhatans lived in a region penetrated by numerous navigable waterways. The English exploited this geographical feature by confining the Indians with lines of fortifications and sailing into their homelands on heavily armed ships to burn their villages and crops. A central weakness of Indian societies was slender food reserves and the inability to replace lost provisions by imports. The English sought to force them to choose between an open field battle against armored musketeers or starvation. Naval power gave the English the ability to strike deeply and unexpectedly. In the Pequot War of 1637 the Connecticut troops exploited their ability to move by sea to carry out their devastating surprise attack against the Pequots' village at Mystic.

Continued challenges by the Powhatan Indians forced Virginia to maintain vigorous militia institutions during the first half of the seventeenth century. There is evidence that the militia began to adapt to the Indian way of war by employing loose order and firing at marks. As the threat waned and social tensions increased in the second half of the century, the militia became smaller, excluding slaves and servants. The militia had become an agency of domestic order

---

[35] William Shea, *The Virginia Militia in the Seventeenth Century* (Baton Rouge: Louisiana University Press, 1983), p. 140. For Elizabethan military institutions and practices see C.G. Cruikshank, *Elizabeth's Army*, 2nd ed. (Oxford: Oxford University Press, 1966); Lindsay Boynton, *The Elizabethan Militia* (London, 1967); and John S. Nolan, "The militarization of the Elizabethan state", *The Journal of Military History*, Vol. 58, No. 3 (July, 1994), 391–420.

[36] Cyril Falls, *Elizabeth's Irish Wars* (New York: Barnes and Noble, 1970), 341; Nicholas P. Canny *The Elizabethan Conquest of Ireland: A Pattern Established 1565–1576* (New York: Harper and Row, 1976), p. 160.

and the colony now relied on imperial forces or diplomacy for external defense. The middle colonies, insulated until the mid-eighteenth century from threats from Canada, also allowed their militias to decay. South Carolina's militia remained active in the face of a three fold threat: Spanish and Indian enemies on the frontier and a large slave population within the colony's borders. Indian fighting during the eighteenth century seems to have influenced the partisan war carried out by militia veterans against British and loyalist forces during the War of Independence. However, in normal circumstances, South Carolina's unique situation made it difficult to assemble a large force, for militiamen were reluctant to leave their homes unguarded against potentially rebellious slaves. The militia's military potential was neutralized by the demands of domestic order.[37]

The New England militia, recruited from towns governed by elected officials and faced with a long term threat from hostile Indians and their French allies, remained a vigorous institution throughout most of the colonial period. During King Philip's War, 1675–1676, the militia provided adequate local defense, but was continually outmatched by an enemy skilled in the use of firearms and in woodcraft. Trained in close order and volley fire, the militia suffered a series of stinging defeats at the hands of an enemy who seemed always to have the advantage of surprise.[38] Massachusetts Bay experienced a wave of anti-Indian hysteria which led colonial authorities to confine even friendly Christian enemies to an island in Boston harbor, thus depriving the English of allies skilled in forest warfare. Connecticut, by contrast, employed non-Christian Pequot and Mohegan warriors and its forces fared much better in the woods. The most famous English soldier in this war was Benjamin Church of Plymouth Colony, who formed a ranger force that ultimately killed the Wampanoag leader Philip. Church's command included a company of Indians, some of whom were recruited from prisoners. He adopted

---

[37] John Shy, "A new look at the colonial militia" in *A People Numerous and Armed, Reflections on the Military Struggle for American Independence* (New York: Oxford University Press, 1976), Chapter 2. For the Quebec militia see W.J. Eccles, "The French forces in North America during the Seven Years War", *The Dictionary of Canadian Biography*, III, *1741–1770*, ed. Francis G. Halpenny (Toronto: University of Toronto Press, 1974), p. xvii.

[38] Douglas Leach, *Flintlock and Tomahawk: New England in King Philip's War* (New York: Macmillan, 1958, particularly chapter 6. See also the same author's "The military system of Plymouth Colony", *The New England Quarterly*, XXIV (1951), pp. 342–364.

Indian skulking tactics and proved capable of pursuing hostile Indians in the forest.[39] Church's success occurred while the Indian war effort was in decline. After a successful offensive against Massachusetts and Plymouth settlements in the spring of 1676, the Indian effort collapsed. Food and ammunition shortages, Indian disunity, battle casualties, disease and exposure made it impossible for the Indians to continue. Indian losses were horrific. One estimate is that out of a southern New England Indian population of 11,600 in 1675, 7,900 were dead, enslaved or homeless by the end of 1676. The English probably lost at least 1,000 dead out of a population of 50,000. Of 52 towns, 17 had been destroyed and 25 pillaged. The New England economy was virtually bankrupt at war's end.[40]

By the end of the seventeenth century, English-Indian conflicts in New England merged with the great imperial struggles between Britain and France. These wars presented a challenge of new dimensions for New Englanders. Having destroyed Indian independence in southern New England, English settlers now encountered warlike new enemies in the Abenakis of the more remote regions of Vermont, New Hampshire, and Maine. For decades the Abenakis were able to mount destructive raids against English settlements and retire into the remote fastnesses of the north. While New Englanders destroyed the eastern Abenaki settlement at Norridgewock, their punitive expeditions could not even find the villages of the elusive western Abenakis of Vermont. French support for the Abenakis provided them with reliable supplies and ammunition and Canadian sanctuaries for their families. They therefore were able to conduct their war against English settlers from a more secure base than had Philip's followers. However, the Abenakis fought to protect their land and homes, not as French mercenaries. Even during the period of Anglo-French peace in the 1720's, the western Abenaki chief Grey Lock waged an independent and successful frontier war against English settlers.[41]

English militia performed poorly in these campaigns. They lacked adequate training and tactics to match Abenaki warriors in the forest. Furthermore, as part-time soldiers they could not afford to desert

---

[39] See Benjamin Church, *Diary of King Philip's War 1675–1676*, ed. Alan and Mary Simpson (Chester, Conn.: Pequot Press, 1975).

[40] Axtell, *Beyond 1492*, p. 239; Russell Bourne, *The Red King's Rebellion: Racial Politics in New England 1675–1678* (New York: Athenaeum, 1990), p. 36.

[41] Colin Calloway, *The Western Abenakis of Vermont, 1600–1800* (Norman: University of Oklahoma Press, 1990), pp. 113–115.

their fields for lengthy campaigns fought at a long distance. New sources of manpower and new measures were needed to meet the challenge. Colonial governments turned to the recruitment of volunteers who served for pay or the promise of loot. Volunteers came from elements of the population not represented in the militia: Indians, free Blacks, white servants and apprentices, and others who lacked deep ties to settler communities. By the eighteenth century, most frontier warfare was conducted by these soldiers while the militia constituted a part-time home guard with limited training. The New England strategic response to the challenge of border raids was to launch major naval-military expeditions against the Canadian sanctuary. This allowed the English to exchange unconventional border wars in which they were weak for conventional campaigns in which they possessed advantages in ships, men, and materials. However, the strategy did not bear full fruit until the fall of Quebec in 1759.

The tactical superiority of the Indian opponents and their French allies thus required a major imperial response. British naval forces participated in early campaigns against Quebec or its outlying defenses at Louisbourg and Port Royal. Unsuccessful expeditions were launched against Quebec in 1690 and 1711 before it fell in 1759. Port Royal was captured in 1710 and Louisbourg twice in 1745 and 1758. But British regulars did not play a significant role in Indian warfare until Braddock's army arrived to drive the French from the Ohio Valley in 1755. Braddock's campaign was compromised from the beginning when colonial authorities failed to secure him Indian allies who could protect his column in the woods. Braddock may have sealed his fate when he spurned a Delaware chief who asked that the British guarantee the Ohio Indians possession of their lands.[42] The Delawares would be among his opponents on the Monongahela. Although Braddock followed standard march discipline employed against light troops in Europe, his mixed force of regulars and Virginia militia were almost totally without forest experience. When they encountered a numerically inferior party of French and Indians near Fort Duquesne, they were quickly surrounded on three sides by enemy marksmen and shot to pieces. Out of Braddock's defeat came the myth that colonials understood woodland combat better than the regulars, but it was not founded on reality. A few weeks later a colo-

---

[42] McConnell, *The Middle Ground*, pp. 119–120.

nial commander, Colonel Ephraim Williams, led New England troops into an Indian ambush near Lake George without taking even Braddock's precautions.[43]

European commanders learned the value of rangers trained in forest warfare. Many ranger units included Indian scouts. All great frontier commanders including the Anglo-Americans Benjamin Church and Robert Rogers and the French-Canadians La Corne St. Luc and Chaussegros de Lery gained success because of their ability to lead mixed forces of European rangers and Indians. British general John Forbes lamented his lack of Indian support in his march on Fort Duquesne. He experimented with what he called the Indians' "cousins", the Highlanders, as light troops to screen his army, but his able subordinate, the Swiss professional Henry Bouquet, later complained that Highlanders became lost as soon as they stepped off the path.[44] Forbes and Bouquet avoided Braddock's fate by exercising great caution. Forbes moved carefully from one fortified post to another, but even so Colonel James Grant carelessly led an advanced party into a defeat at the hands of the Indians. In 1763, Bouquet also had to command a relief expedition to Fort Pitt, on the site of the former Fort Duquesne. He fought a bloody two day battle with Indians at Bushy Run in which he succeeded in beating off the enemy with a surprise bayonet attack, but suffered such severe losses that he was unable to continue his campaign after the fort was relieved. Bouquet seems to have believed that regular troops could not match the Indians in loose order woodland fighting. His plans for an advance on the Ohio Indian towns in the following year called for the troops to form a square and engage in volley fire if attacked.[45]

During the 1770's English settlers west of the Appalachian mountains adopted styles of warfare similar to that practiced by Indian opponents. This was especially true of the fampous "long hunters"

---

[43] For reports of the Battle of lake George see *Documents Relative to the Colonial History of New York*, ed. E.B. O'Callaghan, VI, pp. 1003–1013, and X, pp. 316–399 and pp. 422–423.

[44] *Writings of General John Forbes*, pp. 117, 191, 198; Douglas Brymer, *Report on the Canadian Archives*, 1889, Note D (Ottawa, 1890), pp. 61–61.

[45] "Disposition for march and to receive attack", Sept. 15, 1764, Bouquet Papers, British Museum, Add. Mss. 21, 653, 316–320. For a discussion of the manner in which the British army adapted to frontier conditions see Steve Brumwell, "'A service truly critical': The British Army and warfare with the North American Indians, 1755–1764", *War in History*, V, No. 2 (April, 1998), pp. 146–175.

whose way of life came more and more to resemble that of the Indians of the region. Frontiersmen such as George Rogers Clark and Daniel Boone wore Indian dress and fought as mounted riflemen. Clark did not hesitate to scalp Indian prisoners. Still, they were often unable to outmatch the Indians in this sort of war. Frontiersmen were plagued by what has been called "fool bravery" which led them into ambushes set by more cautious Indians. The most famous example of this flaw was the defeat of a party of 180 experienced Kentucky woodsmen including Boone who rushed heedless into an Indian ambush at the Battle of Blue Licks in 1782.[46] This incident counters the myth of the natural superiority of the frontier partisan over regulars such as the unfortunate Braddock. Nevertheless, there was a clear evolution from traditional militia training toward the Indian way of war.

During the American War of Independence, American authorities were unable to protect the frontier from raids by Indian warriors supplied from British bases at Niagara and Detroit. American armies launched punitive expeditions against Indian homelands in 1778, most notably General Sullivan's campaign against the Iroquois. Sullivan invaded Iroquoia with an army of 4,000 men including Oneida scouts and troops drawn from Daniel Morgan's famous rifle corps. Sullivan wreaked great destruction on the towns and fields of the enemy Senecas and Cayugas, but fought only one inconclusive skirmish with Indians and Tory Rangers. The expedition was forced to withdraw because of its own logistical problems and the onset of cold weather. The western Iroquois had been rendered dependents on the British, but were still formidable enemies in the field. The inability of the Americans to capture Niagara and Detroit meant that the western Indians retained the military initiative until the end of the war.[47]

The Anglo-American peace treaty presented the western Indians with a situation similar to the one they had encountered in 1763. Even though they had not been defeated, their ally had surrendered title to their homeland without consultation. British officers on the

---

[46] John Mack Faragher, *Daniel Boone: The Life and Legend of an American Pioneer* (New York: Henry Holt, 1992), pp. 214–224

[47] *Journals of the Military Expedition of Major General John Sullivan against the Six Nations of Indians in 1779*, ed. Frederick Cook (Auburn, N.Y.: Knapp, Peck and Thomson, 1887); Calloway, *American Revolution*, pp. 51–51; Swiggett, *War Out of Niagara*, pp. 194–199.

scene were humiliated by this betrayal of those whom they had encouraged to pursue the war. While the new government of the United States looked upon the Ohio lands as a solution to its financial problems, it did not want an Indian war. Its hand was forced by a stream of settlers determined to establish themselves in lands north of the Ohio River. This led to the new republic's first major war in which two American armies were defeated by an Indian confederacy determined to defend its rights by force of arms. Most notably, an Indian confederate army defeated General Arthur St. Clair on November 4, 1791, killing 600 of his 1450 men. It was the worst defeat ever suffered by a United States army at the hands of the Indians. In a manner reminiscent of earlier European-Native American conflicts, Indian riflemen enjoyed the advantages of surprise and cover as they slaughtered the Americans drawn up in close order. St. Clair was avenged by General Anthony Wayne at Fallen Timbers in 1794, but his "decisive" victory owed as much to divisions among the Indians and British failure to provide timely aid as it did to American military prowess. Fallen Timbers led to Indian recognition of American claims north of the Ohio.[48]

However, Indian resistance to American expansion revived after 1809 in the wake of the imposition of new treaties resulting in additional land cessions. Tecumseh and his brother, the Shawnee Prophet, combined nativist spirtualism with an appeal for a great north-south Indian alliance. Tecumseh's attempt to rally the southern Indians met with little success and the Prophet's followers were dispersed by Indiana Governor William Henry Harrison at the Battle of Tippecanoe in 1811. The outbreak of the War of 1812 breathed new life into native resistance. During 1812, the British and their Indian allies swept all before them in the Northwest, capturing Michilimackinac and Detroit. Indians made up the majority of the allied forces and, under Tecumseh's leadership, they retained the initiative in forest warfare. However, American fortunes revived in the following year when the American fleet gained control of Lake Erie. Fearing isolation in upper Canada, the British commander General Procter abandoned the Northwest and his Indian allies. Overtaken by William Henry Harrison in his retreat, Procter made a stand in what became known as the Battle of the Thames. The British troops were routed

---

[48] Wiley Sword, *President Washington's Indian War: The Struggle for the Old Northwest, 1790–1795* (Norman: University of Oklahoma Press, 1985).

by Harrison's Kentucky mounted riflemen and Tecumseh was killed while leading Procter's remaining Indian allies. With Tecumseh's death, the dream of united Indian resistance to American expansion was extinguished.[49]

I have attempted in this brief essay to portray the complexity of European-Native American conflict. Indians and Europeans borrowed from one another and adapted their military efforts to new conditions. Successful European commanders seldom ventured into the forests without Indian allies. On the other hand, Native American societies could seldom sustain long term resistance to European "invasions" without European allies. Neither European professionals nor English colonial militias drawn from settled agricultural districts adapted well to forest warfare. As often happens professional or social conventions had priorities over military realities. Those who best adapted were men of the frontier such as the French Canadian militia, inured to the hardships of the fur trade and accustomed to the Indian way of life. Here, particularly in the latter part of the eighteenth century, the lives of settlers began to resemble those of their Native American neighbors and with that their military practices. The settlers had experienced a military evolution which allowed them to complete the invasion of eastern North America. In this respect, conflict on the frontier may be viewed as a synthesis of two military cultures.

Bibliography

R. Allen, *His Majesty's Indian Allies: British Indian Policy in the Defence of Canada, 1774–1815* (Toronto: Dundurn, 1992).
J. Axtell, *Beyond 1492: Encounters in Colonial North America* (New York: Oxford University Press, 1992).
———— *European and Indian: Essays in the Ethnohistory of Colonial America* (New York: Oxford University Press, 1981).

---

[49] For biographies of Tecumseh and his brother, see R. David Edmunds, *The Shawnee Prophet* (Lincoln: University of Nebraska Press, 1983), and *Tecumseh and the Quest for Indian Leadership* (Boston: Little Brown and Co., 1984). The combination of spiritualism and resistance is best explored by Gregory Evans Dowd, *A Spirited Resistance: The Struggle for North American Unity, 1745–1815* (Baltimore: Johns Hopkins University Press, 1992). For the War of 1812, see Reginald Horsman, *The War of 1812* (New York: Knopf, 1969), and Harry L. Coles, *The War of 1812* (Chicago: University of Chicago Press, 1965).

———— *The Invasion Within: The Contest of Cultures in Colonial North America* (New York: Oxford University Press, 1985).

R. Bourne, *The Red King's Rebellion: Racial Politics in New England, 1675–1678* (New York: Atheneum, 1990).

C. Calloway, *The American Revolution in the Indian Country: Crisis and Diversity in Native American Communities* (Cambridge: Cambridge University Press, 1995).

———— *The Western Abenakis of Vermont, 1600–1800* (Norman: University of Oklahoma Press, 1990).

B. Church, *Diary of King Philip's War, 1675–1676*, ed. A. and M. Simpson (Chester, Conn.: The Pequot Press, 1975).

H. Coles, *The War of 1812* (Chicago: University of Chicago Press, 1965).

D. Delage, *Bitter Feast: Amerindians and Europeans in Northeastern North America, 1660–1664*, trans. Jane Brierly (Vancouver: UBC Press, 1993).

G. Dowd, *A Spirited Resistance: The North American Struggle for Indian Unity, 1745–1815* (Baltimore: Johns Hopkins University Press, 1992).

W.J. Eccles, *The Canadian Frontier, 1534–1760* (New York: Holt, Rinehart and Winston, 1969).

———— *Frontenac: The Courtier Governor* (Toronto: McClelland and Stewart, 1959).

R.D. Edmunds, *The Potawatomis: Keepers of the Fire* (Norman: University of Oklahoma Press, 1978).

———— *The Shawnee Prophet* (Norman: University of Oklahoma Press, 1983).

———— *Tecumseh and the Quest for Indian Leadership* (Boston: Little, Browm, 1984).

L.V. Eid, "A Kind of Running Fight: Indian Battlefield Tactics in the Late Eighteenth Century", *The Western Pennsylvania Historical Magazine*, LXXI (1988), 147–171.

J.M. Faragher, *Daniel Boone: The Life and Legend of an American Pioneer* (New York: Henry Holt, 1992).

J. Ferling, *A Wilderness of Miseries: War and Warriors in Early America* (Westport, Conn.: Greenwood Press, 1980).

G. Fregault, *Canada: the war of the conquest*, trans. Margaret M. Cameron (Toronto: Oxford University Press, 1969).

L.H. Gipson, *The British Empire before the American revolution*, 15 vols. (Caldwell, Id.: Caxton Printers, 1936–1970).

B. Graymont, "The Six Nations Indians in the Revolutionary War", *The Iroquois in the American Revolution* (Rochester: Rochester Museum and Science Center, 1981).

R. Horsman, *Expansion and American Indian Policy, 1783–1812* (East Lansing: Michigan State University Press, 1967).

———— *The War of 1812* (New York: Knopf, 1969).

R.D. Hurt, *The Ohio Frontier: Crucible of the Old Northwest, 1720–1830* (Bloomington: Indiana University Press, 1996).

F. Jennings, *The Ambiguous Iroquois Empire* (New York: Norton, 1984).

———— *Empire of Fortune: Crowns, Colonies, and Tribes in the Seven Years War* (New York: Norton, 1988).

———— *The Invasion of America: Indians, Colonialism, and the Cant of Conquest* (Chapel Hill: University of North Carolina Press, 1975).

I. Kelsay, *Joseph Brant, 1743–1807: Man of Two Worlds* (Syracuse: Syracuse University Press, 1984).

R. Kohn, *Eagle and Sword: The Federalists and the Creation of the Military Establishment in America, 1783–1802* (New York: the Free Press, 1975).

P. Kopperman, *Braddock at the Monongahela* (Pittsburgh: University of Pittsburgh Press, 1977).

D. Leach, *Flintlock and Tomahawk: New England in King Philip's War* (New York: Macmillan, 1958).

P. Malone, *The Skulking Way of War: Technology and Tactics Among the New England Indians* (Lanham, Md.: Madison Books, 1991).

M. McConnell, *A Country Between: The Upper Ohio Valley and Its Peoples, 1724–1774* (Lincoln: University of Nebraska Press, 1992).

J. Merrell, *The Indians' New World: Catawbas and Their Neighbors from European Contact through the Era of Removal* (Chapel Hill: University of North Carolina Press, 1989).

P. Nelson, *Anthony Wayne: Soldier of the Early Republic* (Bloomington: Indiana University Press, 1985).

J. O'Donnell, *Southern Indians in the American Revolution* (Knoxville: University of Tennessee Press, 1973).

S. Pargellis, *Military Affairs in North America, 1748–1765* (1936, repr, Archon Books, 1969).

F. Parkman, *France and England in North America*, 2 vols. (New York, 1983).

H. Peckham, *The Colonial Wars 1689–1762* (Chicago: University of Chicago Press, 1964).

———— *Pontiac and the Indian Uprising* (Princeton: Princeton University Press, 1947).

F. Prucha, *The Sword of the Republic: The United States Army on the Frontier, 1783–1846* (Toronto: Collier-Macmillan, 1969).

D. Richter, *The Ordeal of the Longhouse: Peoples of the Iroquois League in the Era of European Colonization* (Chapel Hill: University of North Carolina Press, 1992).

N. Salisbury, *Manitou and Providence: Indians, Europeans and the Making of New England, 1500–1643* (New York: Oxford University Press, 1982).

W. Shea, *The Virginia Militia in the Seventeenth Century* (Baton Rouge: Louisiana State University Press, 1983).

J. Shy, *A People Numerous and Armed; Reflections on the Military Struggle for American Independence* (New York: Oxford University Press, 1976).

R. Slotkin, *Regeneration Through Violence: Mythology of the American Frontier, 1600–1860* (Middletown, Conn.: Wesleyan University Press, 1973).

J. Soison, *The Revolutionary Frontier, 1763–1783* (New York: Holt, Rinehart and Winston, 1967).

I. Steele, *Betrayals: Fort William Henry and the "Massacre"* (New York: Oxford University Press, 1990).

———— *Guerrillas and Grenadiers, The Struggle for Canada, 1689–1760* (Toronto: Ryerson Press, 1969).

———— *Warpaths: Invasions of North America* (New York: Oxford University Press, 1994).

H. Swiggert, *War out of Niagara: Walter Butler and the Tory Rangers* (New York: Columbia University Press, 1933).

W. Sword, *President Washington's Indian War: The Struggle for the Old Northwest, 1790–1795* (Norman: University of Oklahoma Press, 1985).

B. Trigger, *The Children of Aataentsic: A History of the Huron People to 1660*, 2 vols. (Montreal: McGill-Queen's University Press, 1976).

A. Vaughn, *The New England Frontier: Puritans and Indians, 1620–1675* (Boston: Little, Brown, 1965).

R. White, *The Middle Ground: Indians, Empires, and Republics in the Great Lakes Region, 1650–1815* (Cambridge: Cambridge University Press, 1991).

J. L. Wright, Jr., *Britain and the American Frontier, 1783–1815* (Athens: University of Georgia Press, 1975)

———— *The Only Land They Knew: The Tragic Story of the American Indians in the Old South* (New York: The Free Press, 1981).

4. THE LONG CONQUEST:
COLLABORATION BY NATIVE ANDEAN ELITES
IN THE COLONIAL SYSTEM, 1532–1825

David Cahill

Divide and conquer is the conventional ploy of imperial powers bent upon conquest. Indeed, it is almost a metaphor for conquest. Famously, it was the leitmotiv of the Spanish conquest of the Incan empire, as it had been of the Aztec domains. Beyond the immediate conquest campaigns, and their sequel in the implementation of imperial bureaucratic frameworks—military, administrative, fiscal, judicial, civic and ecclesiastical—and the wider colonization process, the trope of divide and conquer may be extended to embrace, *grosso modo*, some three centuries of colonial rule in Spanish America. To be sure, the implementation of colonial rule appeared less stark in the "mature" colonial period than during the early decades of conquest and settlement, simply because Spanish institutions had by then long taken root on American soil. Historical studies on the colonial Andes have hitherto focussed more on resistance movements against Spanish rule than on the bases of the *pax hispana*. The sixteenth century neo-Inca insurgencies and related chiliastic uprisings gave way to a century in which anti-imperial sentiment, such as it was, appears to have been almost entirely dormant.[1] This was, though, just the calm before the storm. As the eighteenth century wore on, an unremitting avalanche of Bourbon reforms sought to restructure the very foundations of the colonial system, a governmental upheaval not witnessed since the sixteenth century. The turmoil of the initial decades of conquest finally spent itself, the overture to the reform programme of Viceroy Francisco de Toledo (1569–81), which established an institutional template for colonialism in the Andes. The swingeing reforms of the Bourbons, most notably spent under the aegis of Charles III (1759–1788),

---

[1] On the conquest period, see especially Hemming (1970) and Espinoza Soriano (1981). For the resistance and/or chiliastic movements see the articles in Ossio (1973), which also carries through such themes into the modern period, and Stern (1982). The study of this poorly-understood phase of early colonial resistance is now undergoing considerable revision: see, e.g., Ramos (1993).

effected a governmental revolution in the Andes, wound back colonists'
rights and privileges, witnessed an almost exponential increase in
colonial resources accruing to the Crown, pressed especially hard
upon the indigenous communities, alienated the several tiers of colonial society, and paradoxically undermined the imperial control the
reformists had sought to enhance.

Commencing in the 1730s, and gathering pace from the 1770s,
an upsurge of protests, revolts, conspiracies and rebellions represented
merely the most emphatic Andean response to this root-and-branch
overhaul of the colonial compact, the implementation of a swathe
of legislation known as the "Bourbon reforms". This eighteenth-
century conjuncture of violent protest, as indeed the entire Andean
repertoire of contention and "weapons of the weak", has long been
a favorite stamping ground for historians.[2] Yet to focus unduly on
these often spectacular resistance movements, small as well as great,
rather obscures the circumstance that by far the greater part of the
three centuries of colonial rule was peaceful. While much effort has
been expended on the institutions, social arrangements, and economic life in the colonial Andes, little attention has been directed
to the key question of how and why peace was maintained for so
long in such an inequitable colonial system. There was never a time
when the causes of discontent were lacking; indeed, those selfsame
grievances that underlay the open, violent protest of the late colonial era had for the most part always existed. The obverse of the
question as to why rebellion was mainly confined to the late eighteenth century is that of how and why the colonial settlement endured
for so long unchallenged. Rebellion and protest were exceptions to
the rule. Yet to set rebellion against quiescence is to frame the historical problem too starkly. Between accommodation and resistance
were myriad nuances that variously described the colonial relationship, and which fluctuated over time according to a wide array of
local, regional and international circumstances. These shadings of
colonial power shifted and evolved as the wider imperial context
fluctuated, and the continuous flow of metropolitan laws, decrees
and orders were articulated through all the colonial levels of governance, from a Viceroy and Audiencia down to a village mayor or
petty chieftain.

---

[2] Stern (1987) reviews the historiography, while Lewin (1957) and O'Phelan (1985)
address the entire, late colonial "age of insurgency" in the southern Andes.

This essay will deal with the latter type of indigenous "élites". It will focus on the structure of indigenous officeholders and their post-conquest functions, circumscribed though these were. These officials were heirs to the complex, hierarchical Incan bureaucracy. While on the face of it the structure of native Andean local government embraced a less elaborate hierarchy of officeholders than that to be found in colonial Mesoamerica, it is likely that this was a matter of semantics: the same functions in the Andes were performed by local officials sporting a smaller and therefore less splendid array of titles. We know from the chronicler Felipe Guaman Poma de Ayala that in the pre-conquest era there had been a wide variety of petty officials at village level, a sophisticated division of labour that was collapsed into a handful of offices soon after the conquest. In the colonial Andes, these sorted into four groups: the several tiers of the "chief-tain" office of *kuraka* a.k.a. *cacique*; the village municipal authorities (*alcalde, regidor, alguacil et al.*); ecclesiastical minor officials, confrater-nity and ritual sponsors (*cantor, fiscal, mayordomo, prioste, alférez*); with, finally, the comparatively patrician officeholders representing the sur-viving Inca nobility of Cuzco, erstwhile capital of the Inca empire, and a few scattered indigenous nobles elsewhere in the Viceroyalty. This chapter will discuss the manner in which the first of these indigenous offices—the several variations on the theme of the generic cacique—dovetailed into comparable Hispanic institutions and the overarching governmental *cum* bureaucratic colonial system. As a nec-essary point of departure, however, it will first sketch the structure of prehistoric chiefdoms and their subsequent reorganization into the encompassing Incan decimal structure. It will then analyse the ramifications of the Spanish conquest for indigenous governmental structures, above all for the ranks of the *kurakas*, a catch-all category applied (usually indiscriminately) to village headmen and headwomen (*cacicas*), moiety rulers, provincial lords, and even to those rulers rec-ognized by first Incan then Spanish conquerors to have been bona-fide monarchs. The discussion has two overriding goals: to indicate the ways in which these native Andean élites directly and indirectly contributed to the initial and continuing Spanish conquest of Andean lands and their subject peoples, and to explore the evolution of the chiefly office, the kuraka or cacique, over the three centuries of colo-nial rule. It will focus especially on the network of caciques in the southern Peruvian highlands, heartland of the Inca empire, and the region for which extant colonial documentation is most abundant.

Indeed, it was there that caciques were also most abundant: in the 1754 census, there were 1512 "caciques principales" in the Viceroyalty, plus another 566 in the neighbouring Charcas region, largely co-terminus with present-day Bolivia; 639 (42%) of the former were located in the Archdiocese of Cuzco.[3]

It is, then, a study in collaborationism, a word that in its contemporary usage carries overtones of treason, of Quislings rushing to do the bidding of occupying forces. It would be a crass anachronism to cast indigenous élites in such an unfavourable light. Those élites were for the most part not betrayers of their peoples, but rather intermediaries or brokers mediating between the colonial State and the communities they ruled or for which they were otherwise responsible. This was a thankless rôle that rarely satisfied either their communities or the colonial officials to whom the native élites reported. Many, perhaps most, exploited their communities and communal resources shamelessly, employing high-handed and even violent methods in their expropriations. Colonial archives abound with detailed accounts of exploitative kurakas/caciques, yet such illicit behaviour is usually all of a piece with the pre-conquest modus operandi of these local authorities: privileged access to communal resources; marshalling a labour corvée from willing or unwilling communities; extraction of taxes in kind or in cash; using such resources to buy allies within and without a community; controlling the flow and distribution of scarce produce or sumptuary goods; the use of force to compel loyalty or just subservience; pre-eminence in village justice and policing; insertion in religious and sacerdotal networks; mediating with overlords from provincial ruler to even the Inca lords themselves—all these functions were features of the exercise of many pre-1532 kurakazgos.

It follows from this commonplace that what often appears in colonial documentation as overweening arrogance and unconscionable exploitation on the part of kurakas, may represent little more than incumbents exercising their functions, rights and privileges in the traditional manner. Put another way, such behaviour, extraordinary to outsiders, may have fitted easily into a kind of traditional, political "moral economy". However, whether a kuraka's hapless victims nec-

---

[3] These figures are drawn from the viceregal census of 1754, compiled under the aegis of Viceroy José A. Manso de Velasco, Conde de Superunda—see Moreno Cebrián (1983).

essarily accepted despoliation or mishandling is another matter entirely, manifestly so in view of the abundant documentary evidence of judicial complaints against colonial *kurakas*.[4] Individual or group bucking of traditional practice does not disprove the existence of such a moral economy, but merely indicates that not everyone was prepared passively to accept victimhood or that an existing, perhaps implicit, moral economy was breaking down under the impact of colonialism, a colonialism far more disintegrative and burdensome in its extraction of resources than its Incan forerunner had been. Moreover, what may at first sight appear overbearing behaviour may be no more than a kuraka attempting to force communal compliance in order to meet State, Church or local Hispanic élite demands for taxes and labour prestations. Colonial kurakas, great and small, had to straddle two worlds.

Chiefs and Chiefdoms

What comprised "great" and "small" chiefdoms or *kurakazgos* is a problem of definition, on which anthropologists and archaeologists on the one hand, and historians on the other, tend to take diametrically opposed positions. The former base their approach (in the Andean case) largely on a reading of the conquest chronicles combined with the archaeological method, while the latter rely especially upon archival documentation on native Andean society stretching across five centuries. The former present a basically static and synchronic picture, while the latter seek to trace developments in the several levels of "chiefdom" office over time. There is little crossover, perhaps reflecting a demarcation of Andean history into pre-Columbian—monopolized by archaeologists and anthropologists—and colonial and republican eras, which are dominated by pedigreed historians. The upshot of this academic artificiality is that each side seems to be talking about a different world. The positive outcome, however, is that the social science approach is heavily and usefully theoretical, while historians bring an abundance of new archival data

---

[4] These documentary materials form the principal basis for studies of caciques/kurakas, cf. Spalding (1970, 1973, 1984); Stern (1982); O'Phelan (1985); Cahill (1984, 1990, 1993); Larson (1988); Rasnake (1988); Sempat Assadourian (1994); Powers (1995); Sala i Vila (1996).

to the discussion (such as it is). While this essay will be heavily empirical, a brief glance at the theory of chiefdoms developed by anthropologists, on which there is a good deal of common ground, will
provide a framework for what follows.

A landmark 1988 conference on chiefdoms aimed to reach an
anthropological consensus on the nature and evolution of the institution across several culture areas.[5] It sought to construct a typology
that would hold true across cultures and timeframes. The broad premise on which the anthropological *cum* archaeological approach relies
is that "[a] chiefdom is a regional polity with institutional governance and some social stratification organizing a population of a few
thousand to tens of thousands of people" and that "[c]hiefdoms are
intermediate polities, bridging the evolutionary gap between small,
village-based polities and large, bureaucratic states".[6] Chiefdoms, however, sort into "simple" and "complex", according to the size of the
subject population under the command of a chieftain. Simple chiefdoms embrace populations in the "low thousands"; complex chiefdoms have "polity sizes in the tens of thousands". The former is
"one level in the political hierarchy above the local community"; the
latter two levels above. Dispensing entirely with the possibility that
chiefdoms of less than a few thousand subjects might exist at all,
Timothy Earle contends that "the fundamental dynamics of chiefdoms are essentially the same as those of states, and that the origin
of states is to be understood in the emergence and development of
chiefdoms".[7] These are complex polities indeed, much closer to states
than to "small, village-based polities". How well does this typology
or conceptualization fit the Andean case?

The first thing that strikes one is the sheer arbitrariness of its
assumptions. On what grounds are polities measuring two or three
thousand inhabitants considered to be chiefdoms, while those with
less than, say, two thousand are not only regarded as less than chiefdoms but as lower on the evolutionary scale of political formation
that runs from hunter-gatherers to full-blown state? Chiefdoms defined as "complex" exist on a higher evolutionary rung than do their
"simple" counterparts. There appears to be no provision within this
hierarchic "model" for a political entity located somewhere between

---

[5] Earle (1991) is, effectively, a record of the proceedings of the conference, with
an acute summary by the editor.
[6] Earle (1991); also Earle (1997).
[7] Ibid.

village-based and intermediate polities, though presumably there are simple and complex models of village-based polities, encompassing many villages rather than just a few. Nor, for that matter, does it take into account the experience of rapid depopulation in the colonial Americas. In the sixteenth century, polities the size of both complex and simple chiefdoms declined vertiginously, well below the benchmark 2000 figure. Did they therefore cease being chiefdoms? And when their populations later recovered and came to exceed 2000 inhabitants, was their chiefdom status restored? The gap between complex and simple chiefdom status is, theoretically, presumably a transition or "evolutionary" phase, but the theory appears to make no provision for historical cases such as the demographic devastation in the chiefdoms of the Americas. Chiefdoms with widely fluctuating populations, in the light of this model, appear to be maverick or pathological cases. This immediately raises the question of what the leaders of these complex and simple village-based polities are to be called: headman and headwoman, "big man", petty chief, foreman, bureaucrat, or just leader (as in "take me to your leader")? To pose the question thus is to highlight the extent to which the word "chief" is a construct, and an English-language one at that. Moreover, while the 1988 conference ranged across cultures and chronological periods, its outcome does appear to reflect the academic *status quo* concerning prehistoric chiefdoms.

Chiefdoms and Cadres under the Incas

The picture that emerges does indeed involve a hierarchy of chiefdoms. These range from powerful ethnic lords to humble village officials, the latter often just one remove from the hewers of wood and drawers of water, yet all are subsumed within the one category of "kuraka" or the later colonial "cacique". This generic designation is warranted for all, because they depended on each other and to a large extent developed from one another—a chieftain magnified several times over, like a set of Russian dolls that fit snugly within one another. The most vivid and perhaps the best metaphor for the structure of the Andean chiefdoms is Karen Spalding's image of a "nested tier".[8] This almost perfectly describes the hierarchy of Incan imperial

---

[8] Spalding (1984).

officials ordered in terms of the Incan decimal scheme of imperial administration, and remains a useful short-hand characterization of the several tiers of indigenous governance in the colonial era. The decimal structure, moreover, was based upon earlier Andean polities that had been similarly organized in hierarchies, for all that these were less complex than the Incan arrangement in the "mature" imperial phase. As the idea of a "nested tier" implies, the respective powers of the several chieftains overlapped, with the higher supervising the lower, and so on down the chain of command. The following representation of the Incan decimal organization illustrates the simplicity of the system, though this should not obscure the complexity of its operation.[9]

The leaders of these entities, great and small, were called *"camáyoc"*, not kuraka, and the alternative terminology was perhaps indicative of the Incan subjugation of local tradition to the imperial ethos, with a corresponding shrinkage of local autonomy. *Camáyoc* was a generic Quechua suffix appended to all manner of offices, from artisans, bureaucrats, settlers, to provincial governors; it indicated function as well as level of authority. The salient point to be made here, however, is that the hierarchy of imperial functionaries bore a strong resemblance to the several tiers of kurakas in the colonial era, indicating that kuraka was likewise a generic term encompassing not only those "decimal" levels but perhaps many besides; those, for example, that reflected remnants of local ethnic autonomy, or an overlapping of chiefly and sacerdotal functions, or perhaps other officially acceptable local élites who continued to function parallel to the imperial decimal organization. The Incas, after all, were prepared to be flexible in their treatment of polities who submitted to the Inca's will without putting up too much of a fight. Moreover, as we know from the northern chiefdoms, the decimal organization and related Incan impositions on the newly conquered were often tentative and gradual in their implementation.[10] It was often one step forward and two steps backward, such that when the Spaniards arrived, the notional decimal system was either absent or incomplete in the northern

---

[9] Bravo (1986), p. 113.
[10] See especially Salomon (1986) for a remarkable historical reconstruction of the transition from pre-Incan to Incan eras in the Quito region (essentially, that co-terminus with present-day Ecuador); see also Powers (1995), who takes the story of evolution of the Quiteño cacicazgos into the colonial era.

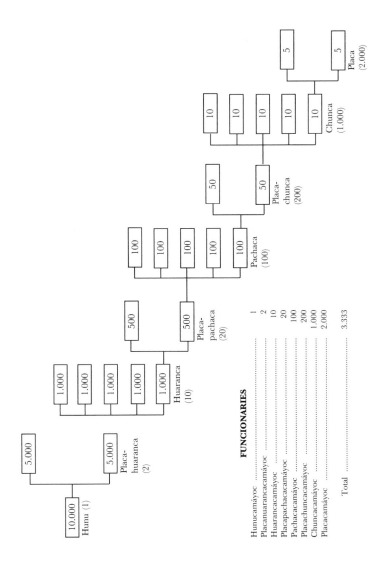

Figure 4.1. The Incan decimal organization.

marches. The empire of Tahuantinsuyu frayed and unravelled at its edges.

The base of the decimal system was the *pachaca*, the unit of one hundred families (*purej*), and this was the fundamental basis for tribute and military levies. The highest unit of ten thousand (*hunu*), was further integrated into a provincial structure of forty thousand (*huamani*), comprising four of the *hunu*, and this greater administrative unit was ruled by a Ttocrícuc, a Cuzqueño noble who was something of a little Inca in his domain. These *huamanís* were in turn integrated into one of the four *suyus*, the quarters of the empire individually ruled by an *Apo*, a great lord closely related to the ruling Sapa Inca himself. The overall structure was something of a bureaucrat's delight, with a putative 3333 officials for each 10,000 tributary families, or 13,342 *camáyoc* for each unit of 40,000 families. In fact, most provinces fell well short of this figure, with some provinces little more than the size of a *hunu*; it is doubtful if more than two provinces met the optimal figure of four *hunus*.[11] Yet this was far from being the extent of the administrative hierarchy in the empire (Tahuatinsuyu). It was superimposed upon a vast network of traditional (i.e. pre-Inca) chiefdoms, which continued functioning and operated simultaneously with the somewhat artificial decimal organization. If the *pachaca* was the fundamental building-block of the latter, then the kin-based *ayllu* or lineage group was and remains the cornerstone of native Andean society generally. Under the Incas, though, the *ayllu* ostensibly comprised 300 families or three *pachacas*. Yet they operated "on two different planes": administration of the empire by the *camáyoc* cadres; and the traditional community life and customs controlled by the kurakas who, though, might aspire to any of the *camáyoc* posts up to the *hunu* or 10,000 level. There was of course considerable integration of these two parallel ruling groups, but it was always clear where precedence lay. Local autonomy was wholly subordinated to the imperatives of the empire. It was precisely resentment at this erosion of autonomy that spurred local polities (*etnías*) to cast their lot with the conquistadores. The Spanish incursion represented an opportunity for a recovery of autonomy in partnership with a powerful ally which, to all appearances, seemed only interested in booty. In any case, anyone was better than the

---

[11] Wachtel (1977); Bravo (1986); Zuidema (1989); Pärsinnen (1992).

devil they knew. Insurgent Andean provinces could always settle accounts later with the newcomers, should they prove recalcitrant. From a native Andean viewpoint, the quarrelsome conquistadores, riven by internecine disputes embracing even civil war, were dispensable allies, right from the first moment of contact.

Brokers, Opportunists and Social Climbers: The Early Conquest Era

The Spanish conquest from 1532 ineluctably swept away the decimal system and the hierarchy of *camáyocs* who administered it. The end of decimal administration ordained that in each erstwhile Incan province or *huamaní* of a putative 40,000 tributaries, exactly 13,342 administrators, from the provincial governor or *ttocrícuc* to the lowliest *placacmáyoc* were ostensibly out of a job; even in the smallest province of 10,000, some 3333 officials were affected. In practice, however, the implications of the collapse of the decimal system were undoubtedly less disruptive. Many of the *camáyoc* were drawn from the communities, such that there was logically a significant overlap between not only the two groups of local authorities, but between imperial and traditional governing structures. While the remaining Incan and *mitmaqkuna* who staffed the upper reaches of the *camáyoc* hierarchy may well have found themselves suddenly anachronistic and surplus to requirements, some may have been accepted into traditional communities. The existence of separate *mitmaq* communities throughout the colonial period suggests that this did happen at some remove, but the fact that *mitmaq* groups or *ayllus* remained distinct from the "traditional" or *originario* communities suggests that few of the supernumerary *camáyocs* were welcome in their localities once the decimal system had disintegrated. Presumably many were among those dislocated *vagabundos* who took to the roads in the wake of the conquest, attached themselves to Spaniards as servitors (*yana, yanacona*), or otherwise carved out sundry niches for themselves under the new colonial dispensation.[12]

In what seemed almost a reprise of the conquest of Mexico, Pizarro's host descended on Peru to an enthusiastic welcome from some among the subordinate polities or *etnías* of the Incan empire.

---

[12] Villar Cordova (1966); Murra (1975); Wachtel (1977); Cahill (1995).

The *pax incaica* was an agony for small kingdoms, for kingdoms they were. Chiefdoms such as the Chimu, Huanca, and Chincha had been wealthy kingdoms or "feudal" domains (*reinos, etnías, señorios*)— the designations were coined by the early chroniclers—prior to their subjugation to Inca rule. The Chimu had even consolidated their own empire, which the emergent Incas of the fourteenth century may have sought to emulate as a model for their own, greater empire. The glory of autonomy was in some cases a living memory, such that tribute in kind, labour and army levies, and the imposition of Incan satraps and bureaucrats served only to underscore what had been lost. Once the Spaniards' aggressive intent became apparent, however, the possibility of alleviation or liberation from the reach of Cuzco and its attendant burdens was immediately grasped by the Inca's forced "allies", most of whom reluctantly provided levies for the Incan armies. Disgruntled Andean polities now offered martial and logistical support to the Spanish cause, invaluable and perhaps indispensable help in the inhospitable terrain that the conquistadores had to negotiate along the route to Cuzco.[13] As in Mexico, allies counted.

Their desertion to European ranks correspondingly weakened the Incan defences, not least because they understood Incan warfare from the inside. When the Spaniards laid siege to Cuzco, they were able to count upon the support of several Andean *etnías*, such as the Cañaris from Ecuador—many of whom were already resident in Cuzco—the Chachapoyas from the tropical lowlands of the north-eastern Peru, and the numerous Huanca from the central sierra.[14] Famously, the Spaniards had arrived in the midst of a war of succession to the Incan throne, between the Cuzco- and Quito-centred pretenders, sons of the emperor Huayna Capac. The pretender from Quito, Atahuallpa, had like his father forged strong links with the Cañaris, such that they came to comprise the Inca's bodyguard. Yet, at the last moment, they turned, and became the allies of the new invaders. For this, the Cañaris and especially their chiefs were amply rewarded with lands, servitors (*yana, yanaconas*) and (with their confederates the Chachapoyas) a monopoly of the postillion (*chasqui*) jobs in the colonial postal service. Such was the gratitude of conquistadores and later viceroys alike that these two allied groups were con-

---

[13] Hemming (1970); Espinosa Soriano (1981).
[14] Ibid.

signed effective control of the Cuzco *barrio* of Carmenca, the colonial parish of Santa Ana as it soon became, and the lush Incan lands of Yucay in the "sacred" Vilcanota valley.[15]

When we look at the early colonial documentation on the functioning of the kurakazgo, however, the perspective alters radically. When set against the theory of chiefdoms, the historical reality looks very messy indeed. At the point at which we move from prehistoric to historic Andean chiefdoms—the Spanish conquest itself—these suddenly loom into view as their incumbents speak, as it were, for the first time. Whatever the worth of theories on the nature and size of prehistoric Andean chiefdoms, in the historical era the functions of a cacicazgo and the collateral expectations held of caciques by royal officials were unequivocal. Most extant colonial documentation on succession to cacicazgos stipulated those functions and expectations clearly enough.[16] They were to be guardians of legality and moral police, vigilant against the pernicious alcoholic excesses that, then as now, were the bane of campesino communities. Caciques retained, too, a vaguely defined if minor judicial jurisdiction, which meant little other than acting as an impromptu justice of the peace in mediating minor village squabbles, though many caciques accrued de facto policing powers, behaving much as minor despots. They were tax agents, above all for the royal tribute or capitation tax, for a whole range of ecclesiastical taxes—above all the parochial or sacramental fees that so enriched beneficed rural clergy—and the sale of the several types of indulgences (*bulas de cruzada*) distributed by the cura, but whose proceeds mostly went into royal coffers. Their religious role, however, was not merely passive. It was they who, in the first instance, were responsible for marshalling the community for mass, the *doctrina* and celebration of fiestas, notwithstanding that a range of minor officials and sponsors formally carried out these functions. Moreover, colonial caciques left eloquent testimony to their own piety—syncretic though it may have been—by becoming patrons of chantries, pious works and monasteries, founding chapels and even a béguinage (*beaterio*).[17]

---

[15] Ibid.

[16] Díaz Rementería (1977) is a magisterial juridical treatment of the colonial cacicazgo.

[17] For a range of examples: Gisbert (1980); Gutiérrez (1987); Burga (1988).

Collection of taxes and debts by caciques on behalf of clergy and even corregidors was often extra-official, but unavoidable. The collection of tribute was the caciques' principal task, one which enhanced their power in much the same way that pre-1532 caciques had buttressed their own through control and redistribution of resources and labour prestations.[18] Successful administration of tribute was crucial for communities, for the combination of royal and ecclesiastical taxes was a fiscal screw that tightened coeval with the onset of European diseases, and the subsequent depopulation and the alienation of indigenous lands in the sixteenth and seventeenth centuries; in the late eighteenth century, tribute revenues increased exponentially as a result of the enhanced efficiency of the overhauled Bourbon bureaucracy. Successful management of tribute collection was vital even to the very reproduction of a community, but on a lesser scale made a world of difference to individuals. It was the role of a cacique to assign lands within a community on the basis of need, to those eighteen years and older, as consideration for their tributary status. Even with the best will in the world, this was difficult for caciques to manage, for while in some provinces and communities there was sufficient land to distribute, elsewhere there was a serious shortfall. Much of a cacique's de facto power derived from this land-redistribution faculty, the counterpart of the cacical function of organizing and overseeing a community's agricultural cycle; there was of course favoritism and corruption. So, too, many caciques commonly falsified the tribute lists, causing a shortfall in Crown revenues that, across the board, ran into hundreds of thousands of pesos each year. Yet what appears to be mere peculation, what was called corruption by treasury officials, was often a cacique just easing the pressure on the community within his remit. It was not just an individual who was liable for tribute, but a corporate responsibility for the entire community, though legal responsibility for the most part was borne by the cacique. Not a few caciques landed in jail when takings fell below the stipulated tribute quota.

Tribute was often in kind, but the tax itself was expressed in monetary terms. The products assembled to meet tribute assessments had therefore to be commercialized, either by the responsible cacique— yet a further and unofficial burden—or more commonly by the avari-

---

[18] For the pre-colonial arrangements, see Wachtel (1977); Falk Moore (1958).

cious figure of the corregidor, who arbitrarily set the exchange rates for tributary produce and thereby profited handsomely. Yet this was a minor defalcation compared with the administration of the infamous *repartimientos de mercancías*, the forced sale of goods on credit to individual comuneros and underclasses generally.[19] Some corregidors distributed and collected, either peacefully through a cacique or increasingly by the forceful deployment of their own private collectors, hundreds of thousands of pesos of merchandise within their five-year tenure. The extent of this licit but abusive institution was widespread and the pressure on communities so severe that it constituted a prime structural cause of the Andean rebellion of 1780–83, essentially two great insurrections, north and south, each led by a minor provincial cacique, for all that one boasted Incan antecedents.[20] The uprising failed, but the Crown had finally responded to peasant misery by abolishing repartos immediately following the onset of insurgency.

The colonial cacique was, too, a labour agent and foreman. Under the Incas, the kuraka had provided labour gangs for cultivation of the lands of the Inca and the Sun in each province, and for work on the roads and canals and in the mines. This labour service, however, fell under the rubric of tribute, and was in any case part of an overreaching system of reciprocity and redistribution involving the Sapa Inca himself. After the Spanish conquest, however, communal labour obligations became a separate demand. As with tribute extractions, calls on labour now increased markedly, this occurring *pari passu* with a rapid decline in the indigenous population; withal, many communities ceased to exist altogether. Quite apart from maintenance of local infrastructure, comuneros found themselves obliged to till the soil, pastor the herds and man the sweatshop looms of colonial officials, encomenderos, hacendados and priests. Moreover, because tribute demands fell on the community as a collectivity, caciques marshalled (by choice or by force) working parties paid at token daily rates in the obrajes and on haciendas and estancias, in order to raise funds to pay the community's *repartos*, royal imposts, and ecclesiastical fees. More economically and socially destructive— legendarily so—was the mining corvée for gold and silver at Potosí

[19] Moreno Cebrián (1977); Golte (1980).
[20] See n. 2.

and elsewhere, or for the indispensable mercury of Huancavelica.[21]
Adult males (*mitayos, septimas*) in each community were obliged to
work in the mines for one year in each seven; a team went each
year under a "captain", usually a cacique. The mines were usually
a long distance from the home community, and manpower demands
and depopulation were such that many were forced to serve at least
twice within the mandatory seven-year span. While many died in
the mines, many more simply did not return. A hatred of the *mita*,
freer and perhaps more lucrative working opportunities, and not least
a newly acquired family in the mining town all conspired to dis-
suade *mitayos* from returning to their base communities. Caciques
were involved at every stage of the *mita* process, as ever victims
themselves of the exploitative processes they were forced to admin-
ister. Nonetheless, not a few caciques profited from the commercial
opportunities that involvement in the internal trade circuits of the
Viceroyalty offered. Some native and mestizo caciques, notably José
Gabriel Túpac Amaru, the leader of the northern insurrection of
1780–83, even became *arrieros*, owners of fleets of mules that provided the commercial transport of the era. Many more indigenes
plied those same trade circuits, whether as mitayos, in paid employment with the muleteers, or as grudging participants in a corregidor's
private commercial interests. Some caciques, upwardly mobile after
the conquest, revelled in the role of the corregidor's troubleshooter.

The celebrated case of the Cañari kuraka, Francisco Chilche, is
the best if atypical case-study of how an upstart chieftain might profit
from Spanish conquest and colonization. His is the exemplary case
of the phenomenon of the parvenu cacique, the native as "social
climber".[22] Chilche's long, post-conquest career described an arc that
went from the immediate rewards that fell to him through his close
collaboration with the Pizarros, to a middle period in which he exercised an almost untrammelled local despotism largely devoid of traditional Andean forms of reciprocity, to a period of decline starting
in the 1550s in which his power and resources were wound back
by a succession of royal administrators, and which culminated in the
Toledan attenuation of the powers of "over-mighty" indigenous lead-

---

[21] There is now a large bibliography on colonial mining and its labour arrangements; the best place to start is Bakewell (1984).
[22] Spalding (1970).

ers in the 1570s.[23] Chilche was an immediate beneficiary of the dislocation of indigenous society in the Cuzco region in the immediate aftermath of the Spanish conquest of the Inca capital. Serving the Spaniards as he had served Atahuallpa, he was awarded the overlordship of the several indigenous groups in the Yucay area of the Vilcanota Valley, the so-called "Sacred Valley". There, he moved quickly to usurp the vast estates of the Inca and the land dedicated to the Sun cult. He thus possessed most of the premium valley lands, such that he was able to bind indigenous groups to him by granting them access to these lands. He thereby carved out a new kind of polity, one in which his power was based not on the traditional *ayllu* but on a "vast clientele" of servitors (*yana*). Chilche had, according to Nathan Wachtel, "deflected the ancient system of reciprocity to his own advantage".[24] Chilche's career was extraordinary, but points the moral that for all the indigenous authorities brought low by the onset of colonialism, there were still others who profited mightily. However, notwithstanding that some kurakas enjoyed despotic power in certain microregions, unburdened now by an Incan *camáyoc* at their shoulder, the authority of kurakas progessively unravelled and declined once the colonial system was bedded down by Viceroy Toledo. By the eighteenth century, the colonial kuraka appears as a much diminished figure, notwithstanding the elaborate pomp and ceremony that flattered some of their more illustrious brethren in the public sphere.[25]

Many were opportunists, most were cultural brokers or "hinge men", mediating between new overlords hungry for gain and the financially and socially besieged communities, reeling under the impact of exponential tribute and labour demands. Prestigious kurakas were soon brought low, while the opportunistic and unscrupulous floated to the top. The traditional Andean cycle of reciprocity and redistribution was broken, as production now flowed in one direction only; Spanish demand for basic and sumptuary goods was insatiable. Communities endeavoured to pay monetary and labour tribute by stepping up production and commercialization of agricultural, pastoral, textile and craft goods. Incessant Spanish demands for increased production and corvée labour took place, paradoxically and

---

[23] On Chilche, see especially Wachtel (1977); Heffernan (1995); Farrington (1995).
[24] Wachtel (1995).
[25] Dean (1990); Cahill (1998).

tragically, against a backcloth of devastating population decline and its attendant social disintegration. The ingenious archipelago system, the exploitation of several ecological zones by single communities, crumbled under the weight of disease, social dislocation, and the introduction of the *encomienda* system.[26] This last entailed the carving out of large, quasi-feudal grants of tributaries to individuals. Ostensibly, it involved no grant of land, but in practice many of its beneficiaries were able to carve out large estates within their remit. It affected the cacicazgos in an immediate and adverse manner. Encomienda grants often cut across existing archipelago units and thereby severed or obstructed many communities' access to a wide array of products not available in their own microregion. The attendant reduction in the range of available foodstuffs can only have exacerbated existing demographic trends. Many significant cacicazgos lost much of their resources and wealth, and with it, the prestige of their incumbents. The unquenchable demands of the corregidores and the avaricious *encomenderos* for tribute and labour were stridently parroted by the settlers and bureaucrats who followed close upon their heels.

It was the kurakas who rode to the corregidors' rescue, they and the tiny phalanx of indigenous officials who clustered around them. Even without the effects of disease and depopulation, any thoroughgoing exploitation of the communities was only possible through a hierarchical organization staffed by native speakers familiar with traditional means of making the best of an inhospitable terrain. There were, to be sure, footdraggers among the indigenous élites, but for the most part they cooperated in accentuating the extraction of resources for Spanish consumption and commercialization. Acknowledged local authorities or not, their jobs depended on it. By and large, accession to a cacicazgo was through inheritance, though appointment through communal acclamation for want of an heir was possible, always supposing that the corregidor, a kind of provincial satrap or governor, concurred with a community's choice. Frequently he did not, and disputes over succession to cacicazgos or over the termination and replacement of a legitimate cacique were a staple of colonial litigation. These disputes usually turned upon the intersection of Spanish administrative process, consuetudinarian law, and pecuniary interest. Corregidors, and the subdelegates who replaced

---

[26] Murra (1975); Trelles (1982); de la Puente Brunke (1992).

them in the late eighteenth century, had their own interests to pursue, and these were often at variance with their official functions. When a conflict arose between the King's interest and those of his financial backers, a corregidor usually invested his energies in pursuit of the latter.

Nevertheless, these often coincided. Whether guarding the royal prerogative, extracting taxes or feathering his own nest, a corregidor had need of the services of several caciques and "principals", a catch-all category that embraced several levels of native Andean authorities, from the caciques' traditional alter ego (*segunda*) down to a handful of minions.[27] Sometimes a corregidor sought wholly or partly to bypass this petty hierarchy by relying on a group of private employees. These comprised his scriveners (*escribanos*), his cashier or "bag-man" (*cajero*), and the collectors (*cobradores, recaudadores*) whose pecuniary interests and social provenance rarely dovetailed with those of the communities on whom they preyed. Indeed, this very lack of coincidence enhanced their efficiency, for tribute and repartimiento collections were conventionally shot through with peculations, falsifications and sometimes violence. Yet even where reliance was placed on outsiders, full exploitation of communal and individual resources was possible only through mediation by, and reliance upon, the caciques. Their range of functions was synergistic, such that concentration of those functions in the hands of one (locally powerful) individual optimized the functioning of one or several communities in a pueblo or on an *estancia* or hacienda. The obverse of this optimally efficient community was that extraction of its resources was correspondingly optimized, always to its detriment.

The colonial cacique, then, performed a range of functions more vital to Crown coffers, the enrichment of corregidors and their lackeys, and maintenance of the *pax hispana*, than to the welfare of their communities. A pivotal figure nonetheless, many caciques were by a range of subterfuges able to ameliorate the fiscal and forced labour burdens of their communities, in a way that enabled their reproduction while simultaneously responding to claims on communal resources, whether from within the communities or from without, whether for the livelihood of a family or the avarice of a corregidor, an hacendado or cura.

---

[27] See especially the literature on Mesoamerica, e.g., Haskett (1991).

Bourbon Reforms, Rebellion, and Crisis in the Cacicazgos

The colonial kurakazgo or cacicazgo remained fundamentally unchanged from the 1570s, when its defining colonial character and
functions were set fast by the watershed Toledan reforms, until the
second half of the eighteenth century, when the equally landmark
Bourbon reform programme began to be implemented in earnest.
The great kurakas whom the conquistadors encountered in 1532,
and who for a brief time exercised authoritarian powers in their
regions, had long passed their heyday by the time the Bourbon
dynasty ascended the throne. Notwithstanding the surface impres-
sion of continuing glory suggested by the dazzling raiment displayed
by colonial Cuzco's Inca nobles on civic occasions, the typical kuraka
of the Bourbon age was a much diminished figure, more akin to a
village headman than to the regional chieftains or *señores naturales*
who had so exercised the imagination of the early chroniclers of the
Indies. The late colonial cacique, furthermore, was more than ever
a vital cog in the colonial bureaucracy, his juridically defined powers placing him—or her, for the presence of female kurakas or *cacicas* was not uncommon in late colonial southern Peru—right at the
centre of official life. The institution of the kuraka persisted after
Andean emancipation from Spanish rule in the 1820s, and continues to exist today. It is, though, a vastly different office, one perhaps more akin to the pre-1532 local headman than to the colonial
office.[28] Indeed, the colonial cacicazgo *per se* rapidly disappeared after
Independence, the office losing its fiscal responsibilities which, at least
in the eyes of governing officials, had comprised much of its *raison
d'être*. The taxes did not disappear, but the cacique as collector
assuredly did. Others willingly took up that rôle.

The colonial cacicazgo underwent a process of radical transformation in the wake of the great uprising of 1780–83, so much so
that it is appropriate to speak of a degeneration of the office, barely
recognizable as a continuation of the early colonial or Toledan cacicazgo, much less of its pre-Columbian analogue. After 1780 it all
too often appeared to be a bastardized institution, a canker from
within rather than a mediator of demands from without. The rebel-

---

[28] Rasnake (1988) is the only study to bridge colonial and republican eras to any
significant extent. The native élites of the post-Independence period have attracted
little scholarly attention.

lion itself focussed the minds of royalist authorities wonderfully, given that both the northern and southern movements, only very loosely allied, had been led by provincial "Indian" caciques. Similarly, caciques in the southern Andes split into those supporting the insurgency, and those who remained steadfastly loyal to the Crown.[29] In fact, lines were often blurred, with caciques bending now this way, now that, according to the relative proximity of royalist and rebel forces and sometimes prompted by the express preference of one or more communities for one or other. Many caciques had been introduced to a certain military discipline through their participation—not always willingly—in the proliferation of militias that were established from the 1760s; this initiative was of uncertain value for the Crown, given the enthusiastic martial participation of indigenes in the 1780 rebellion and especially the abortive 1814–15 revolution.[30] The Crown responded to the equivocal loyalty of native Andean leaders by ordering in 1783 that hereditary caciques were no longer to succeed to vacant cacicazgos, save for those cases where it could be demonstrated that a cacical family had remained loyal to the King under rebel provocation.[31] There were enough examples of this exception to the rule to provide a new generation of native Andean leaders, but these were rapidly diminishing in number. Appointment was now through direct nomination by the corregidors and later subdelegates, save for the limited application of the hereditary principle.

This was not itself a particularly radical break with tradition, for during the entire colonial period, and perhaps especially from the mid-eighteenth century when the corregidors increased their regional economic influence, there had been examples of outsider "intruder caciques" or "interim caciques" inserted into cacicazgos by corregidores, the better to control communities and thus maximize a corregidor's profit margins. Venality in cacical appointments was hardly new. What was new was the widespread appointment of non-indigenes to cacical office. It thus becomes possible to refer to a switch from the traditional kuraka to a new cacique, one with scant ties to the communities within the cacicazgo's remit. While it is clear that some of the ante-bellum caciques were indigenous outsiders (*indios*

---

[29] Vega (1969); Mörner and Trelles (1987); Cahill (1985, 1990).
[30] Campbell (1978); Cahill (1988); Cahill and O'Phelan (1991).
[31] Díaz Rementería (1977) discusses the 1783 decree and the subsequent, related, 1790 *cédula*.

forasteros) and a few were castes, perhaps even creoles (*españoles*), some
of the "interim caciques" had replaced deceased caciques and did
indeed have the right to an hereditary cacicazgo. Others had been
in office on an interim basis for many years, but did not care, or
did not know how, to arrange to obtain their cacicazgos *en propiedad*.
Prior to the establishment of a Royal Audiencia in the southern
highlands, in Cuzco in 1787, cacical titles were awarded by the
Royal Audiencia in Lima, and in many cases a cacique lacking an
apoderado had to travel to Lima to obtain just title, often after years
of litigation or just bureaucratic delay. But there is no doubt that
on the eve of the great uprising some caciques held office solely by
favour of a corregidor, rather than by hereditary right or acclamation by a community. The rebellion itself considerably worsened this
phenomenon.

José Gabriel Túpac Amaru, the eponymous leader of the northern insurrection, appears to have launched his movement without
the support of the caciques of the southern highlands. Few caciques
gave unwavering allegiance to his cause but, where they did so, they
tended not to be individuals of substance or prestige; as the Bishop
of Cuzco, Juan Manuel Moscoso y Peralta was to remark, with just
one exception, no "cacique of honour" supported the rebel leader.[32]
It is of note that in the Collao provinces, well to the south of Cuzco
and the principal theatre of conflict after the failed siege of Cuzco
in January, 1781, many of the caciques who did pledge fealty to
him appear to have done so because they had no alternative. They
were caught up in the vortex of rebellion; others had taken a last
chance to escape south to Chucuito, some to the city of Arequipa.[33]
There appears to have been a high rate of attrition among these
refugee caciques, especially around Lake Titicaca. Similarly, most of
the caciques who supported Túpac Amaru were either killed in battle, executed by their captors, or at best removed from their cacicazgos upon restoration of royalist order. So, too, some royalist

---

[32] *Colección* (1971), Tomo II, Vol. 3, p. 334: ". . . with the exception of Tomasa
Tito Condemayta, cacica of Acoz . . . it was notable that no cacique of honour followed the standard of the insurgent José Gabriel". Moscoso went on to remark that
had it not been for the loyalty to the Crown of the principal caciques of the southern highlands, the rebellion would have been irresistible. Historians remain divided
on this issue.

[33] The vicissitudes of the caciques in the rebellion are based on the testimonies
in: Archivo General de Indias (AGI), Audiencia de Lima, Legajo 1052.

caciques, such as the Inca noble Pedro Sahuaraura, were killed in combat. Many refugee caciques either lost their position while in exile, lost the papers necessary to defend possession of their cacicazgos from pretenders once peace had been restored, or else had their properties and chattels destroyed or stolen by insurgents, and thus were unable to provide the collateral (*fianza*) necessary to fulfil their tribute responsibilities or else lacked that degree of wealth indispensable for the maintenance of their de facto authority within the communities. In such manner, the attrition attendant upon the rebellion severely weakened the structure of indigenous self-government in the southern Peruvian highlands, as well as undermining the ability of communities to defend their resources from the incursions of outsiders in the aftermath of the great uprising.

This debilitation of indigenous governmental authority occasioned by the rebellion was exacerbated by the Crown policy to abolish eventually hereditary cacicazgos and to appoint, at least on an interim basis, non-indigenes—mainly creoles (*españoles*)[34] and mestizos—in order to facilitate the restoration of royal control over the communities. This policy sought, too, the financial recovery of the local exchequer by way of a more efficient and rapid collection of tribute, which had ceased almost entirely as a consequence of the uprising. Some *españoles*, though, had already entered the cacicazgos prior to the rebellion. Quite apart from the interim or "intruder" caciques installed by corregidors to do their bidding, yet another group, and an influential group at that, gravitated into hereditary cacicazgos through marriage. Such cases are instructive for what they reveal of the ambivalently pivotal function of female incumbents in the overall structure of indigenous governmental authority, of the mechanisms of reproduction of a cacicazgo, and of the dire consequences of poor marital choice for those communities within the remit of a *cacica*. Moreover, such cases illustrate the ways in which collaboration by native Andean élites might serve the interests of the State on several different planes, not least that of cauterizing the spread of sedition and rebellion.

---

[34] In the eighteenth century, the designation *españoles* referred to Creoles (Americans of Spanish descent) and occasionally also to the mestizos, but rarely to peninsular Spaniards. The latter were usually referred to as "de los reynos de España" or simply "gallego", "catalán" etc., or even in the pejorative terms of "chapeton", "gachupín", "cotenses", "pucacuncas". See Cahill (1994), pp. 325–346. The point is crucial for disentangling the social provenance of participants, and not a few interpretations

Case Histories

Cameos of two cacicazgos illustrate nicely a structural weakness associated with distaff incumbency.[35] Females held cacicazgos in fifteen
of the sixteen provinces (*partidos*) of the southern highlands. These
cacicas were crucial to maintaining continuity in hereditary cacicazgos, in compensating for the loss of fathers and brothers who fell
victim to the recurrent epidemics or were just absent long-term in
the mines or on trade journeys; cacicazgos belonged to families, at
least until such time as a family could no longer provide a legitimate heir. It is also possible that, in the immediate wake of the great
uprising, the number of *cacicas* was abnormally high due to the attrition among proprietary caciques during the rebellion. Notwithstanding,
a significant number of females had held office prior to 1780. In
some cases, females obtained office because they were the only surviving issue of an hereditary cacique; a few widows of caciques served
only until their sons attained their majority; some others were *cacicas* in name only, because their spouses carried out the duties of
office; there are also a few isolated cases in which the wife of a *de
jure* cacique was called "cacica" by custom, though this may have
reflected common usage.[36] Nonetheless, it is clear that the majority
of *cacicas* undertook all of the responsibilities of the cacicazgo. In the
context of changes in the system of cacicazgos in the aftermath of
the rebellion, the presence of female incumbents assumes especial
importance because they paradoxically provided, through marriage,
a conduit for the entry of male, non-indigenous outsiders into key
cacicazgos. The examples of the prestigious cacicazgos of Anta and
Pisac/Taray, in the Cuzco region, highlight the phenomenon and
the deleterious results it could have for the affected communities.

Colonel Nicolás de Rosas is well known as the royalist leader who,
with Indian noble leader Mateo García de Pumacahua, did most to
impede the advance of the *tupamarista* army in 1780 prior to the
arrival of the royalist regulars from Lima. Then described as cacique
of Anta, he was creole, and rose to prominence through marriage
(sometime before 1780) to Doña María Dominga Quispe Huamán,

---

of the rebellion are unreliable precisely because their authors have failed to com-
prehend it.

[35] Cahill (1986).
[36] Ibid.

daughter of Mateo Quispe Huamán, hereditary cacique of the four Anta *ayllus*, whose succession went back beyond the Incanato. There was family testimony to the effect that Rosas came to the marriage "devoid of wealth", but that his wife brought with her "a considerable dowry". Above all, it was she who inherited the cacicazgo, and she who carried out its duties, such as collecting tribute and organizing the harvests. By 1794, however, it is Rosas who is described as *cacique gobernador* of Anta and neighbouring Pucyura. By then, he was also mayordomo of the principal confraternity of the two churches of the *doctrina* of Anta and the owner of several haciendas and a small coca plantation (*cocal*), whereby he was heavily indebted to the convents and monasteries of the city of Cuzco, which in that era functioned as banks within the viceregal economy. The couple had one daughter, who also married a creole, Sergeant-major Ramón Riquelme. Upon the death of Rosas c. 1798, Riquelme paid one thousand pesos as a "sweetener" to the subdelegate of Abancay for succession to the Anta cacicazgo—it was worth far more—whereupon he and his henchmen proceeded systematically to usurp community lands.

The Unzueta family more closely approximates a mini-dynasty. Sebastián Unzueta y Mendoza, a creole, won a certain notoriety in early 1780 when he betrayed his brother-in-law Bernardo Tambohuacso, cacique of Pisac and a ringleader of an abortive conspiracy that variously bears his name. Unzueta was married to the cacica Rita Tambohuacso, who had succeeded to the cacicazgo of Taray upon the death of father, quite as her brother had succeeded to the contiguous cacicazgo of Pisac. As a reward for his betrayal of Tambohuacso, Unzueta on July 18, 1780 was appointed to the cacicazgo of Pisac, in any case to become emphatically vacant following the judicial execution of its quondam incumbent. The father of Rita and Bernardo, Don Joseph Tambohuacso, had earlier succeeded to the two cacicazgos through marriage to the *cacica* Doña Agustina Suta Sayritupa Chachona, though the Tambohuacso family had earlier been the proprietary caciques of Pisac, How it came to lose possession of its inheritance is not clear, but appears to have stemmed from a transgression of an earlier incumbent.

From this base, the Unzueta fortunes flourished. During the 1790s, Sebastián Unzeuta served as *subdelegado* or provincial governor of the provinces of Calca y Lares and Urubamba. As early as 1784, Hermenegildo Unzueta, brother of Sebastián, is described as having

succeeded to the cacicazgo of nearby Coya through marriage to the
noble *cacica* Doña María Inga Paucar, who had also inherited from
her father. In 1793, one Felipe Unzueta, probably their son, is cacique
and alcalde of Coya. Meanwhile, Sebastián had sired two sons, Juan
de Dios Unzueta y Tambohuacso and the illegitimate Ildefonso
Unzueta, who succeeded to the cacicazgos of Taray and Pisac respectively, though the former was challenged by his aunt Marcosa
Tambohuacso, who curiously and anachronistically argued that as a
mestizo he could not occupy any cacicazgo. Both brothers owned
small coca plantations in the province of Calca y Lares, whence they
sent the *ayllus* under their jurisdiction to work in fearful conditions;
many returned gravely ill, some not at all. Ildefonso, in particular,
was noted for his brutality towards the comuneros of Pisac, whose
lands he forcibly usurped, working some for his own benefit and
renting others to creoles and mestizos. Many comuneros remained
without any land at all, whether on the heights or the valley floor,
such was the scale of his misappropriation. Collectively the Unzueta
family, from obscure beginnings, came to own extensive lands in the
rich terrains of Pisac, Taray, Calca, Yucay and Paucartambo.

The case histories of the Rosas and Unzueta families have mer-
ited extensive treatment because, though they were more prominent
than most and their cacicazgos more prestigious and lucrative than
the norm, their examples serve to illustrate starkly some wider processes
affecting the cacicazgos after 1780: outsiders, particularly creoles and
mestizos, entering the cacicazgos by way of marriage to incumbent
cacicas; the widespread phenomenon of both native and creole caciques
as hacendados, for all that their holdings were modest in size; and
the consequent demands on land and labour with scant regard to
traditional notions of reciprocity between caciques and communities.
The pernicious outcome of these tendencies can be seen in the cases
of the eventual successors, Riquelme and the sons of Sebastián
Unzueta; if Rosas and Sebastián Unzueta appear to have been fair
and responsible governors within their respective fiefs, the second
generation was quite the opposite.

Stemming the Tide

It is worth reiterating that this flood of creoles and mestizos into the
cacicazgos was a phenomenon that touched every province of the

southern Peruvian highlands. Few towns, villages or *ayllus* appear to have escaped hosting a creole or mestizo as cacique at some time during the four decades between the failed rebellion of 1780–83 and Independence in the 1820s. Moreover, once a creole or mestizo had taken possession of a cacicazgo, he was almost always followed by another. Here is the 1798 testimony of the subdelegate of Calca y Lares: "upon my entry into this province I found all the towns and ayllus with their respective *español* caciques occupying this office with just title".[37] The response of the indigenous communities was to swamp first the Intendency of Cuzco and then (from 1787) the Royal Audiencia there with appeals against the machinations of this new breed of exploiter. During the 1790s the Audiencia made a belated attempt to halt what it called "this pernicious abuse . . . of naming españoles and other castes as *caciques gobernadores* of the Indian towns or ayllus",[38] and the concomitant exploitation of indigenous lands and labour. However as the subdelegates were quick to point out, there was a royal provision of 1783 instructing royal officials to give preference to *españoles* over native Andeans in the appointment of caciques and tribute collectors (these were no longer necessarily one and the same). Furthermore, the law of 1783 had been reinforced by yet another in 1790. A survey by the Royal Audiencia of all sub-delegates of the southern highlands revealed that they had indeed followed such practice.[39] The Audiencia knew, of course, of the exis-tence of the 1783 and 1790 provisions, but grappled with the appalling consequences of their implementation. They did so ineffectually.

The Royal Audiencia failed to control the manifold abuses atten-dant upon creole capture of the cacicazgos because, in the final analysis, its belief that *españoles* should not be awarded cacicazgos was in conflict not only with existing royal provisions, but more

---

[37] Archivo Departamental del Cuzco (ADC), Real Audiencia: Asuntos Adminis-trativos, Leg. 160, "Expediente sobre el Auto Acordado para que se recojen los nombramientos de casiques de todos los partidos del distrito", 26 April, 1798.

[38] Ibid.

[39] Ibid.; ADC, Real Audiencia: Causas Ordinarias, Leg. 34, "Casicazgos: Exp[edien]te . . . a nombre de Don Pedro Mendoza Solorzano Tapara . . .", 19 November, 1799. For the *real cédula* (Aranjuéz) of 9 May, 1790, and its interpreta-tion and implementation at local level, see especially ADC, Real Audiencia: Asuntos Administrativos, Leg. 154, "Expediente formado a instancias de Don Luis Farfan . . .", 10 November, 1791; *idem*, Leg. 153, "Expediente por el que Lucas Huamanpuco solisita el Casicasgo de Santa Rosa . . .", 21 November, 1791.

importantly with the fiscal imperative of the Crown. Successive Bourbon administrations were perennially short of revenue and laden with debt, above all because Spain was at war in each and every decade of the eighteenth century. The ostensible justification for having creoles and mestizos as caciques was that they were "persons of means", but the Audiencia held this to be a "subterfuge, or false pretext".[40] Nevertheless, subdelegate after subdelegate continued to insist that the level of tribute revenue would be deleteriously affected were they obliged to rely once more on native caciques. They argued that the *españoles* were necessary to control the communities which, they alleged, would not pay tribute of their own volition and, further, that indigenous caciques "have to look out for their own caste".[41] A more serious objection to permitting indigenes to retain or return to cacicazgos lay in the inability of many indigenous aspirants to pay the financial guarantee demanded from each tribute collector, although this regulation ostensibly had always obtained. At any rate, the Royal Audiencia, faced with such financial logic and specious argument, contented itself with its fiat that the subdelegates could appoint whomsoever they liked as tribute collectors, providing that these bore the title of "collector" (*recaudador, cobrador*) rather than "cacique". Notwithstanding this caveat, these collectors continued to refer to themselves as "caciques recaudadores" and, for better or worse, were thus recognized by the communities. Subdelegates insisted that as they alone were responsible for tribute revenues in their respective provinces, it stood to reason that the Intendants, their immediate superiors, should have no say in the appointment of collectors. This spurious claim, eroding the effective power of Intendants vis-à-vis subdelegates, was astonishingly ratified by the Royal Audiencia. In such manner, social justice—"the Spanish struggle for justice", in Lewis Hanke's famous phrase[42]—was swept away by a combination of fiscal imperative and cynical legal sophistry.

Thus, after an administrative and jurisdictional struggle lasting several years, the Royal Audiencia ended by capitulating to the subdelegates, who in all other facets of their office were weaker than their nominal predecessors, the corregidores. Moreover, in so doing,

---

[40] Ibid.
[41] Ibid. See also ADC, Real Audiencia: Asuntos Administrativos, Leg. 162, "Expediente sobre caciques de sangre en la Intendencia de Puno", 29 June, 1800.
[42] Hanke (1949).

the Audiencia undermined the Intendants, ironically established in order to coordinate and oversee the actions of the subdelegates, lest the latter become as overmighty and avaricious as their predecessors, the corregidores, who by their exercise of despotic power had sparked a major rebellion. As so often, the Crown's good intentions, expressed in an infinity of royal laws and provisions, to protect its indigenous subjects from excessive exploitation—though never exploitation as such—foundered on its own fiscal imperative. It had been the same story with the *mita de minas*, land grants, encomiendas, the *repartos*, and so many other issues. To a large extent, the history of Spanish America may be written in the interstices of the inherent conflict between the paternalism of the Crown and its fiscal imperative. From around 1800, then, local creoles were effectively given a green light to enter into the cacicazgos without hindrance from judicial authorities, a euphemism for official permission to exploit the indigenous communities however they wished. Though the Audiencia salvaged some pride by endeavouring to protect native Andeans when they lodged claims for judicial redress of specific grievances, on the whole the notorious delays which the legal system permitted malefactors were used by creoles to thwart the orders and decrees of the tribunal.

The New Caciques

Well, what was the point of having one's own cacicazgo? What was the attraction? These were not the chiefdoms of yore, for all that some prestigious and lucrative cacicazgos fell to this new, avaricious dispensation. Most were modest village posts, sometimes more trouble than they were worth for their indigenous incumbents, who often found themselves out of pocket when communal tribute monies had to be handed over to the subdelegate. In the first place, it does not seem to have been a response to market forces, at least with regard to commercial opportunities outside a particular microregion. In the second place, however, it did provide employment for a number of poorer creoles and mestizos. The corregidors had employed considerable numbers of collectors of *reparto* debts. In 1780, several creoles and mestizos are mentioned as collectors of the corregidor of Tinta; he undoubtedly had more. While illicit repartos persisted after their formal abolition in December, 1780, they were infrequent and on a much smaller scale, and tended to be organized from one or two village "shops".[43] The abolition of repartos, then, implied the destruction of a traditional if informal office, that of the reparto collector. The actual collection of tribute monies had been in the hands of the caciques and their helpmates (*segundas, principales, hilacatas*), so that one obvious avenue of alternative employment after 1780 might be found by pushing caciques to one side, with the "new men" functioning as overseers of those selfsame offsiders, who remained responsable for the physical collection of the monies or produce. This explanation of the social origins of the new caciques must remain hypothetical, given the anonymity of most of the pre-abolition reparto collectors. Beyond this social explanation, however, local value systems and behavioural patterns should be taken into account when assessing the attraction of cacicazgos for non-indigenes. Of interest here is the potent combination of *egoísmo, categoría* and *envidia* that have been identified as a permanent source of social conflict in Mexican village life, especially when considered in the light of the "theory of the limited good".[44] Cutting a good figure, throwing one's weight around, simple envy and cupidity—these provided ample motive for coveting village office.

Such social and cultural explanations are of course difficult to substantiate, but are not for that reason any less persuasive than the economic arguments often advanced to explain change in Andean societies. The material goals of the new caciques, however, do emerge with striking force from the extant documentation. As one subdelegate noted, the one per cent of tribute takings allocated as remuneration to collectors usually did not suffice to cover the deceased and absent tributaries for whose payments a cacique was responsible,[45] at least until the next formal review of the tribute rolls. The eagerness with which local creoles sought cacicazgos is in large part explicable in terms of the lands and labour service that attached to the office of cacique, though not, officially at least, to that of "collector". Thus it was that the period from 1780 to 1825 bore witness to an onslaught on community lands unrivalled in intensity since the

---

[43] On post-abolition repartos etc., Fisher (1970); Moreno Cebrián (1977); Cahill (1988).

[44] Romanucci-Ross (1986), especially pp. 93–97; Foster (1965).

[45] ADC, Real Audiencia: Asuntos Administrativos, Leg. 160, "Primer Quaderno de los pertenecientes al Partido de Lampa", 15 August, 1798.

sixteenth century, certainly without parallel since the *reparticiones* of the 1590s, when the first official allocation and register of community lands took place. These were small plots and parcels, for the most part, but they represented livelihoods. It was almost axiomatic that as soon as a creole or mestizo attained office, he proceeded to usurp community lands and make demands upon the communal labour force. In this, he was often aided by individuals and factions within a community, or from contiguous *ayllus* or villages whose lands conjoined those of the hapless victims. It would be misleading to pay too much heed to notions of the "closed corporate community" or any associated presumption of indigenous solidarity. Then as now, there was considerable differentiation and conflict between and among *ayllus*. Divide and conquer starts close to home.

The demand for labour, especially unpaid labour, was perhaps the major attraction of capturing the cacicazgos. Perhaps this is the decisive point, given the prevailing low grain prices of the era, a crisis of sorts in the textile sector, and the high loan, lien and fiscal burdens, with their corollary of shaved profit margins. Unpaid labour might make the world of difference to a struggling hacendado or textile manufacturer (*obrajero, chorrillero*). A cacique's "right" to land and free labour derived in the first instance from the sixteenth-century *Ordenanzas del Perú*. The Crown permitted caciques twelve *topos* of land as a perquisite attaching to their office, as well as the privilege of using unpaid work details (*faenas*) to cultivate those lands. In practice, however, many caciques held far more land, and not a few were hacendados, albeit on a small scale, though for labour on lands in excess of their official allocation they were supposed to pay the standard (and nominal) wage of two *reales* per day. If these land portions do not appear excessive, it was the quality and location of plots that were important: arable land is at a premium in the Andes. In a large sample of land disputes surveyed, only a tiny number pertain to disputes over lands in the infertile *punas*, the high places. The lands that the new breed of cacique coveted were usually maize, wheat or orchard lands, and often near the centre of an *ayllu*, which was a topographical as well as social entity. One further motive for capturing a cacicazgo was to make illicit repartos, sometimes though not invariably as the agent of a subdelegate, though this feature appears to have been of marginal attractiveness compared with land and labour.

Who, finally, were these interlopers? In many cases it is difficult
to locate information on these individuals and their social provenance; even where the documentation is more than fragmentary,
there is nothing in the way of a *relación de méritos y servicios*—the
official curriculum vitae of the time—otherwise so useful in constructing group profiles of key social groups such as clergy, merchants and bureaucrats. Nevertheless, the principal lineaments of this
new, or perhaps merely displaced, social stratum have come into
focus. The two most prominent among what was a motley cluster
of social types were hacendados and officers in the provincial militias; some hacendados, hardly surprisingly, also held a coeval commission in the militia. Indicative perhaps of a wider pattern of change
in local governmental authorities, not a few of these new caciques
simultaneously held office as *alcalde mayor de españoles*, while still others are simply identified as *alcaldes mayores*; there is no specific mention of the office of *alcalde mayor de indígenas* in this period.[46] There
is, though, a maverick case of a manifestly indigenous cacique who
was also the *alcalde mayor de españoles*. It was perhaps the case that
the old caste labels had by this time lost some of their erstwhile
force, and that, away from the *tertulias* and salons of the cities, class
and cultural traits were the determining elements in social stratification,
notwithstanding the continuing close correlation between race and
class. The Hispanic office of *alcalde* variously translated as mayor of
a town or village or as one of the senior deputies of a town or village council with policing and other civic responsibilities. The indigenous *alcaldías* were, however, very much minor offices, with a range
of alcaldes and regidores—comprising the *cabildo de indios*—elected
or appointed each year in the villages. Often they were just helpmates of the caciques, or of the alcalde mayor de españoles. There
is thus detectable a merging of the authority vested in the cacique
and that of the senior official of the local village or town council
(*cabildo*), thereby eroding the independent authority of the caciques
and diminishing even further the relevance of the *cabildo de indios*. In
other words, there had occurred a further contraction of the political distance between the *república de españoles* and the *república de indios*,

---

[46] Espinosa Soriano (1960) is an attempt to reconstruct the history of this little
understood office. The whole question of the functions and importance of the indigenous *alcaldes*, *regidores* and *cabildos* is poorly understood for the Andean regions,
whereas there is a substantial historiography on indigenous élites for Mesoamerica:
for a recent example, see Haskett (1991).

one of the constitutional tenets of Spanish imperial rule in the Americas. Not surprisingly, this partial conflation of the two offices, two jurisdictions, was almost always to the detriment of the indigenous sector.

The rural priests (*curas* or *doctrineros*), those other ubiquitous actors at local level, were also making their influence felt in cacicazgo appointments. Some indigenous caciques had long been in their thrall, but after 1780 some curas managed to capture cacicazgos outright by arranging for one of their relatives, retinue, domestic servants or other dependants to fill a cacicazgo; caciques and curas were often inveterate enemies.[47] Here, too, the principal motives of the curas and their shadows were to gain access to community lands and unpaid labour, though greater control in the extraction of parochial and fiesta fees was assuredly also an aim, as many caciques sought to shelter their charges from priestly avarice; beneficed clergy tended to be wealthy, and that wealth was mainly accrued by appropriating the surplus product of the indigenous peasantry. In this context, it is worth noting that the extraction of parochial fees (*obvenciones*) increased markedly after 1780, presumably because the curas moved into the economic "space" vacated by the corregidors and their lucrative repartos.[48] That is to say, the extraction of native surplus remained much the same before and after the rebellion, the essential differences being the mode of extraction and the principal beneficiaries. There was even one case in which the cura himself was cacique: in 1811 in Marcapata (within the Cuzco jurisdiction), the cura was cacique of two ayllus and his creole brother-in-law was cacique of the other two ayllus of the town.[49] In 1815, as the suppression of the attempted Cuzco revolution was in the offing, there was a major indigenous uprising in Marcapata and environs. This insurrection, which fed into a wider pattern of indigenous insurrection in that year, was in the first instance directed against the exploitative activities of that self-same cura.[50]

---

[47] See, for example, ADC, Real Audiencia: Asuntos Administrativos, Leg. 159, "Expediente de apelación . . . a nombre de Evaristo Delgado . . .", 16 January, 1797.
[48] Cahill (1984).
[49] ADC, Real Audiencia: Pedimentos, Leg. 184, Pedimento de Manuel Champa *et al.*, 25 June, 1811.
[50] Cahill (1988); Cahill and O'Phelan (1992).

Seven cases of textile workshop owners (*obrajeros, chorrilleros*) in just two provinces have been detected among these new caciques.[51] In the province of Quispicanchis, the cacicazgo of Pomacanche was transferred with the sale of the *obraje* of that name, from one *obrajero* to another.[52] In 1798, Domingo de la Mar died after six years as incumbent of the cacicazgo of Accha (Paruro province); he too was a *chorrillero*, and remarkably had also been a corregidor prior to the 1780 rebellion.[53] Two prominent functionaries of the city of Cuzco, the scrivener of the Royal Audiencia, notary and eventual revolutionary of 1814, José Agustín Chacón y Becerra, and procurator of the Audiencia, Pablo del Mar y Tapia, were respectively caciques of the towns of Colquepata (1791–94) and Poroy (1815).[54] Other categories of outsiders, including some *indios forasteros*, also attained office in this period. Perhaps most extraordinary of all, a notable white hacendado from the far-flung city of Arequipa somehow managed to succeed to three hereditary cacicazgos simultaneously; in Llaulli (province of Azángaro) in 1811, both caciques were creoles from the equally far-flung La Paz.[55] To give the kaleidoscope one final twist, a cacique of the city of Cuzco was described as being a "free black", but the Dean of the cathedral chapter insisted that this cacique was still his slave.[56]

A Colonial Heritage

This decapitation of indigenous society was the final, parting gesture of the Crown to native Andeans, the capstone of their colonial heritage. Quite as such instruments of colonial exploitation as the repartos and the mita attacked the indigenous community from without, these 'new men' in the cacicazgos constituted a canker from within.

---

[51] Cahill (1986).

[52] ADC, Real Audiencia: Asuntos Administrativos, Leg. 160, "Expediente sobre el casicazgo de Pomacanche", 1799.

[53] ADC, Real Audiencia: Causas Ordinarias, Leg. 29, "Testamento de Domingo de la Mar", 1798.

[54] ADC, Real Audiencia: Pedimentos, Leg. 184, "Pedimento de Ancelmo Cusilloclla", 24 December, 1815; ADC, Real Audiencia: Causas Ordinarias, Leg. 9, "2° Quaderno sobre la solicitud . . . a el Cacicazgo de Coya . . .", 1791–94.

[55] ADC, Real Audiencia: Asuntos Administrativos, Leg. 174, "Expediente seguido por la comunidad . . . del Pueblo de San Jose de Llaulli . . .", 12 August, 1811.

[56] ADC, Real Audiencia: Causas Ordinarias, Leg. 15, Petition of Francisco Xavier Pineda, 1794.

The office of hereditary cacique, in any case, was formally abolished in the immediate aftermath of Independence, along with all other hereditary titles. As the incipient republic unfurled following Independence from Spain in 1824, the tax base was widened to include non-natives. The new republican fiscal arrangements provided employment for yet another type of "collector", responsible for the shadowy non-indigenous *castas*, though there was inevitably some degree of overlap between old and new collectors. At once, the "white" and mixed-race underclasses, largely lost to view in colonial documentation, come sharply into focus for the very first time, however elusive they were for tax collectors, many of these *castas* being transient artisans, petty traders and others of no fixed abode.

The documentation of the 1820s and 1830s is further remarkable for the vivid images of rural poverty that it conveys. Already in 1791 the subdelegate of Tinta had underscored the absolute poverty of his province, the worst of which was experienced by the mestizos and other castes, for the indigenes had at least their meagre subsistence plots (*topos*) to cultivate.[57] After Independence, the hard-pressed subprefects (the successors to the subdelegates) by way of explaining their inability to collect the new tax called the *contribución de castas*, sang a unanimous descant to that earlier, abject assessment. So miserable was the prevailing standard of material culture in some provinces that even the pitiless collectors themselves had no compunction in admitting that they stripped the ponchos and shawls from creole and mestizo women in the streets as part payment of poll-tax.

The ruthlessness of those collectors brings into focus the end product of the process of the capture and despoliation of the cacicazgos by creoles and castes. At Independence in 1824 these *españoles* appear to have been in full control of the new *contribución de indígenas* (the old tribute repackaged), though as before the actual collection of monies and produce was in the first instance in the hands of the *segundas*. Thus in the province of Abancay in 1825, eight collectors listed for seven towns all bear Spanish surnames; in the town of Limatambo, the *recaudador* was assisted by three native caciques, as good an index as any of the decline in authority and prestige of the indigenous cacique.[58] In the province of Calca y Lares in 1830 there were twenty-five *recaudadores de indígenas*, only four of whom bore

---

[57] See in Cahill (1988).
[58] ADC, Administración Tesoro Público: Asuntos Contenciosos, Leg. 76, "Sobre la administración del ex Intendente . . . de Abancay Don Antonio Leefdael", 1825.

Quechua surnames; of the twelve whose occupation it has been possible to identify, all were hacendados or owners of coca plantations
(cocaleros).[59] The trend is most evident in the province of Paruro, also
in 1830. There were only five collectors for the entire province, all
of whom were hacendados, two of them also being textile producers.[60] Other data from adjoining provinces of Chumbivilcas, Quispicanchis and Tinta accord with these findings.[61]

There remains the wider question of correlating the social provenance of the collectors of the new indigenous poll-tax with the identity of the financial backers or guarantors (fiadores) of the subdelegates
and subprefects. In 1820, six of the eight guarantors of the subdelegate of Urubamba were hacendados, the remaining two also
property owners.[62] In 1830, the fiadores of all eight subprefects in
the Cuzco region are listed: all were property owners, a majority of
whom possessed haciendas, coca plantations, pastoral estancias, or
sugar-producing haciendas (cañaverales, ingenios).[63] However, in Paruro
in 1830, only one of the five collectors was simultaneously one of
the subprefect's guarantors.[64] Clearly, there was a community of interest, expressed in financial terms, between large agricultural, pastoral
and textile producers, on the one hand, and district governors, on
the other. These intersect with the incumbents of the new "collector" posts—indeed they were sometimes one and the same—often
conflated with caciques or simply replacing them. Sandwiched between
the two were the indigenous communities and the mixed-race or
caste underclasses. This was hardly what the rhetoric of the Independence era had promised them. This disillusionment was well expressed

---

[59] Idem, Leg. 67, "Exp[edien]te de la Matrícula General de Indíjenas . . . en esta
Provincia de Calca Lares y sus valles . . .", 1830; "Exp[edien]te de la Matrícula
General de Castas Industrias y Capitales . . . en la Provincia de Calca, Lares y sus
valles . . .", 1830.

[60] ADC, Administración Tesoro Público: Asuntos Contenciosos, Leg. 77,
"Exp[edien]te sobre la justificación de no haber podido cobrar la Contribución de
castas . . .", 2 January, 1830.

[61] Idem, Leg. 76, "Contra . . . Don Juan Manuel Pinelo y Torre", 1830; Leg. 78,
"Trata sobre rebaja de Contribución . . .", 1833; Leg. 78, "Sobre . . . DD Mariano
Noriega . . .", 1821–47; ADC, Intendencia: Real Hacienda, Leg. 189, "Exp[edien]te
sobre . . . Donativo dado por los vecinos del Partido de Tinta . . .", 23 March, 1791.

[62] ADC, Administración del Tesoro Público: Contenciosos, Leg. 78, "Sobre . . .
Don Jose Maria de la Torre . . .", 1822–53.

[63] Idem, Leg. 77, Testimony of the fianzas of the subprefects of the Department
of Cuzco, 28 July, 1830.

[64] Idem, "Exp[edien]te sobre la justificación de no haber podido cobrar la Contribución de castas . . .", 2 January, 1830.

in 1826 by the community of Marcaconga (province of Quispicanchis), in complaining to the Prefect of Cuzco (and future President of Peru), Agustín de Gamarra, of the depredations of their creole cacique, who had built a textile sweatshop with free labour on lands he had usurped at the centre of the ayllu:

> All tyranny and despotic oppression should have ended, especially for the miserable indigenes under the protection of the beneficial laws of the beloved Independence, but that has not been our experience . . . because they have still not left behind the erroneous Spanish maxim of dealing harshly with the Indian, and American.[65]

That mordant judgement, delivered just two years after Peruvian Independence from Spain, well expresses the essence of the subsequent history of the indigenous communities, little different under creole rule than it had been under the Spanish imperial hegemony. In the final analysis, the colonial heritage meant just more of the same for the indigenous communities.

Conclusion

The three centuries of collaboration by the several levels of Andean chieftains in the Spanish colonial project throw into stark relief the long-run degeneration of the kurakazgo or cacicazgo. The great kurakas, the *señores* who had ruled over vast domains, had been conquered by the Incas and incorporated into Tahuantinsuyu, just as the Incas, at the outset of their imperial march, had earlier crushed the smaller, independent warrior chieftains (*sinchis*) in the south. Those once great lords, whom the Sapa Inca permitted to remain as provincial suzereigns, still exercised power albeit in a kind of dominion status, at the point when the conquistadores made their landfall. Availing themselves of the possibility presented by the Spaniards to liberate their polities from the Incan hegemony, a number of them willingly provided martial and logistical assistance which was vital to the eventual conquest. For a time, the provincial lords and their "kingdoms" felt themselves free, but only until such time as the conquerors began to set the parameters of colonial domination. For a time some of

---

[65] ADC, Administración del Tesoro Público: Asuntos Contenciosos, Leg. 76, "Los indígenas del pueblo de Marcaconga contra la (*sic*) Recaudador Don Mariano Luna", July, 1826.

them flourished, most notably in the fief established in the "Sacred Valley of the Incas" by the Cañari chieftain Francisco Chilche; yet after two decades presiding over the richest land in the old empire and with numerous personal retainers, his power also began to ebb rapidly. It followed that of other great lords whose hold on their provinces had quickly disintegrated, not least because their subjects were quick to realize that the new overlords would insist upon direct rule, rather than on the maintenance of a loose alliance with the *señores naturales*. Their day had long passed by the time the radical reformist administration of Viceroy Francisco de Toledo finally established the definitive colonial system, one destined to prevail until successive Bourbon administrations clumsily overhauled it, from around the middle of the eighteenth century.

A network of local caciques, the so-called "nested tier", remained in place as intermediaries of the colonial State, effectively negotiating between that State and the communities. Many, probably most, of these small-time caciques were traditional office-holders, whose predecessors had held office in much the same way even before Incan domination. Some of these had no doubt been integrated into the Incan decimal system among that army of *camáyocs*, while the more senior of the ex-decimal functionaries often had little alternative but to win Spanish favour or take to the roads in search of new livelihoods. The colonial caciques who remained, large and small alike, were the main conduits of wealth for the Spaniards; the real wealth in Andes was its manpower, available either free or heavily subsidized to Spanish colonists. The caciques, on their behalf, extracted tribute in coin and kind; gathered taxes, royal and ecclesiastical; organized chainless labour gangs for mine, hacienda, estancia and sweatshop; and, finally, operated the often illicit commerce of venal corregidors, subdelegates, and subprefects.

Yet there was a bright side to their activities. While cooperating in the extraction of indigenous wealth and the bullying of those who produced it, many were able to ameliorate the colonial condition of the peasantry in their charge. They were frequently able to soften the harsher edges of colonial exploitation. They organized their charges in accord with communal tactics and strategies of survival, arranging manpower in a variety of (low) wage-earning activities. They struck deals with hacendados, curas and other local notables, deals buttressed by the ties of ritual kinship (*compadrazgo*), and further reinforced by the ephemeral comradeship of the numerous fiestas of the Andean highlands. Some were cruel, some corrupt, some tyrannical, most high-handed, but as a corps they were collectively able to mediate their communities' interests and soften the blows. Moreover, it was usually they, often at great cost to themselves, who led judicial appeals and more rowdy, "moral economy" protests and village riots against the district satraps and abusive village élites such as the curas. That their endeavours were not fruitless was to be demonstrated by the assiduity with which such local élites and their lackeys assailed the cacicazgos when the Crown lifted, in the wake of the great uprising of 1780–83, legal bars and the obstacles of custom to the incumbency of non-indigenes.

The flood of creoles and mestizos into the cacicazgos after 1780 was devastating for indigenous communities, as well as for their displaced caciques. The conquest had ushered in sweeping, usually deleterious changes for native Andeans—epidemics, depopulation, exponential tribute and labour demands, expropriation of lands—yet this capture of the upper tiers of indigenous authority by non-indigenes was perhaps the greatest structural change to confront the communities since the turmoil of the sixteenth century. The intensified exploitation implied by this assault upon the resources of the communities, led by the new breed of cacique, ostensibly only a "collector", is somewhat obscured by the relatively small losses of land in each community. Yet these plots were scarce, not least because in many communities land was at a premium; in economic parlance, they were "positional goods" Nevertheless, the main attraction for the new intruders appears to have been the access, untrammelled by any need to negotiate with indigenous caciques, to the manpower of the communities, otherwise available to outsiders only for wages, however token, or in repayment of a communal debt. Tribute earnings were an added attraction, because of the opportunity for fraudulent gain; after all, indigenous caciques had honed their own manipulation of the tribute system to an art.

Yet whatever the motives of the new and unofficial "caciques" or "collectors", the end result of the process may be seen in the tribute records of the early republican years. There it is manifest that creoles controlled every aspect of the post-colonial tribute (now called "contribución") collections. Starting with their monopoly of the financial guarantees for subprefects, they either occupied or controlled most of the collector (*recaudador*) positions in the provinces, at least those for which records are available. Acting as guarantors, controlling the collectors, they also controlled the subprefects. Given this community of interest, it is hardly surprising that these interested parties were mostly hacendados and textile producers, who could therefore rely on subprefects and the new caciques to supply them with free labour, by force or through debt. Traditional ties of reciprocity between cacique and community unravelled even further, quite as the brokering roles of the native cacique as mediator and ameliorator became increasingly ineffectual. This was only made possible, at least on a large scale, by the effective degeneration of the office of colonial cacique, through the imposition of incumbents from without where they had once emerged from within. The traditional village kuraka—now more than ever akin to its pre-conquest counterparts—continues to exist in the less acculturated communities, but stripped of most of the functions that had tied the community to the colonial State. The destructiveness implicit in the three century-long process of evolution of the colonial cacique and colonial cacicazgo was of fundamental importance for the nature of the new republican State in Peru. That process was so detrimental to indigenous communities that the century after Independence from Spain in 1824 was perhaps even more exploitative than the Bourbon century that had preceded it. The key to that exploitation, now by Peruvian nationals rather than Spanish overlords, lay in the capture of the upper tiers of indigenous authority by non-indigenous outsiders, a phenomenon explicable not just in terms of creole cupidity, but above all by the Crown's fiscal imperative, its political weakness, and the cynicism and pusillanimity of its royal officials and judges. Thus ended the Spanish struggle for justice in the Andes.

Bibliography

Bakewell, Peter, "Mining in colonial Spanish America", in *The Cambridge History of Latin America*, Vol. 2 (Cambridge: Cambridge University Press, 1984), pp. 110–51.
Bravo Guerreira, Concepción, *El tiempo de los incas* (Madrid: Alhambra, 1986).
Burga, Manuel, *Nacimiento de una utopía* (Lima: Instituto de Apoyo Agrario, 1988).
Cahill, David, "Curas and social conflict in the *Doctrinas* of Cuzco, 1780–1814", *Journal of Latin American Studies*, Vol. 16, No. 2, 1984, 241–276.
———— "Una visión andina: El levantimiento de Ocongate de 1815", *Histórica* (Lima), Vol. XII, No. 2, 1988, 133–159.
———— "Independencia, sociedad y fiscalidad: El Sur Andino, 1780–1880", in *América: encuentro y asimilación* (2ª Jornada de Historiadores Americanistas, Santa Fe de Granada, 1989), comp. Joaquín Muñoz Mendoza (Granada: Diputación Provincial de Granada, 1990), pp. 141–156.

——— "Independencia, sociedad y fiscalidad: El Sur Andino (1780–1880)", *Revista Complutense de Historia de América*, Vol. 19, 1993, 249–268.

——— "Colour by numbers: Racial and ethnic categories in the Viceroyalty of Peru, 1532–1824", *Journal of Latin American Studies*, Vol. 26, No. 2, 1994, 325–346.

——— "After the fall: Constructing Incan identity in late Colonial Cuzco", in *Constructing Collective Identities and Shaping Public Spheres: Latin American Paths*, eds. Luis Roniger and Mario Sznajder (Sussex Academic Press, London), pp. 65–99.

Cahill, David, and Scarlett O'Phelan Godoy, "Forging their own identity: Indian insurgency in the Southern Peruvian Sierra, 1815", *Bulletin of Latin American Research*, Vol. 11, No. 2, 1992, 125–167.

Campbell, Leon G., *The Military and Society in Colonial Peru 1750–1810* (Philadelphia: The American Philosophical Society, 1978).

Colección documental de la Independencia del Perú, ed. Carlos Daniel Valcárcel (Lima: Comisión Nacional del Sesquicentenario de la Independencia del Perú, 1971) Tomo II, Vol. 3.

Dean, Carolyn Sue. *Painted Images of Cuzco's Corpus Christi: Social Conflict and Cultural Strategy in Viceregal Peru* (doctoral dissertation, Los Angeles: UCLA, 1990).

De la Puente Brunke, José, *Encomienda y Encomenderos en el Perú* (Sevilla: Diputación Provincial de Sevilla, 1992).

Díaz Rementería, Carlos J., *El cacique en el Virreinato del Perú: Estudio histórico-jurídico* (Sevilla: Universidad de Sevilla, 1977).

Earle, Timothy (ed.), *Chiefdoms, Power, Economy, and Ideology* (Cambridge: Cambridge University Press, 1991).

———, *How Chiefs Come to Power* (Stanford University Press: Stanford, 1997).

Espinosa Soriano, Waldemar, *La destrucción del imperio de los incas* (3rd edn., Lima: Amaru Editores, 1981).

Falk Moore, Sally, *Power and Property in Inca Peru* (New York: Columbia University Press, 1958).

Farrington, Ian, "The mummy, palace and estate of Inka Huayna Capac at Quispeguanca", *Tawantinsuyu*, Vol. 1, 1995, 55–65.

Fisher, John, *Government and Society in Colonial Peru: The Intendant System 1784–1814* (London: The Athlone Press, 1970).

Foster, George M., "Peasant society and the image of the limited good", *American Anthropologist*, Vol. 67, 1965, 293–315.

Gisbert, Teresa, *Iconografía y mitos indígenas en el Arte* (La Paz: Gisbert & Cia., 1980).

Golte, Jürgen, *Repartos y rebeliones: Túpac Amaru y las contradicciones de la economía colonial* (Lima: Instituto de Estudios Peruanos, 1980).

Gutiérrez, Ramón, *Arquitectura virreynal en Cuzco y su región* (Cuzco: UNSAAC, 1987).

Hanke, Lewis, *The Spanish struggle for justice in the conquest of America* (Philadelphia, 1949).

Haskett, Robert G., *Indigenous Rulers: An Ethnohistory of Town Government in Colonial Cuernavaca* (Albuquerque: University of New Mexico Press, 1991).

Heffernan, Ken, "Paullu, Tocto Usica and Chilche in the Royal Lands of Limatambo and Quispeguanca", *Tawantinsuyu*, Vol. 1, 1995, 66–85.

Hemming, John, *The Conquest of the Incas* (London: Macmillan, 1970).

Larson, Brooke, *Colonialism and Agrarian Transformation in Bolivia: Cochabamba, 1550–1900* (Princeton: Princeton University Press, 1988).

Lewin, Boleslao, *La rebelión de Túpac Amaru y los orígenes de la Independencia de Hispanoamérica* (3rd edn., Buenos Aires: Sociedad Editora Latino Americana, 1957).

Moreno Cebrián, Alfredo, *El corregidor de indios y la economía peruana en el siglo XVIII: Los repartos forsosos de mercancías)* (Madrid: CSIC, Instituto "Gonzalo Fernández de Oviedo", 1977).

Moreno Cebrián, Alfredo (ed.), *Conde de Superunda: Relación de Gobierno (1745–1761)* (Madrid: CSIC, Instituto "Gonzalo Fernández de Oviedo", 1983).

Mörner, Magnus, and Efraín Trelles, "A test of causal interpretations of the Túpac
    Amaru rebellion", in Steve J. Stern (ed.), *Resistance, Rebellion, and Consciousness
    in the Andean Peasant World, 18th to 20th Centuries* (Madison: University of Wisconsin
    Press, 1987).
Murra, John V., *Formaciones económicas y políticas del mundo andino* (Lima: Instituto de
    Estudios Peruanos, 1975).
O'Phelan Godoy, Scarlett, *Rebellions and Revolts in Eighteenth Century Peru and Upper
    Peru* (Cologne and Vienna: Böhlau Verlag, 1985).
Ossio A., Juan M. (ed.), *Ideología mesiánico del mundo andino* (Lima: Ignacio Prado
    Pastor, 1973).
Pärsinnen, Marti, *Tawantinsuyu: The Inca State and its Political Organization* (Helsinki:
    Societas Historica Finlandiae, 1992).
Powers, Karen Vieira, *Andean Journeys: Migration, Ethnogenesis, and the State in Colonial
    Quito* (Albuquerque: University of New Mexico Press, 1995).
Ramos, Gabriela, and Henrique Urbano (eds.), *Catolicismo and extirpación de idolatrías
    siglos XVI–XVIII* (Cusco: Centro de Estudios Regionales Andinos "Bartolomé
    de Las Casas", 1993).
Rasnake, Roger Neil, *Domination and Cultural Resistance: Authority and Power among an
    Andean People* (Durham and London: Duke University Press, 1988).
Romanucci-Ross, Lola, *Conflict, Morality, and Violence in a Mexican Village* (Chicago and
    London: University of Chicago Press, 1986 [1973]).
Sala i Vila, Núria, *Y se armó el tole tole: Tributo indígena y movimientos sociales en el
    Virreinato del Perú, 1784–1814)* (Ayacucho: IER José María Arguedas, 1996).
Salomon, Frank, *Native Lords of Quito in the Age of the Incas: The Political Economy of
    North Andean Chiefdoms* (Cambridge: Cambridge University Press, 1986).
Sempat Assadourian, Carlos, *Transiciones hacia el sistema colonial andino* (Lima: Instituto
    de Estudios Peruanos, 1994).
Spalding, Karen, "Social climbers: Changing patterns of mobility among the Indians
    of colonial Peru", *Hispanic American Historical Review*, Vol. 50, No. 4, 1970,
    645–664.
———— "Kurakas and commerce: A chapter in the evolution of Andean society",
    Hispanic American Historical Review, Vol. 54, No. 4, 1973, 581–599.
———— *Huarochirí: An Andean Society under Inca and Spanish Rule* (Stanford: Stanford
    University Press, 1984).
Stern, Steve J., *Peru's Indian Peoples and the Challenge of Spanish Conquest: Huamanga to
    1640* (Madison: University of Wisconsin Press, 1982).
———— (ed.), *Resistance, Rebellion, and Consciousness in the Andean Peasant World, 18th to
    20th Centuries* (Madison: University of Wisconsin Press, 1987).
Trelles Aréstegui, Efraín, *Lucas Martínez Vegazo: Funcionamiento de una encomienda peru-
    ana inicial* (Lima: Pontificia Universidad Católica del Perú, 1982).
Villar Córdova,, Socrates, *La institución del yanacona en el Incanato* (Lima, Universidad
    Nacional Mayor de San Marcos, 1966).
Wachtel, Nathan, *The Vision of the Vanquished: The Spanish Conquest of Peru through Indian
    Eyes* (trans. Ben and Siân Reynolds, Hassocks, Sussex: The Harvester Press,
    1977 [1971]).
Zuidema, R. Tom, *Reyes y Guerreros: Ensayos de cultura andina* (Lima: Fomciencias,
    1989).

5. THE IMPACT OF DISEASE

Francis Brooks

European Hegemony

The question that each of the essays in this book sets out to examine has been put in many ways. Most recently, Jared Diamond reports it being asked by a remarkable local politician in New Guinea named Yali. Charismatic, energetic and self-confident, Yali was also immensely interested in Diamond's biological research and archaeo-biological interests and what that knowledge might tell him of the history of his own ancestors. As the conversation developed it turned to the differences between his ancestors and Diamond's and the fact that white colonialists enjoyed so many more of the material objects such as steel axes, matches, medicines, soft drinks and umbrellas—collectively referred to as "cargo"—than did even the most prosperous New Guineans. So he asked Diamond, "Why is it that you white people developed so much cargo and brought it to New Guinea, but we black people had little cargo of our own?".[1] Diamond's answer takes him far back in time and all over the earth. It comes down to explaining why it was that, around 1500 AD, a few people located far out on the edge of the Euro-Asian-African landmass that was to its inhabitants the known world were able to impose themselves on a large number of other people—whose very existence was not known to them until just before 1500—and use the land and labour of those people to make a great deal of cargo for themselves.

It was the Spaniards and the Portuguese—the furthest out of all on this far-flung periphery—who first explored and then made for themselves small settlements close to the shores of these new found lands. Their first 25 years grubbing around gave little hint that the course of world history was about to change. The turning point was not October 12, 1492 when Columbus made his landfall but November 9, 1519 when, on the causeway between Iztapalapa and Tenochtitlán, Hernán Cortés met Motecuzoma Xocoyotl, the *Uei Tlatoani*, or Great

---

[1] Diamond (1998).

Speaker, of the Colhua-Mexica people. Just under two years after that meeting Cortés and his motley band completed the destruction of the island city. That moment, August 13, 1521 is the climacteric. It is the inaugural moment of European imperialism, the moment when they definitively set in place the process of imposing themselves on the previous inhabitants of those lands. The crux of any explanation which would provide an answer to Yali's question is what Europeans came to call the Conquest of Mexico and the Conquest of Peru. So another form of Yali's question is: "how did 500 men conquer an empire of millions, and how did they do so in less than two years"?[2]

Most answers to that question start with a list of the possible factors: guns, ships, horses, literacy, money and, these days, germs. Yet it is as well first to examine the question itself. Built into it are implicit assumptions that need to be made explicit. There were about 500 men in Cortés' original band. But what about the thousands of indigenes who did much of the fighting? What about the reinforcements from the Narváez and Garay expeditions? What about the network of human and material resources stretching back into the Old World? And, anyway, what do we mean by "conquer"? There were many conquests and some of them were less total than the more popular accounts would have it. Many indigenes were not subdued until much later, some not until the nineteenth century.[3] Better to ask the less dramatically formulated question: how did the Europeans come to establish hegemony in the continent they discovered to the west of the Atlantic Ocean which they soon came to call America.

Of the various answers to that question from the early sixteenth century to the present, most have asserted or implied that Europeans were so superior that the result was inevitable. Whether it was by innate character, in obedience to the decrees of Providence or through the evolution of their genes, Europeans had from their Civilization or from their God the right, and from evolution and technology the power that made the outcome inevitable. Gonzalo Fernández de Oviedo y Valdés and Juan Ginés de Sepúlveda in the sixteenth cen-

---

[2] Clendinnen (1991). It is perhaps worth observing that in the case of Peru the question could be asked: How did 168 men conquer an empire of millions in one afternoon? But that form suggests rather different answers from those given to the question as usually asked.

[3] Hennessy (1993), pp. 5–36.

tury;[4] the Comte de Buffon, Cornelius de Pauw and William Robertson in the eighteenth;[5] Tsvetan Todorov and Jared Diamond at the end of the twentieth[6] are unanimous at least in this. European power was irresistible.

Criticism of the morality of European behaviour has, of course, not been lacking. From the earliest years there have been those who have denounced as "the destruction of the Indies" what Spaniards did. Fray Antonio de Montesinos in his famous sermon of Advent, 1511 is the first of whom we have record.[7] Fray Bartolomé de las Casas gave the genre definitive form.[8] The Franciscan Fray Toribio de Benavente (who called himself "Motolinía", Nahuatl for "small and weak") and the Augustinian Fray Alonso de la Vera Cruz, were only slightly less vocal than Las Casas.[9] Alonso de Zorita showed that clerics did not hold a monopoly on the denunciation of injustice.[10] Those who today denounce European moral depravity are legion. All the polemicists—the "White Legend" defenders of the civilizing mission and the "Black Legend" castigators of "the destruction of the Indies"—simply assume the reality of Europeans' greater material strength.

Yet that assumption should, perhaps, not be so quickly or so easily made. The indigenes, it is true, had a Stone Age technology. They lacked any metal harder than bronze. They had no wheels or beasts of burden. Their forms of writing and recording made it difficult to maintain the continuities of social and government forms apart from the personalities who temporarily administered them. But it is not clear that European weapons or skills were so superior as to make the outcome inevitable. Moreover guns depended on a problematic supply of gunpowder. Horses were so expensive as to be very rare in the New World until after the conquistadors had laid their hands on that world's booty. Writing had existed in the Old World for over 3,000 years. But it is printing rather than writing that makes possible the uniformity and anonymity which is the

---

[4] Oviedo y Valdés (1959); Sepúlveda (1951).
[5] Gerbi (1973).
[6] Todorov (1984); Diamond (1998).
[7] On Montesinos, see Lewis Hanke (1949). For a different perspective on the Dominicans' motives, see Seed (1993).
[8] Las Casas (1992).
[9] Motolinia (1971); Alonso de la Vera Cruz (1971).
[10] Zorita (1963); Vigil (1987).

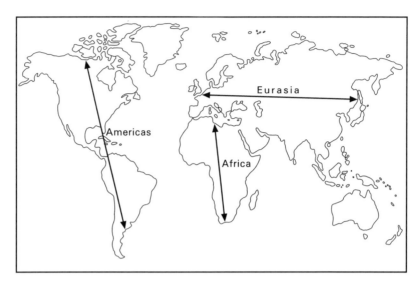

Figure 5.1. Major axes of the continents. From *Guns, Germs, and Steel: The Fates of Human Societies* by Jared Diamond. Copyright © 1997 by Jared Diamond. Used by permission of W.W. Norton & Company, Inc.

strength of bureaucratic rule and printing had been in western Europe for less than forty years at the time of Columbus' landfall. The technical edge, except on quite rare occasions, did not by itself determine the outcome.[11]

But the moment of conquest, if moment it was, is less important than the long haul. From Yali's perspective, the question is what was it in the culture of Europeans that for several hundred years made them apparently irresistible and in point of fact not during all that time effectively resisted. Diamond's enquiry into Yali's question leads him to assert that guns, germs and steel determined the outcome. His answer reaches back to the ultimate structures of the planet Earth, the shape of its landmasses and the struggles of each of its lifeforms to find an habitable niche thereon. Life forms proliferated and diversified along lines of latitude rather than of longitude. It was easier to move east and west where climates remain much the same than it is north and south where they change to an extent which is literally intolerable. So it was along those axes and especially along the zone of temperate climate stretching from China

---

[11] Elliott (1984), pp. 175–176.

to the Atlantic coast of Europe that all the major civilizations of the world arose. When it came to breaking out of the Euro-Asian-African landmass it was natural that the process should continue the same trend out into the ocean and across to the one continent which had not until then been connected to the others.

Diamond's maps and his ecological explanation are very persuasive. Cultivated plants and domesticated animals which are the material elements of life evolve through diversification. The swirling interaction of life forms across the temperate latitudes allowed the best adapted, the most diverse and the most adaptable to thrive. In Africa and the Americas the east-west axes are shorter than are the north-south. Interaction, and hence diversity and enrichment, of life forms were more restricted. The technologies for producing, extracting, exchanging and defending the resources needed to sustain life were much stronger in the Old World than in the New. Tools and techniques and materials were less strong in America. As a result, argues Diamond, the life-forms of the Americas were more fragile than those of Europe and Asia. In any contest—or simply in a chance encounter—American life forms were always likely to yield.

Yet another set of maps would make Diamond's argument less compelling. Felipe Fernández-Armesto argues that geography did not necessarily determine the outcome.[12] A galactic observer of planet Earth in the time interval that most of its inhabitants have come to call the fifteenth century might well have concluded that disparate parts of the globe would become connected. But he (it?) would probably not have concluded that the unifying force would have come from the area of Latin Christendom, sometimes dismissed by better placed cultures as "a promontory on the edge of Asia."

Throughout the world of the fifteenth century we can identify eight exploring cultures: the Polynesians, Japan, China, India, Islam, Latin Christendom, the Aztecs and the Incas. Each was a contender for the role of world unifier. All had the technical resources to undertake long journeys and to return home. All had the skills to sustain life in unfamiliar places. All had some means of recording and communicating these two vital pieces of information. Since they were all

---

[12] *The Times Atlas of World Exploration*, ed. Felipe Fernández-Armesto (London: Times Books, 1991), pp. 16–17. *The Times History of the World*, new edition ed. by Richard Overy (London: Times Books, 1999), pp. 154–155.

explorers all, we presume, had motives for further exploration. But not all were equally well placed.

The Chinese were the best equipped to mount large expeditions but in the fifteenth century they turned their gaze inward. India and Islam had the most adaptable ships and the best navigators but were not attracted by any potential beyond their known world. The Japanese, who ventured little further than to Korea, appear to have lacked curiosity. The Aztecs and the Incas were the least equipped for ocean-going. They lacked suitable ships and had no means of navigating over long distances. The Aztecs had inchoate map-making skills but the Incas of Peru, as far as we can tell, lacked such techniques entirely. The Polynesians, who had advanced further proportional to their more limited resources than any others, do seem to us now to have reached the limit of their technology.

Yet, as Fernández-Armesto points out, technology does not sufficiently explain the outcome. They had all achieved more than a determinist view of their potential might have predicted. That the move came from western Europe was not pre-determined. "At a crucial time, Latin Christendom was to develop a unique combination of exploring impetus and technical prowess that enabled explorers rapidly to catch up with and surpass the achievements of their counterparts elsewhere."[13]

What was achieved by that "unique combination of exploring impetus and technical prowess" came to be called the Discovery of America. Whatever that meant it was a curiously protracted affair the pivotal nature of which took a long time to become clear.[14] Capitalism might have been born around 1500 (although much earlier birth days have been suggested) but it did not come to dominate the world until the nineteenth century.[15] If there was a "spiritual conquest of America" the Christianity it spread was a different breed (if not creed) from Christendom in Europe.[16] The destruction of Tenochtitlán or the capture of Atahuallpa were important but they were not all that was involved in conquest; still less were they the sole cause for the setting up of European hegemony in the Americas. The conquest was

---

[13] Ibid. See also Fernández-Armesto (1995).
[14] Elliott (1970).
[15] Fernández-Armesto (1995), pp. 364–371.
[16] MacCormack (1991); Farriss (1984); Gruzinski (1993); Harris (1993); Millones (1979); Mills (1994); Cervantes (1994).

much more complex, multi-layered and longer in being achieved
than many historians think. And the establishment of European cap-
italist empires happened in a context much larger than the square
at Cajamarca or the shores of Lake Texcoco. We need to keep in
mind a dual perspective of the short-term victory and defeat and of
the long term establishment of the instruments of power and economic profit.

Other essays in this collection will consider many of the proffered
explanations for the establishment of European hegemony in the
Americas. Until quite recently diseases have not loomed large among
them. Of course, from the beginning reports of diseases have been
part of the story. Yet almost until the twentieth century little more
was made of them. That disease has come to occupy a more central role—for many historians today disease is the principal explanation of the European victory—is the result of two other changes
to the scholarship. In the first place estimates of the numbers of indigenes involved have increased by a factor of six or more, in central
Mexico from about three million to 25 million. Disease, it is argued,
must have cleared away the vast majority of that population. In
the second, the model of "virgin-soil populations", peoples who have
never previously experienced a particular disease and thus have no
immunity to it, has come to dominate the discussion of the historical
epidemiology.

So many Indians are now thought to have died as a result of the
Conquest that the superior European arms and technology are hope-
lessly inadequate to account for those numbers. They did make the
Spaniards more efficient killers but not by such orders of magnitude
that explain hecatombs. We know, too, that the Indians did not
superstitiously abandon themselves to an irresistible fate. The enor-
mous numbers who must have died are explicable in terms not of
technical backwardness or cultural feebleness but of virulent and pandemic disease. Disease as explanation of the conquest both affects,
and is affected by, all other explanations.

The Explanations

For the most part those explanations have been couched in terms
of the disparity between the newcomers and the native inhabitants.
A dynamic, entrepreneurial, energetic, expanding and prosperous

civilization, albeit represented by only a handful of men, was able to overwhelm effete, self-absorbed, listless, fatalistic and superstitious tribes. The antithesis is embodied in the personalities of Cortés and Motecuzoma: Cortés machiavellian, resourceful, manipulative and intrepid; Motecuzoma fearful of his gods, crippled by superstition and unable to make up his mind whether to welcome the strangers or push them back into the sea. The starkness of the contrast thus drawn has not infrequently occasioned some scepticism. Many historians today discount it almost entirely. We have come to see that this study in contrasts is a complex construct, of Cortés writing to the King of success when he had just suffered humiliating defeat; of chroniclers and historians all too ready to fashion the icon of the invincible European; and not least of the defeated Indians who consoled themselves that subjugation was the will of their gods.[17]

In one respect, however, Europeans did possess complete superiority over all the indigenous people of the new found continent. This was their command of the sea. Once the Portuguese had rounded the Cape of Good Hope and Columbus had found for the Castilians a route across the Atlantic, their seafaring skills and the power of the guns on their ships proved irresistible. No non-European power successfully challenged European naval power until the Russo-Japanese war of 1905. Yet sea-power, while it built trade, did not of itself build colonial empires. Significantly, almost all early European settlements overseas were close to the sea. Ships gave the adventurers access to foreign lands but ships had to be left at the sea shore.

And on land the story was different. The psychological shock of both guns and horses—the trope which is paraded with such glee in so many early accounts—was very short-lived. Most indigenes not only quickly recovered but almost as quickly devised strategies to counter the dangers. Many learned to use horses to such effect that they were virtually uncatchable until nineteenth century rifles could pick them off at a distance. Cannon procured none but the rarest strategic advantage against massed armies of Indians and against fortified cities. Horses have been described as the tanks of the conquest. But their military superiority came into its own only in pitched battles in open country. And few of the conquistadors' important victories were such.

---

[17] Fernández-Armesto (1992).

European adventurers are, of course, said to have had an advantage in ruthlessness. Like Alexander the Great it was their preferred strategy to capture the ruler, and use him as a puppet through whom they could rule. In America, this was the strategy adopted in the Caribbean and in the isthmus of Panamá. Yet, these early campaigns did not set up European hegemony. It was in Mexico and in Peru that lasting European power was established and in both regions capturing the chief was not as simple as the storybooks told it. In Mexico Cortés reports that he captured Motecuzoma.[18] Whatever the truth of his claim it was not the success he was looking for. In the six months and more from November 1519 to June 1520 that the Spaniards were in Tenochtitlán they did not advance their control of the country one bit. Even with Motecuzoma—and his immediate successor—dead, the Aztecs were able to mount a fierce resistance to the Spaniards as well as to the several thousands of the native allies who fought with them. In Peru the strategy worked with the capture of Atahuallpa. Yet even there it took another seven years after November 16th, 1532 before the Spaniards finally defeated the Inca state.

The real superiority of the Spaniards lay in communications: ships that could go and return; writing carried in those ships which could communicate the power of the State; the bullion and credit instruments which were profits for that State and orders for supplies for the adventurers; wheels and mules (eventually so much more important than horses) that could transport goods and money from production centres to population centres and from landed centres to ports; and a network of commercial agencies that stretched from Seville to Vera Cruz and Panamá and back into the merchant and banking operations in Europe. Above all, it lay in the institutions of the bureaucratic state that could maintain these system of communications and enforce power along their lines. It was especially those impersonal agents of state power, no longer dependent on the vagaries of succession and the charisma of the ruler, that concentrated and made effective European power.

The disunity and fragility of indigenous state systems has come to loom larger in explanations of the conquest.[19] It has been argued

---

[18] Brooks (1995).
[19] Elliott (1984), p. 174.

that the economic structure and religious ideology of both the Aztec and the Inca state forced them into colonialist expansion to prevent collapse from within by an overextended state structure. Civil war was always a likely accompaniment to a succession struggle. In both empires the leader died at a critical moment. Motecuzoma died in Tenochtitlán as the Spaniards struggled to escape. He was followed within a short while by Cuitlahuac. In Peru, Huayana Capac died sometime between 1524 and 1526. Conrad and Demarest argue that the war between Huascar and Atahuallpa left the empire "shattered and all the Spaniards had to do was to pick up the pieces." To which John Guilmartin comments that "though perhaps overstated for effect [it] aptly highlights the pivotal underlying political realities".[20] And those realities were that the structures of the indigenous empires could not guarantee unchallenged succession.

For this reason the importance of native allies has become clearer. Nathan Wachtel notes that "it was the Indians themselves who provided Cortés and Pizarro with the bulk of their conquering armies, which were as large as the Aztec and Inca armies against which they fought".[21] In the past that participation of other natives—often dismissed as "collaborators"—has been depreciated. The natives were "porters". They were "auxiliaries" led by the Spaniards. Tlaxcala, of course, provided the Spaniards a refuge in their extremity without which they must surely have been annihilated. The Tlaxcalans, too, carried some 150 kilometres the brigantines upon which the siege of Tenochtitlán depended. Yet they are still thought of as "allies" associated with the conquering Spaniards. And within a few generations the vital role they had played would be forgotten. The allies, whether necessary or merely auxiliary, were soon as much subject to the new State as the enemies whom they had made it possible for the Spaniards to defeat.

The Role of Disease

It is the insufficiency of all the standard arguments that makes disease as the explanation for the "few hundred who conquered millions" so cogent. None of the "guns and sails" explanations is persuasive

---

[20] Conrad and Demarest (1984), p. 138; Guilmartin (1991).
[21] Wachtel (1984), pp. 210–211.

when examined in detail except at the margins of the argument. The cooperation of the other natives is convincing but it leaves intact the need to show why those native collaborators themselves then fell under the European jackboot. Only pandemic disease and the almost instant destruction of millions before the onslaught of European diseases seems to be able to account for the otherwise incomprehensible victory.

An extensive scholarship on the history of disease in the colonial Americas has arisen in the last thirty years. On the effect of the first impact it remains speculative. A generation after contact, that is to say about 1545–1550 in Mexico, somewhat later elsewhere, repeated studies have shown that diseases killed millions of the indigenes, possibly more proportionally than died in even the worst epidemics in Europe. There were at least 5 million, possibly 10 million people living in Mexico in 1518. By 1600 there were about 1 million of their descendants alive. That is catastrophe. Within 100 years 80 to 90 percent of the people died without reproducing themselves. But to say that is not the same as saying that disease in general and pandemic smallpox in particular was the principal cause of the conquest and the consolidation of the conquest.

Over the centuries, the role assigned by historians to diseases in the European conquest has varied somewhat but it was not until quite recently that diseases have come to loom large. Sixteenth century chroniclers mention disease but none give it pride of place as an explanation of the conquest. Motolinía, the Franciscan friar, who first wrote of the culture of the Indians, constructed an extended *mythos* comparing the Spanish conquest to the Exodus of the children of Israel out of Egypt and Hernán Cortés to Moses.[22] Within this allegory he likened smallpox to one of the ten plagues of Egypt. There are, as Robert McCaa has pointed out, a considerable number of references to smallpox, some by eyewitnesses, some by contemporaries or near-contemporaries and a great many by subsequent historians.[23] But comments on the wide extent of the epidemic come from two other sources, Cortés' secretary and biographer, Francisco López de Gómara, and Bernal Díaz del Castillo which will be considered below.

---

[22] Phelan (1970), pp. 29–38.
[23] McCaa (1995).

In the eighteenth century, the exiled Jesuit Francisco Xavier Clavijero and the Scottish historian William Robertson both refer to smallpox. Clavijero uses the epidemic as an occasion to illustrate the charisma of Cortés.

> The conquests of the Spaniards, and the number of their allies, so aggrandised their name, and procured such authority to Cortes among those people, that he was the umpire in all their differences, and they repaired to him as if he had been the sovereign lord of all the region, to obtain confirmation of the investiture of vacant states, and in particular those of Cholula and Ocotelelco in Tlascala, both vacant by deaths occasioned by the small-pox. This scourge of the human race, totally unknown hitherto in the new world, was brought there by a Moorish slave belonging to Narvaez.[24]

From there the infection spread throughout "to the irremediable destruction of those nations". Many thousands died, including Cuitlahuatzin in Tenochtitlán, after a reign of three or four months, and Maxixcatzin in Tlaxcala. Thereafter, Clavijero makes no further mention of smallpox or of depopulation as a result of disease.

Robertson mentions smallpox twice. On the first occasion he refers to the untimely death of Cuitlahuac, Motecuzoma's successor. In the last three months of 1519 he was busy preparing himself for the return of Cortés from Tlaxcala "with a degree of foresight uncommon in an American" when his days were cut short by the smallpox which raged at that time in New Spain with fatal malignity.

Robertson makes no further comment on the effect of smallpox on the outcome of the Spanish conquest. The second occasion he mentions the disease is in reference to the outbreak in New England, 100 or so years later. Here he is aware of the interpretation that smallpox cleared the way for English settlement. "It swept away such multitudes of the natives, that some whole tribes disappeared". He is no less aware of the providential slant of such interpretations, but his enlightened sensitivity has little sympathy with such superstition. "Heaven, by thus evacuating a country in which the English might settle without molestation, was supposed to declare its intention that they should occupy it."[25]

---

[24] Clavigero (1979).
[25] Robertson (1843), pp. 243, 433. The Providential argument receives much shorter shrift in the 18th century.

In the nineteenth century, vaccination against smallpox was the great triumph of European medicine. Historians like Macaulay were at pains to emphasize the horrors of "the most terrible of all the ministers of death" over which modern science had triumphed.[26] Prescott echoed Macaulay's portentous style. According to Prescott, smallpox swept over the land "like fire over the prairie, smiting down prince and peasant". Its path was strewn with the dead bodies of the natives "who, in the strong language of a contemporary [Motolinía], perished in heaps like cattle stricken with the murrain."[27] But Prescott, too, ascribes no further role to the disease.

The first to hint at some more significant role was Hubert Howe Bancroft. In the moment of the Spaniards' greatest peril after the *Noche Triste*, it is smallpox that wards off the danger of annihilation.

> At hand even now, coming to the assistance of the magnificent Cortés, civilization's pride and pet for the moment, is another ally of civilization, more terrible than horses, bloodhounds, gunpowder or steel.... The terrible force of the first attacks of epidemics is well known, and it has been advocated, with apparent truth, that the diseases of a strong people fall with particular force on weaker races. [The disease crossed from the Atlantic to the Pacific] smiting high and low, rich and poor. For sixty days, according to the native records, the hueyzahuatl, or great pest, raged here with such violence as to fix itself a central point in their chronology. In most districts, says Motolinía, over half the population died, leaving towns almost deserted and in other the mortality was appalling.[28]

In the first half of the twentieth century E.W. and A.E. Stearn, physicians turned historians, pointed to the importance of the impact of smallpox. E. Wagner Stearn collected material on a number of diseases and his son Allen E. published it in 1945 as *The Effect of Smallpox on the Destiny of the Amerindian*.[29] For the most part the book is carefully researched material mostly from the history of the North American Indians. The first chapter, however, reviews some accounts of diseases in Spanish America in the sixteenth century. For the most part he relies on Bancroft but he does include other comments. His own: "Smallpox decimated the native population for four centuries and 'so demoralized the tribes through the terror it spread among them

---

[26] Macaulay (1889), Vol. II, p. 498.
[27] Prescott (1970), p. 482.
[28] Bancroft (1883), Vol. I, pp. 541–542.
[29] Ashburn (1947); Stearn, E.A. and Stearn, A.E. (1945).

that it has been considered by many authorities to have been an important factor in their comparatively easy subjugation by the whites'".[30] Other physician-historians had been inclined to be no less apocalyptic.

> The Spaniards brought small pox with them to the West Indies in 1507 and to Mexico in 1520, resulting in devastating epidemics which decimated the Indians. The phenomenal success of a few conquistadores in subjugating the Aztec and Inca kingdoms may well have been abetted by an advancing pandemic of smallpox which is estimated to have caused the death of 3 1/2 million people within a few years.[31]

Professional historians came to the question at the urging of geographers and ecologists. During the 1930s and 1940s Carl Sauer, of the University of California at Berkeley, was re-writing much of the historical geography of the Caribbean to take account of the biological effects of the coming of the Europeans.[32] He was joined by Sherburne F. Cook, who applied his biological and medical knowledge to the early history of European America. Among other things Cook examined the record for human sacrifice and made the startling, but on his figures and calculations not preposterous, claim that human sacrifice as practised by the Aztecs was a method of culling a population which had grown too large.[33] He further suggested, although his evidence suggested that population might have been pressing on resources, that the population was remarkably free of epidemic diseases.[34]

Until after the end of World War 2 it was possible to talk about the impact of disease without assigning it any very crucial role. The assumption generally was that while educated guesses might be made by analyzing the carrying capacity of the land or by extrapolation from post-conquest figures, we cannot know precise numbers. So a consensus that the pre-contact population of Mexico was within the range of three million to six million was rarely contested. Then, in 1948, Cook and Lesley Byrd Simpson published calculations the conclusion of which was that the population of central Mexico was of the order of eleven million, double or more the accepted figure.

---

[30] Stearn, E.A. and Stearn, A.E. (1945), p. 13.
[31] Simpson (1954) quoted in Beneson (1989), p. 634.
[32] A large number of biological and ecological studies published between 1936 and the early 1960s were made available to a much wider audience in Sauer (1966).
[33] Cook (1946: i), pp. 81–102.
[34] Cook (1946: ii).

In the next fifteen years that number was again to be more than doubled. Cook and Woodrow Wilson Borah systematically examined the statistical evidence for the Indian population of Mexico and, especially, for its decline in the years after the arrival of the Spaniards. Their first conclusions were published in 1957 when they showed that for the non-epidemic years of 1550 to 1570 the annual depopulation rate of Indians in Central Mexico was of the order of 3%.[35] Cook and Borah also published three papers in the Ibero-Americana series of the University of California culminating in the conclusion that the population of Mexico in 1518 had been 25.2 million. Further, they had found that the population in 1532, eleven years after the Conquest, had fallen to about sixteen million and in 1548 it had fallen to 6.3 million. The population continued to drop throughout the rest of the sixteenth century so that by about 1600 there were rather less than one million living descendants of the twenty-five million in 1518.[36] There had been a 96% decline in the population in about eighty years. Such a collapse was, at that time, literally unheard of. If it was true, it was, for such a large initial population, unique in the history of the world. By the early 1960s, then, the role of disease and depopulation in the establishment of European hegemony was in urgent need of re-definition.

The biggest question was what had precipitated this catastrophic collapse. The Black Legend had always had it that it was the Spaniards who had caused—in Las Casas' celebrated phrase—"la destrucción de las Indias". Yet, the sheer enormity of the collapse as it stood revealed by the Californian historical demographers made that conclusion somewhat problematical. Even after the glamour of Mexico had been revealed in Cortés' letters, Spanish migrants were numbered only in the few thousands. If they had all done little else except kill Indians they would have had their work cut out to have destroyed so many. Brutal treatment there was and cynical disregard for alien life but the Spaniards wanted the Indians alive, not dead. What killed the Indians, it seemed apparent, was not just Spanish ill-treatment but disease, epidemic disease and, above all, pandemic smallpox. In 1966, coincidentally, but with an almost dramatic sense of timing, the World Health Organization announced a campaign to

---

[35] Cook and Borah (1957).
[36] Cook and Simpson (1948); Borah and Cook (1960); Cook and Borah (1960); Borah and Cook (1963).

eradicate smallpox from the world. It provided a fitting backdrop to
the gruesome story of the devastating effect of the disease in the
Conquest of Mexico.

In 1963 and in 1966 Henry F. Dobyns, an anthropologist, published two articles which placed the discussion in a different and a
much wider context. He argued that depopulation of the indigenes
often began far in advance of the first contact with Europeans. He
based his argument on epidemics in the Andes, some of which
occurred several years before Pizarro arrived there. Infected Indians
in one area carried diseases to other areas far away from any European
contact. This was the basis of the conclusions to a more general discussion he published in 1966. In this he reviewed the techniques of
the Berkeley historical demographers and suggested further applica-
tions. He argued that European diseases and Indian depopulation
had preceded the arrival of the Europeans. The Cook and Borah
ratio of depopulation, from zenith to nadir, was too low. A more
plausible estimate would be something of the order of thirty to one.
With this reasoning and estimating a low point in the seventeenth
century of three to four millions, he calculated that the population
of the hemisphere in 1492 had been between ninety million and 112
million. This was, in a quite special sense, a new world.[37]

In 1967 A.W. Crosby published a seminal article on the role of
smallpox in the Conquest of Mexico. He cast Dobyns' somewhat
general argument into a much more rigorous epidemiological framework. He showed that the unique epidemiology of smallpox was the
reason why there had been a delay of twenty-seven years between
1492 and the first appearance of the disease in the New World. The
course of an attack of smallpox is comparatively shortlived. An infected
person incubates the multiplying virus for ten to fifteen days, suffers
the appalling symptoms for a period of up to four weeks at the end
of which time he is either dead or recovered. Only in the three to
four weeks when the pustules are erupting can he infect someone
else. The recovered victim is thereafter immune from the disease for
the rest of his life.

One result of this epidemiology was that it was very difficult for
the virus to be transported across the ocean by sailing ship. The
voyage rarely took less than six weeks. Many adults would already

---

[37] Dobyns (1963); Dobyns (1966).

be immune as a result of childhood attacks. Anyone aboard who had not had the disease before and who had been infected even immediately prior to boarding would go through the whole course of the disease during the crossing. When they arrived in the New World they would no longer be infectious. By the time a ship got to the Caribbean there was no longer any infectious agent on board. That is why it took so long for the disease to migrate.

But, as Crosby pointed out, it was, of course, only delayed. When it did finally arrive, it infected a population which had been biologically isolated from the pathogens of the Old World for perhaps thirty thousand years. That population had no acquired immunity so that when hitherto unknown diseases struck they did so with a violence unknown in Europe. Mild diseases like measles became virulent killers. Childhood diseases struck young adults whose immune system's reaction could perhaps have overwhelmed them. From a small beginning in 1519–1520 the pandemic appears to have spread throughout the continent often wiping out whole tribes of indigenes before any European was present. Bacteria and viruses might well have been carried by natives far in advance of the Europeans' presence so that the disease would have seemed to have leap-frogged vast distances and to have whipsawed up and down the continent.[38]

Crosby made two further substantial additions to the historiography of epidemic disease in the achievement of European hegemony in America. First, in 1976, he generalised the concept of "virgin-soil epidemics". Human societies geographically isolated from the pathogens which have attacked the rest of the human race will have evolved no acquired immunity or resistance to them. When the experienced come into contact with the inexperienced they will inevitably bring with them the microorganisms with which they have learned to live. The previously untouched group will suffer all the more violently for having been free of the disease in the past.[39] A "virgin soil" population is an explosion waiting to happen.

Crosby subsequently went on, in 1986, to extend the whole concept to what he called, unprepossessingly, *Ecological Imperialism*.[40] In this he universalised the phenomenon of virgin-soil populations. It is not just the people and their germs who arrive in a hitherto untouched

[38] Crosby (1967).
[39] Crosby (1976).
[40] Crosby (1986).

land. They bring with them their animals, their plants, and their weeds, as well as their ills. Human colonisation is but one part of the spread of new life forms, vegetable and animal as well as human, into the unhandselled, defenceless new lands. That spread spelt catastrophe for the previously inviolate lands and societies. But the catastrophe was not instantaneous. It was not a Wellsian invasion from outer space. It was the assertion of superiority by compatible but aggressively stronger life-forms. Crosby's story, for the most part, told of sheep and oranges and viruses which eventually took over the ecologies they had invaded.

In one respect, though, the story is, literally, catastrophic. "Smallpox may have ranged from the Great Lakes to the pampa in the 1520s and 1530s".[41] In the extent and in the rapidity of its spread it exactly corresponded to the dictionary definition of catastrophe as a "sudden, noteworthy and signal disaster".

> Smallpox is a disease with seven-league boots. Its effects are terrifying: the fever and pain; the swift appearance of pustules that sometimes destroy the skin and transform the victim in to a gory horror; the astounding death rates, up to one-fourth, one-half, or more with the worst strains. The healthy flee, leaving the ill behind to face certain death, and often taking the disease with them. The incubation period for small pox is ten to fourteen days, long enough for the ephemerally healthy to flee for long distances on foot, by canoe, or, later, on horseback to people who know nothing of the threat he represents, and there to infect them and inspire others newly charged with the virus to flee to infect new innocents.[42]

As Crosby told the story, smallpox was the one single factor which determined the conquest of Mexico and Peru. "The disease exterminated a large fraction of the Aztecs and cleared a path for the aliens to the heart of Tenochtitlán and to the founding of New Spain ... The miraculous triumphs of [the] *conquistador* ... are in large part the triumphs of the virus of smallpox."[43]

By the early 1970s this reading had become the established account. Such discussion of it as there was was concerned only to demonstrate yet higher figures. Cook and Borah went on to publish several interpretive essays on the Mexican population collapse. Then

---

[41] Crosby (1986), p. 201.
[42] Crosby (1986), p. 200.
[43] Crosby (1986), p. 200.

from 1971 to 1979 they brought out three volumes entitled *Essays in Population History*.[44] For the most part these were discussions of the techniques available to the historical demographer, analyses of the sources, detailed investigations of localities, of migration, of sex and age ratios and examinations of very long term series. They included, however, one piece in which they argued that there was firm evidence and sound logic which pointed to a population of perhaps eight million living on Española in 1492. Given that most earlier historians were extremely sceptical even of Las Casas' apparently absurd estimate of three million, this was grandstanding in the great tradition.[45] But their final conclusion was yet more extraordinary. From eight million people in 1492, the population fell to no more than a few thousand in 1520, that is to say, over 99.9% of the population disappeared in under thirty years.

Questioning the Paradigm

At about the time of the Columbus quincentenary and subsequently, a number of conferences on disease and conquest were held and several books were published.[46] They indicate that this is still the generally accepted version of the story. But now that we are well past 1992 there are signs that it is not the received dogma it was thirty years ago.

Three things have worked to undermine its cogency. In the first place, there has been remarkably little new insight, directly attributable to these new demographic theories, into either pre-conquest society or the structures of Indian society under Spanish rule. There has been a remarkable upsurge of knowledge of Indian life both before and after the arrival of the Spaniards.[47] Historical demography does well—witness the reviews, in 1992 and 1993, by Linda

---

[44] Cook and Borah (1971–1979).

[45] Cook and Borah (1971–1979), Vol. I, pp. 376–410.

[46] No comprehensive bibliography can be given here but any such would include: Cook (1998); Larsen and Milner (1992); Verano and Ubelaker (1992); Cook and Lovell (1992); Whitmore (1992); Alchon (1991). There are, of course, also a large number of scholarly articles.

[47] A sampling from three distinct groups of work give some indication of the richness and the variety of this scholarship and the range of sources on which it is based. From the archaeological investigations into the Templo Mayor in Mexico City have come: Boone (1987); Matos Moctezuma (1988). Several re-examinations

Newson of the most recent scholarship.[48] There are studies about many different parts of the world—Spanish America, of Indian tribes of the United States, southern Africa, Polynesia and Australia.[49] Studies of the impact of western culture on native societies have proliferated. But, in general, studies of the first impact of diseases have not added directly to what we know about pre-contact societies nor about such equilibrium as was eventually worked out between colonial rulers and ruled. They have been, that is to say, somewhat unproductive beyond their own rather special and limited terms.

In the second place, the increasing sophistication of the demographers' mathematical techniques has given rise to criticism of the somewhat cavalier attitude they sometimes display. A number of reviewers expressed some scepticism about the orders of magnitude in the Berkeley demographers' conclusions. Three in particular call in question the whole operation. Sanders, writing the chapter on central Mexico in *The Native Population of the Americas in 1492*, expressed considerable scepticism about the Cook and Borah figures. He had long worked on the Central Mexican Symbiotic Region and concluded that analysis of the carrying capacity of the region suggested a population in the six to twelve million range. On the issue of depopulation he adds that it is difficult to give credence to the early and very catastrophic collapse of the population. Such a collapse is "all the more surprising since the first major epidemic occurred in the 1540s and an equally severe one occurred in the 1570s. One would expect a slow decline between 1519 and 1540 and then a rapid increase in the curve between 1540 and 1595."[50] In 1978, Henige took the analysis by Cook and Borah for the island of Española and showed that the data, so far from pointing to a precontact population of eight million, as they suggest, or even the three

---

have been published of the way in which the chronicles and histories were constructed jointly by native and Spanish chroniclers to provide not so much a history as background to and explanation of the clash between them. The most comprehensive is Lockhart (1992). One of the most exciting is Gillespie (1989). See also Berdan (1982); Clendinnen (1991). Our understanding of the life of the indigenes after the conquest has been revolutionized by James Lockhart and his pupils. See Lockhart (1991); Cline (1986); Haskett (1991).

[48] Newson (1992); Newson (1983); see also Newson (1985) and her definitive studies: Newson (1986) and Newson (1987).

[49] Frost (1994); Denoon (1995); Curtin (1993); Crosby (1992); Jannetta and Preston (1991); Smith (1989); Larocque (1988); Rigau-Perez (1982); Archer (1995).

[50] Sanders (1976).

million that Las Casas suggests, point rather to a figure of the order of 100,000, that is to say, lower than theirs by a factor of eighty.[51] In 1980 Zambardino argued that, for Mexico, the most rigorous conclusion the historical demographer could arrive at with the data available is that the population of Mexico in 1518 numbered somewhere between three million and thirty million. That being so, any kind of averaging would clearly be pointless. His conclusion is that ". . . this method, with the data that are available, does not allow a meaningful quantitative estimate."[52]

While historians continue to be fascinated by the notion of virgin-soil epidemics, of populations unprotected by acquired immunity which are destroyed by pathogens imported by or with Europeans they tend not to build their arguments on precise figures either of pre-contact populations or of the magnitude of the demographic collapse. Figures such as the famous 25.2 million for the 1518 population of Mexico, though widely quoted in more popular accounts, are either heavily discounted or simply ignored by more committed scholars.[53]

The third thing which has undermined their conclusions is the very new place that smallpox has come to occupy in our culture. We have probably learned more about the disease in the last half-century than was known throughout the whole of the previous history of the human race. In the 1950s the electron microscope was developed allowing scientists for the first time actually to see viruses. It became clear that there were not just the two strains *variola major* and *variola minor* but an intermediary strain as well.[54] Moreover, while each of these strains bred true each had a range of virulence, of infectivity and mortality associated with it. The most virulent strains— those with the highest case-fatality rate and which killed most quickly— were actually less dangerous epidemiologically. They could kill by massive toxaemia before any pustules developed thus trapping the viruses before they could escape to infect anyone else. Less virulent strains where the infected were able to come into contact with other susceptibles spread more easily. It also became clear that there was

---

[51] Henige (1978).
[52] Zambardino (1980).
[53] See for instance Denevan (1976), pp. 3–4; Cook (1998), p. 23; McCaa (1995), pp. 398, 429.
[54] Dumbell and Huq (1975).

no such thing as inherited immunity. All populations in which the disease had not appeared for thirty or forty years are "virgin-soil". In that respect most European communities were not very different from those in America. In 1962 the standard English language textbook on smallpox was published.[55] Between 1966 and 1977 smallpox was eradicated from the whole world. In 1988 the World Health Organization published what must be the definitive account, 1,500 pages long, of the history, the aetiology and epidemiology of smallpox and of the experience of the eradication of the disease both in the global eradication campaign of 1959–1966 and in the intensified Programme 1966–1977. With the publication of this massive tome, there is now readily available an immense amount of information on smallpox and its history.[56]

That new knowledge revealed some inconsistencies between historical accounts and the experience of epidemiologists in the twentieth century. Smallpox as reported in the Americas in the sixteenth century did not behave like the disease that was known so well in the twentieth. The paradox, once it was pointed out, was quite plain.

> [Smallpox] has indeed slain its millions throughout the ages. Yet smallpox is possibly not a highly infectious disease. When a patient suffers from smallpox, even if he dies from it, he probably does not infect more than two or three people and these are usually members of his own family or household or people he has been in very close contact with. There is thus a paradox somewhere in the behaviour of smallpox, this great disease which can at one time smoulder as a family or village infection yet at another blaze forth as a widespread epidemic.[57]

But so far from querying the historians' accounts, epidemiologists more often adapted their own theories. They noted the large numbers of deaths reported in those first attacks of smallpox in America. That they were familiar with. But they noted too massive infectivity and the rapid spread of the disease. These were different from their own observations, yet they accepted the authority of historians and allowed that in the first attacks infectivity must have been much higher than it was found later to be. Historians, in their turn, found that their own original assertions were now confirmed by the epi-

---

[55] Dixon (1962).
[56] Fenner (1988).
[57] Christie (1977).

demiologists and could therefore be made authoritatively. So the logic came full circle.

There are several possible reasons for the paradox. One of them is that experts in one field sometimes easily, almost naively, accept the still speculative conclusions of experts in a different field. "Epidemiologists engaged in the global smallpox eradication campaign . . . agree with Dixon that smallpox usually spread rather slowly." Nevertheless the accounts of the "devastating effects of smallpox in non-immune populations in the Americas . . . gave rise to the view that it was one of the most infectious of all diseases". Yet, the epidemiologists' conclusion had been that smallpox was "somewhat less infectious than either measles or chickenpox". Even when the number of susceptible persons in casual contact with cases was still large the spread of the disease would halt. Even among household contacts smallpox was not highly contagious; prolonged or intimate exposure was usually necessary.[58] This is in effect what Shea suggests for Peru. For areas with which he was not familiar such as central Mexico he concedes that epidemics may or may not have passed readily from one area to another. But in Peru, he argued, his evidence suggested that this did not happen. "One can still believe, with Dobyns, that Peru was ravaged by smallpox without necessarily accepting a wholesale decline of the population except in the local areas."[59]

Another reason was the widespread willingness in the 1980s and 1990s to accept that new pathogens could be unprecedentedly deadly. A great deal of the more popular literature on the epidemiology of AIDS had made current a view of pathogens sometimes insidiously penetrating other life forms, sometimes rampaging irresistibly across the globe. Stories of the ebola virus and other microorganisms cutting a swathe through the human race were the stuff of television documentaries and Hollywood blockbusters. Smallpox, time and again, has been so described. Yet the reality, we have learned, was different.

Smallpox is not a cloud of infection that descends from on high. It is caused by a virus and there is no other carrier than the human smallpox victim. Only a person in the eruptive stage of the disease can infect someone else. Since such a person is likely to be immobile and even recumbent he cannot carry the disease very far. Virtually

---

[58] Fenner (1988), pp. 199, 200, 204.
[59] Shea (1976), p. 176.

all the viruses which the sick person ejects are attached to droplets coughed, sneezed, breathed or spat out. Anyone in the same room as a smallpox victim will breathe in those viruses and many, if they are not immune, are likely to contract the disease themselves. Viruses, it is true, do adhere to clothes and to scabs shed from dried up pustules, but they will not infect someone else unless they are breathed in. As they tend to fall to the ground, they are a real potential source of new infection but an extremely inefficient one. Aside from droplets breathed in, infection is possible but it is not very probable. There is virtually no other way in which the disease can be passed on.[60]

One observation, suggested previously and confirmed during the eradication campaign, is that people are most infectious in the first week that the rash appears and when virions are being expelled from the oropharynx or nasopharynx. The later stages when the pustules erupted on the external skin were not very infectious. In this stage the expelled virions are enclosed in the inspissated pustular fluid or within scabs. These only rarely come into contact with susceptible cells in a non-immune subject. If such material is breathed in it will usually be caught in the mucus and either swallowed or coughed out again into the atmosphere.[61] Someone who is prostrate with the disease will be very infectious. Someone who is recovering and on his feet is much less so.

In the real world, and despite the language of seven-league boots, whip-sawing up and down the continent, spreading like wildfire or going on the rampage, smallpox tends to infect only people in the same house or in the same hospital. Dr. J.D. Millar, who was head of the Smallpox Surveillance Unit at the Centre for Disease Control from 1962, and director of the Smallpox Eradication Program from January 1967 to April 1970, writes: "The communicability of smallpox is relatively low in comparison to other viral infections such as measles and chicken pox. Perhaps this relates to the rapid settling of the relatively large infective particle."[62] Another reason is the behaviour of the infected person.

---

[60] There is a very small chance of being infected from fomites but, aside from the sick room of a smallpox patient and the special case of launderers who can shake up and breathe in finely powdered and highly infectious scabs, this is epidemiologically almost negligible.
[61] Fenner (1988), pp. 189, 185.
[62] Millar (1972).

... patients in the prodromal stage of variola major, before the rash had appeared and before they could transmit infection were usually quite ill, with toxaemia, headache and backache. Most took to bed, so segregating themselves from the general community although not from their household contacts. In contrast, patients in the early and highly infectious stages of chicken pox and measles have few symptoms and are usually mobile, and thus spread these diseases to school and street contacts as well as to members of the household.[63]

A person infected with measles can usually move around and infect others for a significant time. That is why schools and other public places are such efficient propagators of the disease. A person with smallpox usually does not and often cannot move around. "As a consequence", concludes Millar, "smallpox spreads in two settings: families and hospitals".[64] Clinical descriptions of smallpox and its epidemiology emphasise that it spreads slowly. It, also, does not spread very far.

Comparison of the intrafamilial and extra familial spread of small pox ... demonstrated that the overwhelming majority of secondary infections occurred in close family contacts or overt cases of small pox, especially in those who slept in the same room or the same bed. Next in frequency were those who lived in the same house; residents of other houses, even in the same compound (who would have visited the house of the patient), were much less likely to become infected ... The transmission of smallpox appeared to stop when the number of susceptible individuals in the village who were in casual contact with cases was still large but the supply of such persons in prolonged and intimate contact with cases was virtually exhausted. Even among household contacts smallpox was not highly contagious; prolonged or intimate exposure was usually necessary.[65]

The important factor for determining the epidemiology is not the infectivity nor the case-mortality rate. These will determine the effect of the disease on a local community. Since only a person in the eruptive stage of the disease can infect someone else and since he will usually be prostrate, he is not an efficient mechanism for transmitting the disease beyond his immediate family or household. What determines its movement continent-wide is either the frequency with which infected but asymptomatic people move beyond their local

[63] Millar (1972), p. 815.
[64] Millar (1972), p. 815.
[65] Fenner (1988), p. 191.

community; or it is the presence of means of transportation which can carry the infectious persons into an as yet unaffected locality. Plague—the Black Death—was spread by a network of merchants. Cholera was spread by merchants who soon had railways and steamships to make them more efficient carriers. Influenza in 1919 spread so widely because, uniquely in the history of the world, millions of soldiers, ex-soldiers, camp-followers as well as refugees were on the move. Pandemic diseases are moved by widespread systems of moving people.

One further thing the eradication campaign of 1966–1977 furnished us with which we lack for Mexico in 1520 is a count and it did so in not dissimilar circumstances. Bangladesh in 1972 and 1973 experienced one of the worst outbreaks of smallpox before it finally disappeared. The population of the country was about 70 million. The density was about 485 persons per square kilometre. The density of the population of Mexico in 1519 was of the order of 30 to 50 persons per square kilometre or between 10 and 16 times less dense than was the population of Bangladesh in 1972. We do not know the number of susceptibles in Bangladesh but since the vaccination programme had not been operating for several years it was probably between 10% and 20% of the total, say 10 million, which is about 15% of the total population. The World Health Organization calculated that there were 91,415 cases in 1972 and 81,906 cases in 1973, or rather less than 1% of the susceptible population in each year. There were about 16,000 fatalities due to smallpox in each year or about 0.16% of the susceptible population died of smallpox in each year. It should be noted that Bangladesh has an extremely widespread river system which allows ready communication between all parts of the country. It was also a time of fierce civil war in which mass movements of population occurred. Translating those percentages to Mexico in 1519, 0.16% of even the putative 25 million people living in Mexico in 1520 is about 40,000 not 3.5 million.[66]

The epidemiological conclusions of the report of the Eradication Campaign are quite explicit. Smallpox spreads slowly, it does not spread very far, and epidemics often burn themselves out quite quickly. These findings were not anomalous or peripheral. Rather

---

[66] Fenner (1988), pp. 812, 824, 847.

it was these very characteristics that made the Eradication Campaign feasible. In countries like Nigeria and Ghana, Indonesia and Bangladesh, Somalia and Ethiopia a 100 per cent vaccination rate, on which the original strategy of the campaign had been based, proved to be impossible. But it was not necessary. Widespread surveillance could detect outbreaks of the disease before they had a chance to spread. It was then possible to move quite small teams to areas where the disease was reported quickly enough to throw a ring of vaccinated people around the outbreak. The disease was contained within an enclosure from which it could not break out. Six to eight weeks later it had disappeared.

These are characteristics of a disease very different from what is described by Prescott or Bancroft or for that matter by Motolinía or Gómara. The notion that it was one of the most infectious of all diseases arose because some chroniclers had spoken of devastating epidemics in the Americas. The reason, that is to say, why epidemiologists accepted descriptions of past epidemics contrary to their own present day experience is that they read the record of massive mortality and lightning-swift spread in the first pandemics, and saw no reason to question that record. But it is precisely the function of historians to question the record.

In the light of this knowledge of the epidemiology of smallpox there are difficulties with some of the explanations given for the impact of smallpox on aboriginal America. David Henige has shown that the evidence that smallpox reduced the population of Florida from 700,000 (against more widely held estimates of about one-twentieth of that number) to a few thousand in a matter of a few years is highly suspect.[67] He has also shown up the uncritical subservience to unreliable authority of many historians who assert that smallpox was present in the New World before 1518.[68] A very similar negligence characterises one of the key arguments about the effect of smallpox on "virgin-soil" populations.

Both Crosby and Dobyns contend that we can be certain of the rapid spread and the massive mortality of the first pandemic in America because the same thing happened in Iceland in 1707–1709. "Knowledge of the decimating impact of epidemic smallpox on other

---

[67] Henige (1986); Henige (1986). Both are reviews of Dobyns (1983).
[68] Henige (1987).

susceptible populations requires the assumption of a very high mortality among inhabitants of the Inca Empire." "It is the known smallpox mortality in other populations composed entirely of susceptible persons that leads to the supposition that the Andean population may well have been halved during this epidemic."[69]

Dobyns and Crosby both cite Stearns, *The effect of smallpox*.[70] They, on the page cited, refer only to Sir Harry Johnstone, *The Negro in the New World* published in 1910. Johnstone says nothing about Iceland, but he does say that "it is estimated" that smallpox killed at least three and a half million Amerindians between 1550 and 1850.[71] Then Stearns proceed to cite the case of Iceland without further authority.

The only authoritative source for the Iceland figures is Sir John Simon. In 1857–58 he headed a Parliamentary enquiry into the effect of vaccination on smallpox. The record of the House of Commons, the *Parliamentary Papers*, contains the reply of the Danish Government. It reads, "The annals of Iceland report that smallpox raged in that country . . . [seventeen times before the eighteenth century]." The epidemic of 1707 was the eighteenth. Iceland, that is to say, had experienced smallpox about as frequently as most other countries of Europe. The report goes on: "Of the then population of Iceland, somewhat exceeding 50,000, this disease carried off, according to reports, 18,000. . . . It was no unusual occurrence that persons having once gone through the disease and bearing the marks upon them, were attacked again and died."[72] Unfortunately the document gives no indication what these "reports" were. However, the assertion of second, fatal attacks must call their reliability in question. If this were true, it would be unique in the history of smallpox.

The 1707 epidemic in Iceland was not a "virgin-soil" epidemic. It was one of a number that occurred about every 25 years. It is, however, by a very large margin the worst in the history of Iceland and the worst that Simon had had reported to him by any of the governments of Europe. He highlighted it to indicate just how destruc-

---

[69] Crosby (1967), p. 325; Dobyns (1963), p. 497.
[70] Stearn and Stearn (1945), p. 14.
[71] Johnstone (1910), p. 10.
[72] Extract from an explanatory paper accompanying the official answers from Denmark. *Papers relating to the history and practice of vaccination*, by John Simon. Parliamentary Papers, House of Commons, 1857 (ii) pp. xxxv, 411 (i.e. 173). These papers are not contained in Simon's own account. See Simon (1890).

tive smallpox could be. But he highlighted it precisely because it was not typical. Moreover neither he nor the Danish government give any indication of what the reports to which they refer actually are. It is, says Dobyns, the "annals of Iceland"—and whatever they are they are not reliable on questions of epidemiology—which "requires the assumption of a very high mortality" in America. The logic is less than compelling.

I have elsewhere discussed some of the questions that need to be put to the sources in the light of our modern knowledge of the behaviour of epidemic smallpox.[73] The basis of my argument is what I have outlined above: that only a massive mortality caused by small-pox could explain the very large collapse in population postulated by Cook and Borah and Dobyns. But smallpox, we now know, does not behave like that. Moreover it occurred quite rarely in sixteenth century Europe and usually only in a comparatively mild form.[74] It thus seemed worthwhile, in the light of this knowledge, to re-examine the accounts of the first impact of smallpox.

There are several reports of the disease being present in Mexico between 1519 and 1521 and of specific people, mostly native leaders, dying from the disease.[75] Some of these report "mucho daño" but with no indication of its extent. It is not until the late 1530s that any account is written which suggests that the disease is caus-ing massive and widespread fatalities, that is that it killed up to as many as half the population. The first to do so was written by the Franciscan Motolinía in his *Memoriales*. The next to appear in extended comment are by Francisco López de Gómara, Cortés' secretary and biographer and by Bernal Díaz del Castillo.

Motolinía provides all the basic elements of the story.

> God struck this land with ten cruel plagues on account of the obsti-nacy and hardness of heart of the inhabitants and for having held cap-tive the daughters of Sion, that is their own souls under the yoke of Pharaoh [Satan], the first of which happened at the time when the captain and governor Fernando Cortés had already entered this New Spain with his men. At the time Pánfilo de Narváez landed here and in one of his ships came a negro stricken with smallpox a disease which had never before been seen in this land. At that time the whole of New Spain was extremely full of people. Since the smallpox began

---

[73] Brooks (1993).
[74] Carmichael and Silverstein (1987).
[75] These are conveniently listed in McCaa (1995), pp. 400–401.

to spread to the Indians, there was among them such a great sickness
and a mortal pestilence in all the land that in some provinces half the
people died and in other a little less [*en algunas provincias morían la mitad
de la gente, y en otras poco menos*]. This was because the Indians did not
know the remedy [*remedio*] for smallpox but as was their custom, whether
well or sick, they took frequent baths and for this reason they died
like flies. Many of them died of hunger, because since they all fell sick
at the same time they could not care [*curar*] for each other nor was
there anyone to make bread. In many places it happened that everybody in some of the houses died with almost no one left alive. And
to be rid of the stench, because there was no one to bury the dead,
the houses were pulled down on top of them so that thus their houses
became their sepulchres. They called this the *huey zahuatl* which means
the great leprosy because being covered from their feet to their heads
with the smallpox so that they looked like lepers. And this disease
seemed to signify to them the tribulations and the plagues that all of
them in all parts had to undergo. Today, in some of those who recovered from this sickness its virulence can be seen in the pockmarks
which cover their faces.[76]

Gómara incorporated a great deal of Motolinía's material into his
own history. His account of smallpox is almost identical in its content to the Franciscan friar's adding only a few humanistic touches.

This war cost Diego Velázquez a great deal of money, Pánfilo de
Narváez his eye, and the Indians many dead, who died, not of wounds,
but of disease. It happened that among the men of Narváez was a
Negro sick with the smallpox, and he infected the household in Cempoala
where he was quartered; and it spread from one Indian to another,
and they, being so numerous and eating and sleeping together, quickly
infected the whole country. In most houses all the occupants died, for,
since it was their custom to bathe as a cure for all diseases, they bathed
for the smallpox and were struck down. They had the custom, or vice,
of taking cold baths after hot ones, so a man sick with the smallpox
only escaped by a miracle. Those who did survive, having scratched
themselves, were left in such a condition that they frightened the others with the many deep pock-marks on their faces, hands, and bodies. And then came famine, not because of a want of bread, but of
meal, for the women do nothing but grind maize between two stones
and bake it. The women, then, fell sick of the smallpox, bread failed,
and many died of hunger. The corpses stank so horribly that no one
would bury them; the streets were filled with them; and it is even said
that the officials, in order to remedy this situation, pulled the houses
down to cover the corpses. The Indians called this sickness *huitzahu-*

---

[76] Motolinía (1971), p. 21.

atl, meaning the "great leprosy", and later counted the years from it, as from some famous event. It seems to me that this was how they were repaid for the *bubas* [syphilis] which they gave our men.[77]

Motolinía was not an eyewitness of the epidemic. He arrived in Mexico three or four years later. Gómara never went to America at all. Bernal Díaz, however, was there. It is the central strand of his *Historia verdadera* that he was present, he was an eyewitness. Whatever other people said he describes what he saw. In the light of this his account of the smallpox epidemic is strange.

> Let us now return to Narvaez and a black man whom he brought covered with smallpox, and a very black affair it was for New Spain, for it was owing to him that the whole country was stricken and filled with it, from which there was a great mortality, for according to what the Indians said they had never had such a disease, and, as they did not understand it, they bathed very often, and on that account a great number of them died; so that dark as was the lot of Narvaez, still blacker was the death of so many persons who were not Christians.[78]

It is striking how close these accounts are. There are a few other occasions when Bernal Díaz reports in passing on incidents of the smallpox epidemic but on the widespread effect this is all he has to say and clearly he is copying the gist of either Motolinía's account or of Gómara's. He adds, as is his wont, a couple of slightly jokey comments. Yet the event he is purporting to describe is a catastrophe without precedent in the history of the world. When he comes to describe the suffering in the siege of Tenochtitlán the following year he is heart-rending in his graphic detail. It makes it difficult to imagine that he has actually seen what he is describing here. Gómara was a historian back in Europe but he did have access to other sources. Bernal Díaz however is setting out to write the true account. He was there. He was an eyewitness. That he could describe a cataclysm such as Motolinía recounts—about half the population dying—in words that he has copied from someone else beggars the imagination. If this hecatomb occurred and he saw it he cannot but have described it in his own words. That he chose to copy someone else's words must call in question his authority, not for the existence of the epidemic—of that we are quite certain—but of this massive spread.

---

[77] López de Gómara (1964), pp. 204–205.
[78] Diaz del Castillo, Bernal (1967), Vol. 2, pp. 218–219.

And that is what is crucial. Not the existence of the disease. But
of this rampaging killer. Twenty or thirty thousand deaths might
have been caused by smallpox. That is a disaster. That is a human
tragedy of massive proportions. But it falls short by several orders
of magnitude of the cataclysm which has to be present to account
for millions dying in a few months, one-third of a population of 25
million in a few years.

My critique of the received version received in its turn a massive
rejoinder from Robert McCaa. On several points he shows my argument to be defective. But the crux of his case is my reading of
Motolinía.[79] I quoted the spurious *Historia* rather than the genuine
Memoriales. But on this point there is no real difference between them.
In the *Memoriales* Motolinía writes: "en algunas provincias morían la
mitad de la gente, y en otros poco menos" ["in some provinces a
half of the people died and in other somewhat less"]. In the *Historia*
Motolinía's unofficial editor writes: "en las mas provincias morían
mas de la mitad de la gente, y en otras poco menos" ["in the majority of the provinces more than half the people died and in others
somewhat less"]. There is of course a difference between the two
but it really is so small that it is difficult to see what argument can
be hung on the difference.

Smallpox probably killed Cuitlahuac at some time between September and December 1520. But the Aztecs were already experiencing the trauma of transition with the death of Motecuzoma. If the
Spaniards were spared in July 1520 it was not because the new
Aztec Lord had died nor because smallpox was raging. The reason
was, rather, that the Aztecs could not imagine a siege and especially
that the Spaniards might be able to build boats in order to mount
one. Smallpox killed many, perhaps thousands, of the Aztec population. But it killed as many of the Spaniards' allies as it did their
foes. And the battle when it came never suffered from lack of forces
on either side. The massed fighters, "the brave warriors" on both
sides might have been weakened by the epidemic but there were
still more than enough of them alive to take part in the battle. After
the destruction of Tenochtitlán, and in Peru after the capture of

---

[79] He is quite right that I showed that I did not distinguish between the spurious *Historia* and the genuine *Memoriales*. As a matter of fact I used both versions
but quoted the much more accessible *Historia* rather than the *Memoriales*.

Cuzco diseases added to the difficulties the indigenes had in attempting to recreate a centralized polity. Yet what doomed them from the start was above all the immensely superior centralizing forces and resources available to the Europeans.

That smallpox occurred in Mexico in 1520 is not in contention. Nor that it caused many deaths if by many we mean figures of, say, 30,000 or 40,000 which correspond to those we know occurred in Bangladesh in 1970. But there is no evidence that several million people died within a few months. Motolinía certainly had nothing remotely approximating to a count. If what he says were true, Bernal Díaz must have reported this unbelievably shocking calamity not by copying Motolinía's text but in his own heartfelt words as he did his accounts of the suffering during the siege of Tenochtitlán a year later. If the Mexica of Tenochtitlán suffered and died in that way and in those numbers so too must have the Spaniards' allies. Yet all the accounts of the final campaign are at pains to stress the numbers involved, the numbers who died and even the numbers who in their extremity, but still alive, filed out of the remains of the city when it finally surrendered.[80]

European diseases wreaked a terrible toll on the peoples of the Americas. Since we have only the most approximate estimate of the numbers who were living there before 1492 we cannot say how many died as a result of those diseases. Nor, since we cannot separate the effect of diseases from that of trauma, anomie, malnutrition and direct killing by European weapons (or in their own civil wars) can we give a number to those who succumbed to the imported pathogens. But we can be certain that it was in the millions. Little is served by trying to be any more precise. Eighty percent at least of that original population was gone within a century of the arrival of the Europeans. For Mexico, where we have something approximating to a count within thirty years of the fall of Tenochtitlán, we can be sure that four out of five and possibly nine out of ten did not reproduce themselves. By any reckoning that is total catastrophe.

Such figures allow us to see the story as most of the sources tell it. An original trauma, the product as much of a fissiparous society as of external invaders, was enhanced by a range of new pathogens

---

[80] Clendinnen (1991).

which killed thousands but did not determine the outcome of the clash of the two worlds. Despite the trauma, there was considerable continuity of native peoples who reverted to their age-old foci of community life and of their religion bound to their earth and their localities. But at the centre it was the impersonal European institutions of permanent power and structured communications that prevailed.

It can be argued that diseases played a critical role, that the story would have been very different without them. But whether in the momentary advantage won as the Spaniards escaped disaster, in the protracted civil war and siege of the capital, and in the long haul of three hundred years and more of colonial domination, the sources point to an explanation in which the role of disease, though clearly catastrophic for the indigenes, did not to any significant extent alter the eventual outcome.

Bibliography

Alchon, Suzanne Austin, *Native Society and Disease in Colonial Ecuador*. Cambridge: Cambridge University Press, 1991.

Alonso de la Vera Cruz 1971, *The Writings of Alonso de la Vera Cruz: The Original Texts with English Translation*. Edited and translated by Ernest J. Burrus. 5 Volumes. Rome, St. Louis: Jesuit Historical Institute, St. Louis University, 1967–1975.

Archer, Christon I., "Whose Scourge? Smallpox Epidemics and the Spanish Maritime Expeditions to the Northwest Coast of North America in the Late Eighteenth Century", unpublished paper given at a symposium on the history of small-pox, La Trobe University, August, 1995.

Ashburn, P.M., *The Ranks of Death: A Medical History of the Conquest of America*. New York: Coward-McCann, 1947.

Bancroft, Hubert Howe, *History of Mexico*, 6 volumes. San Francisco, 1883.

Beneson, Abram S., "Smallpox", chapter 24 in *Viral Infections of Humans: Epidemiology and Control*, 3rd edition. New York: Plenum, 1989.

Berdan, Frances F., *The Aztecs of Central Mexico: An Imperial Society. Case Studies in Cultural Anthropology*. New York: Holt, Rinehart & Winston, 1982.

Boone, Elizabeth Hill, ed., *The Aztec Templo Mayor*, A Symposium at Dumbarton Oaks. Washington, DC: Dumbarton Oaks Research Library and Collection, 1987.

Borah, Woodrow W., and Cook, Sherburne F., *The Aboriginal Population of Central Mexico on the Eve of the Spanish Conquest*. Ibero-Americana, 45. Berkeley: University of California Press, 1963.

——— and Cook, Sherburne F., *The Population of Central Mexico in 1548*. Ibero-Americana, 43. Berkeley: University of California Press, 1960.

Brooks, Francis J. "Motecuzoma Xocoyotl, Hernán Cortés, and Bernal Díaz Del Castillo: The Construction of an Arrest", *Hispanic American Historical Review* 75, no. 2 (1995): 149–83.

————, "Revising the Conquest of Mexico: Smallpox, Sources, and Populations", *Journal of Interdisciplinary History* XXIV, no. 1 (Summer, 1993): 1–29.

Carmichael, Ann G. and Silverstein, Arthur M., "Smallpox in Europe before the Seventeenth Century: Virulent Killer or Benign Disease?", *Journal of the History of Medicine and Allied Sciences* 42 (1987): 147–168.

Cervantes, Fernando, *The Devil in the New World. The Impact of Diabolism in New Spain.* New Haven and London: Yale University Press, 1994.

Christie, A.B., "Smallpox" in *A World Geography of Human Disease*, edited by G. Melvin Howe. London: Academic Press, 1977, 255.

Clavigero, Francisco Saverio, *The History of Mexico* (Storia Antica Del Messico). Introduction by Burton Feldman. New York: Garland Publishers, 1979. [Reprint of the 1787 ed. printed for G.G.J. and J. Robinson, London.]

Clendinnen, Inga, *Aztecs: An Interpretation*. New York: Cambridge University Press, 1991.

————, Fierce and Unnatural Cruelty: Cortes and the Conquest of Mexico. *Representations* 33 (Winter, 1991): 65–100.

Cline, Sarah, *Colonial Culhuacan, 1580–1600. A Social History of an Aztec Town.* Albuquerque, New Mexico: University of New Mexico Press, 1986.

Conrad, Geoffrey W., and Demarest, Arthur A., *Religion and Empire: The Dynamics of Aztec and Inca Expansionism*. Cambridge: Cambridge University Press, 1984.

Cook, Noble David, *Born to Die. Disease and New World Conquest, 1492–1650.* Cambridge: Cambridge University Press, 1998.

———— and Lovell, William G., eds., *"Secret Judgments of God": Old World Disease in Colonial Spanish America*. Norman: University of Oklahoma Press, 1992.

Cook, Sherburne F., "Human Sacrifice and Warfare as Factors in the Demography of Pre-Colonial Mexico", *Human Biology* 18 (1946): 81–102.

————, "The Incidence and Significance of Disease among the Aztecs and Related Tribes", *Hispanic American Historical Review* 26 (1946): 320–335.

———— and Borah, Woodrow Wilson, "The Rate of Population Change in Central Mexico, 1550–1570", *Hispanic American Historical Review* 37 (1957): 463–70.

———— and Borah, Woodrow Wilson, *Essays in Population History: Mexico and the Caribbean*, 3 vols. Berkeley and Los Angeles: University of California Press, 1971–1979.

———— and Borah, Woodrow Wilson, *The Indian Population of Central Mexico, 1531–1610.* Ibero-Americana, 44. Berkeley: University of California Press, 1960.

———— and Simpson, Lesley Byrd, *The Population of Central Mexico in the Sixteenth Century*, Ibero-Americana, 31. Berkeley: University of California, 1948.

Crosby, Alfred W., "Hawaiian Depopulation as a Model for the Amerindian Experience", in *Epidemics and Ideas. Essays on the Historical Perception of Pestilence.* Edited by Terence Ranger, and Paul Slack. Cambridge: Cambridge University Press, 1992, pp. 175–201.

————, "'*Conquistador y Pestilencia*': The First New World Pandemic and the Fall of the Great Indian Empires", *Hispanic American Historical Review* 47 (1967): 321–37.

————, "Virgin Soil Epidemics as a Factor in the Aboriginal Depopulation in America," *William and Mary Quarterly*, 3rd Series 33 (1976): 289–99.

————, *Ecological Imperialism. The Biological Expansion of Europe, 900–1900.* Cambridge: Cambridge University Press, 1986.

Curtin, Philip, "Disease Exchange across the Tropical Atlantic", *History and Philosophy of the Life Sciences* 15, no. 3 (1993): 329–56.

Denoon, Donald, "Pacific Island Depopulation: Natural or Un-natural History?" in *New Countries and Old Medicine*, Proceedings of an International Conference on the History of Medicine and Health, Auckland, New Zealand, 1994, edited by Lynda Bryder and Derek A. Dow, Auckland: Pyramid Press, 1995, pp. 324–339.

Diamond, J., *Guns, Germs, and Steel. The Fates of Human Societies*. New York: Norton, 1998.

Diaz del Castillo, Bernal, *Historia Verdadera de la Conquista de la Nueva España*. Introduccion y notas de Joaquin Ramirez Cabanas, Mexico City: Espasa-Calpe Mexicana, 1950.

———, *The True History of the Conquest of New Spain*, translated by Alfred Percival Maudslay, 5 volumes in 4 [London: Hakluyt Society, 1906–1909], Nendeln: Kraus Reprint, 1967.

Dixon, Cyril, *Smallpox*. London: Churchill, 1962.

Dobyns, Henry F., "An Outline of Andean Epidemic History to 1720", *Bulletin of the History of Medicine* 37 (1963): 493–515.

———, "Estimating Aboriginal American Population: An Appraisal of Techniques with a New Hemispheric Estimate", *Current Anthropology* 7 (1966): 395–416.

———, *Their Number Become Thinned: Native American Historical Demography*. Knoxville, 1983.

Dumbell, K.R. and Huq, Farida, "Epidemiological Implications of the Typing of Variola Isolates", *Transactions of the Royal Society of Tropical Medicine and Hygiene* 69:3 (1975): 303–308.

Elliott, John H., "The Spanish Conquest and Settlement of America", in *Cambridge History of Latin America*, Vol. 1: *Colonial Latin America*. Cambridge: Cambridge University Press, 1984.

———, *The Old World and the New 1492–1650*. Cambridge: Cambridge University Press, 1970.

Farriss, Nancy M., *Maya Society under Colonial Rule. The Collective Enterprise of Survival*. Princeton: Princeton University Press, 1984.

Fenner, Frank, et al., *Smallpox and Its Eradication*. Geneva: World Health Organization, 1988.

Fernández-Armesto, Felipe, "'Aztec' Auguries and Memories of the Conquest of Mexico", *Renaissance Studies* 6, nos. 3–4 (1992): 287–305.

———, *Millennium: A History of the Last Thousand Years*. London: Bantam Press, 1995.

Frost, Alan, "The Curse of Cain", in *Botany Bay Mirages. Illusions and Australia's Convict Beginnings*. Melbourne: Melbourne University Press, 1994, pp. 190–210.

Gerbi, A., *The Dispute of the New World. The History of a Polemic, 1750–1900*. Pittsburgh: University of Pittsburgh Press, 1973.

Gillespie, Susan D., *The Aztec Kings. The Construction of Rulership in Mexican History*. Tucson: University of Arizona Press, 1989.

Gruzinski, Serge, *The Conquest of Mexico. The Incorporation of Indian Societies into the Western World, 16th–18th Centuries*. Cambridge: Polity Press, 1993.

Guilmartin, Jr, John F., "The Cutting Edge: An Analysis of the Spanish Invasion and Overthrow of the Inca Empire, 1532–1539", in *Transatlantic Encounters. Europeans and Andeans in the Sixteenth Century*, edited by Kenneth Andrien and Rolena Adorno. Berkeley: University of California Press, 1991.

Hanke, Lewis, *The Spanish Struggle for Justice in the Conquest of America*. Philadelphia: University of Pennsylvania Press, 1949.

Harris, Max. *The Dialogical Theatre: Dramatization of the Conquest of Mexico and the Question of the Other*. New York: St. Martin's, 1993.

Haskett, Robert S. *Indigenous Rulers: An Ethnohistory of Town Government in Colonial Cuernavaca*. Albuquerque, NM: University of New Mexico Press, 1991.

Henige, David, "On the Contact Population of Hispaniola: History as Higher Mathematics", *Hispanic American Historical Review* 58:2 (1978): 217–237.

———, "When Did Smallpox Reach The New World (And Why Does It Matter)?" in Paul E. Lovejoy, ed., *Africans in Bondage*. Madison, Wisc., 1987, pp. 11–26.

————, "If Pigs Could Fly: Timucuan Population and Native American Historical Demography", *Journal of Interdisciplinary History* 16 (1986): 701–720.

————, "Primary Source by Primary Source? On the Role of Epidemics in New World Depopulation", *Ethnohistory* 33 (1986): 293–312.

Hennessy, A., The Nature of the Conquest and the Conquistadors. *Proceedings of The British Academy* 81 (1993): 5–36.

Jannetta, Ann Bowman, and Samuel-H. Preston, "Two Centuries of Mortality Change in Central Japan: The Evidence from a Temple Death Register", *Population Studies* 45, no. 3 (1991): 417–36.

Johnstone, Sir Harry, *The Negro in the New World*, London, 1910.

Larocque, Robert, "Le role de la contagion dans la conquête des Ameriques: Importance exagerée attribuée aux agents infectieux", *Recherches Amerindiennes au Quebec* 18, no. 1 (1988): 5–16.

Larsen, Clark Spencer and Milner, George R., eds., *In the Wake of Contact. Biological Responses to Conquest*. New York: Wiley-Liss, 1994.

Las Casas, Bartolomé de, [*Brevísima Relación de la Destrucción de las Indias*], *A Short Account of the Destruction of the Indies*, Edited and translated by Nigel Giffin with an introduction by Anthony Pagden. Harmondsworth: Penguin, 1992.

Lockhart, James, *The Nahuas after the Conquest: A Social and Cultural History of the Indians of Central Mexico, Sixteenth Through Eighteenth Centuries*. Stanford, CA: Stanford University Press, 1992.

————, *Nahuas and Spaniards: Postconquest Central Mexican History and Philology*. Stanford, CA: Stanford University Press, 1991.

————, Editor and translator, *We People Here: Nahuatl Accounts of the Conquest of Mexico*, Berkeley and Los Angeles: University of California Press, 1992.

López de Gómara, Francisco [*La Conquista de Mexico*] Lesley B. Simpson, *Cortés, The Life of the Conqueror by his Secretary*, translated by Lesley B. Simpson, Berkeley and Los Angeles: University of California Press, 1964.

Macaulay, Thomas Babington, *The History of England from the Accession of James the Second*, 2 volumes. London: Longmans, Green, 1889.

MacCormack, Sabine, *Religion in the Andes. Vision and Imagination in Early Colonial Peru*. Princeton: Princeton University Press, 1991.

Matos Moctezuma, Eduardo, *The Great Temple of the Aztecs: Treasures of Tenochtitlán*. New York: Thames and Hudson, 1988.

McCaa, Robert, Spanish and Nahuatl Views on Smallpox and Demographic Catastrophe in Mexico. *Journal of Interdisciplinary History* 25, no. 3 (1995): 397–431.

Millar, J.D., "Smallpox, Vaccinia and Cowpox" in P.D. Hoeprich, ed., *Infectious Diseases*. Hagerstown, MD, 1972, pp. 815–823.

Millones, Luis, "Religion and Power in the Andes: Idolatrous Curacas on the Central Sierra." *Ethnohistory* 26, no. 3 (1979): 243–63.

Mills, Kenneth, "The Limits of Religious Coercion in Mid-Colonial Peru." *Past and Present*, no. 145 (1994): 84–121.

Motolinía, Fray Toribio de, *Memoriales: o Libro de las cosas de la Nueva Espana y de los naturales de ella por Fr. Toribio de Benavente o Motolinia. Nueva transcripcion paleografica del manuscrito original con insercion de las porciones de la Historia de los Indios de la Nueva Espana que completan el texto de los Memoriales*. Mexico: Universidad Nacional Autonoma de Mexico, 1971.

Newson, Linda A., "Variaciones regionales en el impacto del dominio colonial español en las poblaciones indigenas de Honduras y Nicaragua", *Mesoamérica* 12, no. 24 (1992): 297–312.

————, "Indian Population Patterns in colonial Spanish America", *Latin American Research Review* 20, no. 3 (1985): 41–74.

————, "The Demographic Collapse of Native Peoples of the Americas, 1492–1650", *Proceedings of the British Academy* 81 (1983): 247–288.

————, *Indian Survival in Colonial Nicaragua*, Norman, Okla., 1987.

————, *The Cost of Conquest: Indian Decline in Honduras under Spanish Rule*, Boulder, Colo., 1986.

Oviedo y Valdés, Gonzalo Fernández de, *Historia general y natural de las Indias*, 1959.

Phelan, John Leddy, *The Millennial Kingdom of the Franciscans in the New World*, 2nd ed., Berkeley and Los Angeles: University of California Press, 1970.

Prescott, William Hickling, *History of the Conquest of Mexico* [1843]. New York: Random House, 1970.

Rigau-Perez, Jose G., "Smallpox Epidemics in Puerto Rico During the Prevaccine Era (1518–1803)", *Journal of the History of Medicine and Allied Sciences* 37, no. 4 (1982): 423–38.

Robertson, William, *The History of the Discovery and Settlement of America*, New York: Harper, 1843.

Sanders, William T., "The Population of the Central Mexican Symbiotic Region, the Basin of Mexico, and the Teotihuacan Valley in the Sixteenth Century", in William M. Denevan, ed., *The Native Population of the Americas in 1492* [second edition, 1992]. Madison: University of Wisconsin Press, 1976, pp. 85–150.

Sauer, Carl Ortwin, *The Early Spanish Main*. Berkeley: California University Press, 1966.

Seed, P., "'Are These Not Also Men?': The Indians' Humanity and Capacity for Spanish Civilisation", *Journal of Latin American Studies* 25, no. 3 (1993): 629–652.

Sepúlveda, Juan Ginés de, *Demócrates segundo o De las justas causas de la guerra contra los indios*. Madrid: Consejo Superior de Investigaciones Científicas, Instituto Francisco de Vitoria, 1951.

Shea, Daniel E., "A Defence of Small Population Estimates for the Central Andes in 1520" in Denevan (1976): pp. 157–180.

Simon, Sir John, *English Sanitary Institutions, reviewed in the course of their development and in some of their political and social relations*, London, 1890.

Simpson, H.N., "The Impact of Disease on American History", *New England Journal of Medicine* 250 (1954): 679–682.

Smith, A.B. "Khoikhoi Susceptibility to Virgin Soil Epidemics in the Eighteenth Century", *South African Medical Journal* 75, no. 1 (1989): 25–26.

Stearn, E.A., and Stearn, A.E., *The Effect of Smallpox on the Destiny of the Amerindian*. Boston: Bruce Humphries, 1945.

The Times Atlas of World Exploration, edited by Felipe Fernández-Armesto. London: The Times, 1991.

Todorov, T., *The Conquest of America: The Question of the Other*. New York: Harper and Row, 1984.

Verano, John W. and Ubelaker, Douglas H., *Disease and Demography in the Americas*. Washington: Smithsonian Institution Press, 1992.

Vigil, Ralph H., *Alonso de Zorita. Royal Judge and Christian Humanist, 1512–1585*. Norman and London: University of Oklahoma Press, 1987.

Wachtel, Nathan, "The Indian and the Spanish Conquest" in *Colonial Latin America*, Vol. 1 of *Cambridge History of Latin America*. Cambridge: Cambridge University Press, 1984.

Whitmore, Thomas M., *Disease and Death in Early Colonial Mexico. Simulating Amerindian Depopulation*, Dellplain Latin American Studies 28. Boulder: Westview Press, 1992.

Zambardino, Rudolph A., "Mexico's Population in the Sixteenth Century. Demographic Anomaly or Mathematical Illusion?", *Journal of Interdisciplinary History* XI, no. 1 (Summer, 1980): 1–27.

Zorita, Alonso de, *The Brief and Summary Relation of the Lords of New Spain. Life and Labor in Ancient Mexico [Breve y Sumaria Relación de los Señores de la Nueva España]*. Translated and with an introduction by Benjamin Keen. New Brunswick: Rutgers University Press, 1963.

6. PATHOGENS, PLACES AND PEOPLES: GEOGRAPHICAL VARIATIONS IN THE IMPACT OF DISEASE IN EARLY SPANISH AMERICA AND THE PHILIPPINES

Linda Newson

Demographic disaster accompanied Europeans as they expanded overseas. In the Americas, Australia, New Zealand and the Pacific Islands population losses may have been as high as 80 to 95 per cent within the first 100 to 150 years of contact.[1] These high levels of decline are not universally accepted. They are often dependent on high estimates for pre-contact populations which make assumptions about the impact of Old World diseases on non-immune populations and whether the diseases could have arrived prior to direct contact with Europeans. The significance of disease relative to other factors implicated in the decline has also been an area of controversy. In the absence of complete information these issues have generated heated philosophical, political and methodological debates that show little sign of abatement.[2] While these debates have been raging, regional and local studies of population decline in the wake of European contact have been revealing marked geographical variations in the level of decline.[3] Among the factors deemed important in explaining these variations are differences in the ease of conquest, in the form of control exercised by colonial powers and in the extent of the commodification of land, labour and production that accompanied colonial rule.[4] While these factors clearly differed according to the objectives of European powers,[5] differences within any one empire emanated largely from the diversity of native societies and

---

[1] Borah (1964), pp. 386–87; Butlin (1983), p. 147; Crosby (1992), p. 176; Denevan (1992a), p. xxix; Dobyns (1966), p. 415; Kunitz (1994), pp. 46–49; MacArthur (1967), pp. 345–47; Rullu (1991), pp. 176–77; Stannard (1989), pp. 45–49, 79.

[2] Borah (1992); Cook (1998), pp. 9–13; Henige (1978), (1993), (1998); Roberts (1989); Stannard (1989).

[3] E.g. Kunitz (1994), pp. 46–49; Newson (1993), pp. 247–88; Rullu (1991), pp. 176–77; McArthur (1967), pp. 345–47.

[4] Kunitz (1994), pp. 8–18; Newson (1985), pp. 49–66; Parker (1995), pp. 132–43.

[5] Elliott (1990), pp. 43–54; Meinig (1986, Vol. 1), pp. 65–72; Osterhammel (1997), pp. 4–12, 28–32.

resources encountered. While the significance of local environmental and social conditions on the demographic impact of colonial rule has sometimes been recognised, their role in influencing mortality levels associated with the introduction of Old World diseases has received little attention. Instead scholarly interest in Old World diseases has focused on levels of mortality associated with epidemics and on the ability of diseases to run ahead of direct European contact.[6] While there has been some recognition of environmental influences on the incidence of some diseases, less often recognised are the ways in which the character of native societies and the changes they experienced under colonial rule influenced their spread and impact. There is a tendency to assume that once introduced Old World diseases spread unhindered and that their impact was uniform.[7]

This paper will demonstrate that there are likely to have been significant spatial and temporal variations in the impact of Old World diseases that related to particular environmental and social contexts. Any discussion will necessarily require an examination of the pre-Columbian conditions and the changes that occurred as a result of Spanish contact. The focus on impact of Old World diseases provides a useful window through which to examine broad differences in the impact of colonial rule. At the same time, since the Spanish empire in the Americas and the Philippines encompassed such a diversity of lands and peoples, it can demonstrate very clearly the significance of local circumstances.

The discussion starts from the premise that Old World epidemics were a significant factor in the depopulation of both regions, but argues strongly that disease mortality was highly variable. The implication is that overall levels of disease mortality may not have been as high as is often assumed and that its significance relative to other factors responsible for the decline is also likely to have differed from place to place.

The presence or absence of particular infections and their spread and impact on human populations in terms of morbidity and mortality varies considerably with the pathogen itself, host immunity (whether genetic or acquired) and a wide range of environmental and social factors. The paper will first examine the significance of

---

[6] Roberts (1989), p. 1245.
[7] Cook (1998), p. 209; Dobyns (1983), p. 24.

environmental conditions, but it will focus mainly on social factors, such as population size, settlement patterns, forms of subsistence, socio-political structures and ideologies, which influenced the spread and impact of Old World diseases. It will show how variations in population size and the intensity of contact, in nutrition and susceptibility, in the ability of diseases to become endemic and in the capacity of societies to respond to the crises that epidemics precipitated, all affected levels of disease mortality. Although the essay will stress the complexity of processes at work and suggest reasons why levels of mortality are likely to have been highly variable, the discussion will draw some broad distinctions between state and non-state societies. Before embarking on this task, the paper will consider briefly some genetic differences in pathogens and hosts that may have influenced disease mortality, but are often overlooked in the literature.

The Nature of Hosts and Pathogens

Hosts

Advances in medical science and studies of recent epidemics have demonstrated that immune responses to diseases do not differ significantly between human groups and as such cannot explain the exceptionally high levels of mortality among native Americans in the early colonial period. However, it has recently been suggested that the lack of genetic diversity among a population might enhance disease mortality since pathogens become pre-adapted to successive hosts resulting in increased virulence.[8] Hence diseases transmitted from family members are likely to be more virulent and result in higher mortality than those contracted from strangers.[9] During the initial settlement of the Americas, Asian populations lost genetic traits as they passed through the bottlenecks of the Bering Strait and the Panamanian isthmus. As a result South American populations are genetically more homogeneous than their neighbours to the north or in Asia and they might therefore have been particularly susceptible to the new infections. Other isolated populations with restricted

---

[8] Black (1990).
[9] Black (1992).

gene pools include the Papuans, Australian Aborigines and the Polynesians. This tendency towards genetic homogeneity in isolated populations, however, is countered by random genetic drift and some see its influence as relatively minor compared to environmental and cultural factors.[10]

More often differences in human populations focus on differences in levels of immunity. The devastating impact of Old World diseases on New World peoples that accompanied European expansion is generally attributed to the lack of immunity that they had acquired to acute infections, such as measles, rubella and smallpox, due to their previous isolation. Often the distinction is made between Spanish America and the Philippines where it is generally argued that the lower level of depopulation in the islands was due largely to the immunity that populations there had acquired to Old World diseases in pre-Spanish times as a result of trading contacts with the rest of Asia.[11] However, my own research suggests that disease mortality in the Philippines was moderated in the early colonial period not because communities there had acquired immunity to the acute infections that afflicted New World peoples, though some limited immunities may have been acquired in the larger trading centres, but because of the small size of the population and its distribution through several thousand islands.[12] The distinction between Spanish America and the Philippines in terms of levels of acquired immunity would appear to be untenable and, as will be argued, comparisons in the impact of Old World diseases are better drawn between similar types of society, for example, between those in the Philippines and Amazonia.

Pathogens

While some attention has focused on differences in host immunity, very little cognisance is generally taken of variations in the disease organisms themselves. Not only are pathogens spread in different ways—through direct personal contact, contaminated food or water or by biting insects—but they also vary in the duration of human

---

[10] Svanborg-Eden and Levin (1990), pp. 41–44.
[11] Borah (1964), p. 387; Doeppers (1968), p. 61; Owen (1967a), p. 9; Phelan (1959), pp. 106, 156; Reid (1988), pp. 57–58.
[12] Newson (1999).

infectivity and in their impact in terms of the levels of morbidity and potential mortality, as well as in the degree of immunity they confer.[13] As a consequence, they are affected by different social and environmental conditions. Not only that, but over time pathogens may change. Many viral diseases, particularly influenza, but also smallpox and syphilis, evolve rapidly producing different strains with different levels of virulence to which previous exposure may not provide immunity. Because of the mutual advantages to pathogens and their hosts, it has often been argued that over time some diseases, for example, scarlet fever, plague and smallpox, through repeated infections lost some of their virulence.[14] Outbreaks of smallpox in colonial Mexico generally show a decline in associated mortality,[15] though this may be related to increased immunity. However, more recent biological research suggests that on theoretical grounds the coevolution of parasites and hosts may not necessarily trend toward avirulence but follow many paths, depending on the degree to which parasite transmissibility and recovery rates are linked to rates of host mortality.[16] Whether or not later epidemics in colonial Spanish America can be associated with lower mortality, the key point is that it cannot be assumed that all outbreaks of the same disease will have the same potential morbidity and mortality. Although in most cases other factors were probably more significant in influencing disease mortality than differences in the virulence of pathogens, the point is made to urge caution in extrapolating mortality rates from one epidemic to another even when the same disease is involved.

Environmental Influences

Each disease organism has environmental limits beyond which it is unable to survive. The most commonly recognised environmental influence on the incidence of disease is climate, particularly temperature and humidity, but other aspects of physical geography such as the topography and vegetation cover may also be significant.

---

[13] Fenner (1980), pp. 11–14; Ramenofsky (1987), pp. 146–62.

[14] Appleby (1980), pp. 169–73; McKeown (1988), p. 77; Slack (1981), pp. 471–72.

[15] Solominos D'Ardois (1982), pp. 239–40.

[16] Allison (1982), p. 245; Anderson and May (1991), pp. 649–53; Ewald (1994), pp. 3–6; Levin *et al.* (1982), p. 214; Pimental (1968), p. 1437.

Certain diseases, such as malaria and yellow fever, only thrive in tropical climates, while others such as typhus and pneumonic plague are more commonly associated with cool dry climates. Diseases which are transmitted through the air, such as influenza, smallpox or measles, or are dependent on insect vectors for their propagation, such as malaria or yellow fever, are particularly sensitive to variations in temperature and humidity and are often seasonal in their prevalence.[17] Smallpox, for example, prefers cooler, drier conditions losing its infectivity at temperatures over 30°C and above 55 per cent humidity.[18] Due to the seasonality of temperate climates temporal variations in the incidence and impact of some diseases are likely to be more marked in those regions. It is worth noting, however, that not all seasonal variations in the incidence and spread of diseases can be related directly to climate, rather in many cases the link is indirect through seasonal differences in human activities. For example, seasonal shortages of food may make populations particularly susceptible to infections, while communal gatherings associated with seasonal availability of food might provide the opportunity for the spread of infections.

In the context of Spanish America it is often argued that the greater depopulation of the tropical lowlands was due to higher incidence of disease. Cook and Borah (1971: 82) have estimated that between 1532 and 1608 population losses on the coast of Central Mexico were of the order of 26.0: 1, whereas in the highlands they were 13.1: 1. Similar differences in depopulation between the highlands and lowlands have been noted for Peru[19] and Ecuador.[20] The higher levels of depopulation in the tropical lowlands are often attributed to the presence of the tropical fevers, malaria and yellow fever, and to the greater prevalence of waterborne intestinal infections such as dysentery, typhoid, hookworm and other helminthic infections. Some diseases may also have been more virulent in warmer climates.[21] These explanations generally fall short of providing a complete answer.

---

[17] Fenner (1982), pp. 112–14; Upham (1986), pp. 119–22.
[18] Upham (1986), p. 120.
[19] Smith (1970), p. 459; Cook (1980), p. 94.
[20] Newson (1993b), p. 1188, (1995), p. 341.
[21] Borah and Cook (1963), p. 89; Borah and Cook (1969), pp. 181–82; Denevan (1992a), p. 41; Friedlander (1969), p. 217; McNeill (1976), p. 197.

In the colonial period chronic infections undoubtedly continued to take a heavy toll of populations in the humid lowlands as they had in pre-Columbian times. Chronic infections are found to varying degrees in the earliest human societies and their incidence generally increases with sedentism and increased dependence on agriculture.[22] Skeletal evidence from pre-historic Ecuador confirms this trend, but it also suggests that environmental factors were important. Skeletal remains, which cover the whole pre-Columbian period from 9,000 BP, indicate higher levels of infection among communities on the humid north coast than among groups on the dry southern coast or in the highlands despite the fact that in the last two regions the settlement pattern was more dispersed and the diet more varied.[23] As will be indicated below, changes in the colonial period, which often congregated dispersed populations in settled communities firmly based on agriculture, probably increased the incidence of many chronic infections, but they alone cannot satisfactorily explain the massive depopulation of the coasts in the early colonial period. The charges against yellow fever and malaria are also difficult to sustain.

It is almost certain that yellow fever cannot be implicated in the early depopulation of tropical coasts since the decline pre-dates its arrival in the mid-seventeenth century.[24] The first identifiable outbreak of this distinctive disease probably occurred between 1647 and 1648 and even then epidemics were confined to the towns which possessed populations large enough to sustain the disease.[25] The case against malaria is a little stronger. Malaria, which is now generally agreed to be a post-Columbian introduction to the Americas may have arrived at an earlier date.[26] Spaniards probably introduced the benign form of malaria, *Plasmodium vivax*, whereas the more acute form *P. falciparum*, probably arrived in the blood of apparently healthy African slaves, the demand for which increased significantly towards the end of the sixteenth century following the decline of the native population. Where it became established malaria is likely to have resulted in high levels of pregnancy loss and infant and child

---

[22] Cockburn (1971), pp. 49–50; Cohen (1989), pp. 39–40, 53; Diamond (1998), pp. 204–205; Fenner (1970), pp. 64–65, (1980), pp. 14–16.
[23] Ubelaker and Newson (in press).
[24] Kiple (1984), pp. 17–20; Cooper and Kiple (1993), pp. 1102–1103.
[25] Pineo (1990), p. 614.
[26] Dunn (1965), pp. 85–93, (1993), p. 860.

mortality, in addition to which it had debilitating effects on survivors making demographic recovery difficult to achieve.

How quickly malaria may have become established is difficult to determine. McNeill (1976: 197) suggests that the *Anopheles* mosquitoes would have needed time to adjust to the new plasmodium, but even once they had become adapted, the transmission of malaria would have been highly dependent on the density of insect vectors whose presence or absence depended on specific climatic and habitat conditions. In the Philippines, and indeed in Southeast Asia in general, malaria, which was probably present in pre-Spanish times, is most prevalent in the foothills,[27] whereas in the Americas the mosquito vectors are largely, but not exclusively, concentrated in the lowlands. In Mexico, for example, the Central Plateau is spotted with areas where malaria is endemic, notably in the Valley of Mexico where swamp lands and lake beds constitute attractive breeding grounds for the mosquitoes.[28] Even within the lowlands the incidence of malaria varies widely. For example, in Ecuador the more virulent *P. falciparum* is found in more open environments, whereas the more benign *P. vivax* is more prevalent where the forest is less disturbed.[29] The presence of malaria depends not only on conditions favourable for the insect vectors, but also on human populations or animals to maintain the cycle of infection. Even today the low population density of parts of the Upper Amazon Basin serves to maintain them free of malaria.[30]

In the early colonial period population decline and forest regeneration would have created less favourable conditions for the spread of malaria in many regions. However, in some areas these processes may have been countered by the introduction of livestock, which would have provided alternative sources of blood for the mosquitoes, and by the expansion of irrigation which would have created more favourable conditions for their reproduction. In summary, conditions favouring the spread of malaria would have been much more localised than is often recognised and the chain of infection must have broken down on many occasions before it became established.

---

[27] De Bevoise (1995), pp. 143–44; Kondrashin (1986), p. 645; Zulueta (1956), p. 651.
[28] Watson and Hewitt (1941), pp. 136, 142.
[29] Newson (1993), p. 1190.
[30] Ayala Mora (1957), pp. 58–59, 65; Kroeger *et al.* (1977), p. 161.

The absence of malaria from the desert coast of Peru,[31] which sustained some of the heaviest losses in the early colonial period, also suggests that factors other than tropical fevers were operative.

Within areas suitable for the propagation of particular pathogens, topographic barriers to their spread, such as mountain, forests, deserts or water, might also be significant. For the most part these barriers were relative rather than absolute, their significance depending on the prevailing technology and the need or desire for social interaction. In the early colonial period, however, communications were relatively slow, such that topographic barriers might be significant in discouraging the spread of disease. The dispersion of populations through a large number of islands, such as in the Philippines or the Pacific Ocean, was an important factor determining the impact of an epidemic and whether diseases became endemic. In these circumstances a single epidemic might cause high mortality but it would affect only a small number of islands and communities before it died out. This moderated its impact and meant that many acute infections failed to become endemic in the Philippines until the nineteenth century when population growth and improved communications facilitated their spread.[32] From the perspective of the spread of disease, the narrow valleys of the Andes were similar to islands. Shea (1992) argues that due to topographic barriers to their spread epidemics took a lesser toll of populations in the Andes than in Central Mexico where diseases could diffuse radially. Forested areas might also hinder the spread of disease, to which should be added socially constructed barriers, such as uninhabited buffer zones in the Amazon and the American Southeast.[33]

Before the discussion shifts completely to a consideration of social influences on the spread and impact of disease, it is worth noting that environmental conditions are not constant and often result from human action. Perhaps the most important human-induced changes from the perspective of disease relate to forest clearance and the extension of irrigation systems. Both these activities, which are sometimes linked, have a direct influence on the incidence of malaria, and in the case of the latter in the Philippines, on schistosomiasis.

---

[31] Cook (1980), p. 62.
[32] De Bevoise (1995), p. 27; Newson (1999), p. 1846.
[33] De Boer (1981), p. 365; Myers (1976), pp. 354–65; Thornton, Warren and Miller (1992), pp. 192–93.

At a very general level the colonial environmental histories of Spanish America and the Philippines appear to have followed different trajectories largely as a result of differences in the level of depopulation and the nature and intensity of Spanish activities. In Spanish America the early decline of native populations in many parts of Mexico and the Andes created shortages of labour that led to the collapse of irrigation systems, land abandonment and forest regeneration.[34] In some areas, however, where Spaniards could develop profitable agricultural enterprises or where wood was required in the mining, construction or shipbuilding industries open environments were maintained. Nevertheless, in the early colonial period environmental conditions and the reduced size of human populations in many regions resulted in less favourable conditions for the spread of diseases than had existed in pre-Columbian times. In the Philippines, however, the exigencies of wars with the Dutch (1609–1648) resulted in widespread forest clearance to supply the naval dockyards and led to the extension of wet padi cultivation to enhance food production.[35] These two examples serve to demonstrate that environmental conditions are not constant, but rather they change over time often in response to shifts in the pattern of human activities.

Social Influences on the Spread and Impact of Disease

The nature of the societies the Spanish encountered profoundly affected the impact of Old World diseases. Population size and distribution influenced the introduction, spread and impact of infections and also determined whether or not they became endemic. Where they became endemic societies could develop immunities to them so that levels of adult mortality declined which had important implications for the degree of economic and social disruption they caused. The ability of acute infections to become endemic depended not only on population size but also on the birth rate which generated new susceptibles to maintain the chain of infection. Apart from immunity, disease susceptibility was also influenced by the nutritional status of individuals that depended on diet and work patterns. Once

---

[34] Denevan (1992b), pp. 377–79.
[35] De Bevoise (1995), p. 143; Phelan (1959), pp. 108–110; Schurz (1959), pp. 196–97.

infected, the level of mortality would depend on the ability of societies to respond to the crises that epidemics precipitated. In all of these circumstances broad differences emerge between state and non-state societies and the way in which they were transformed by colonial rule.

In Spanish America the Inca and Aztec states were socially stratified and had centralised governments with leaders who were able to command labour and tribute from their subjects. Their populations ran into millions and their economies were based on intensive forms of agricultural production. Though they were less populous and highly stratified, chiefdoms groups such as the Maya and Chibcha (Muisca), for the purposes of this discussion will be included in this category. Non-state societies on the other hand were based on less permanent forms of cultivation that were supplemented by the exploitation of wild food resources. They were sometimes nomadic or semi-nomadic and formed social groups of several thousand persons that were largely unstratified and lacked strong leadership. Various forms of non-state social organisation characterised Filipino populations.

Most empires have a core and a periphery with areas of difficult terrain—mountains, forests, deserts—and those where native societies were difficult to pacify and economically uninteresting generally evading control.[36] The Spanish empire was no exception. Since Spanish objectives were to generate wealth and to convert and civilise native populations, interest centred on state societies where large populations constituted greater potential sources of tribute and labour as well as souls for conversion.[37] These societies could be controlled relatively easily through alliances with native leaders and the exaction of tribute and labour could be effected by modifying pre-existing structures and mechanisms. Even the commercial activities that the Spanish developed often built on native systems of production.[38] As Carmack (1991: 406) has suggested, economically and politically these societies were "preconditioned to accommodate to the colonial state".

Notwithstanding the devastation caused in the early conquest years, for state societies colonial rule did not constitute such a marked break with the pre-Columbian past. Subsistence patterns changed as demands for tribute and labour altered and as new forms of land

---

[36] Osterhammel (1997), p. 28.
[37] Elliott (1990), p. 56; Newson (1985), pp. 49–51; Service (1955), pp. 416–19.
[38] Melville (1997), pp. 190–91; Patch (1994), pp. 92–94.

holding and production were introduced. Meanwhile, social and political structures weakened by depopulation gradually adjusted to the
new social and political order. For state societies the tempo of change
was slower and colonial objectives could generally be achieved without major restructuring. However, there were important spatial variations in the experience of native societies that were related to the
intensity of Spanish settlement and the demands it made on native
lands, labour and production. While Spanish settlement generally followed the distribution of native populations, particularly attractive
in the early colonial period were regions which possessed gold or
silver or which could produce tropical crops for export or staples
to support growing populations in the towns and mining areas.[39] Lockhart uses the concepts of "trunk lines" and "feeder routes" to describe
differences in the intensity and nature of Spanish settlement and
associated activities.[40] In Mexico the trunk line ran through Vera
Cruz on the Caribbean Coast to Puebla and Mexico City then on
to the mining regions of the north, while feeder routes led up from
Yucatan and Guatemala. In the Andes the "trunk line" was more
diffuse but went from Lima through Arequipa to Potosi, with Cuzco
and Quito involved in more feeder-line activities. Off the trunk lines
the indigenous way of life was less profoundly changed. Hence the
comparative "mildness" of colonial rule in the Philippines has been
attributed to the absence of minerals and, due to distance, the paucity
of Spanish colonists and their concentration in Manila.[41] The precise way in which the distribution of Spanish settlers and economic
activities impacted on native societies and indirectly influenced populations losses from disease will be explored in more detail below.

Non-state societies proved less attractive to the Spanish Crown
and settlers alike. Being small societies of less than a few thousand,
they offered few opportunities for wealth creation in the form of
tribute and labour. Moreover their semi-nomadic or nomadic existence and the absence of effective leadership provided fewer opportunities for control through political alliances. The lack of incentive
to expend resources in bringing such groups under effective colonial
administration meant that the missionary orders were often entrusted

---

[39] Altman and Lockhart (1976), p. 5; Grieshaber (1979), pp. 107–108; Taylor
(1972), p. 8.
[40] Lockhart (1991), pp. 107–110.
[41] Corpuz (1988), p. 535; Phelan (1959), pp. 105–107.

with their preliminary conversion and civilisation that would pave the way for their full incorporation into colonial society. Although the number of missionaries involved in this task were few, the process of missionisation often resulted in extensive restructuring of subsistence patterns and social relations that threatened their cultural and biological survival.[42] Even those societies, such as the Mapuche, Chichimeca or Guaycuran groups of the Chaco, who in the early colonial period remained outside Spanish control, experienced major changes as a result of population losses in warfare and epidemics and as a consequence of the adoption of horses.[43]

The extent of change under colonial rule is important in understanding the economic and social conditions that might have affected factors influencing the introduction, spread and impact of disease. Changes to subsistence patterns and labour demands impacted on nutrition, but not always, as will be seen, in a negative way. Similarly, the impact of social and demographic changes, some of them induced by epidemics, affected fertility rates, levels of immunity and the ability of diseases to become endemic. They also affected the capacity of groups to respond to crises thereby affecting mortality levels. What the study aims to show is that the introduction, spread and impact of diseases were highly variable and depended to a large extent on socio-economic conditions stemming from the character of native societies themselves and the changes they experienced under colonial rule.

Population Size and Distribution

Differences in the impact of diseases in the Old World and the New are seen to derive largely from the introduction of acute infections, whose introduction, spread and impact was determined to a considerable degree by population size and distribution. Since the following discussion will concentrate on acute infections, it is worth noting these factors also influenced the incidence of chronic infections. For example, the incidence of intestinal and respiratory diseases most likely increased where Spaniards congregated dispersed

---

[42] Newson (1985), pp. 58–60.
[43] Ganson (1989), pp. 473–79, 487; Jara (1961), p. 63; Powell (1975), pp. 47–50, 172.

populations into nucleated settlements to facilitate their control and administration. Population size and distribution influenced the introduction of diseases, since for the most part Spaniards settled where there were large populations, whose size and distribution in turn facilitated their spread. These factors also influenced whether diseases could become endemic, but the latter also depended on population dynamics, especially the birth rate.

The Introduction and Spread of Diseases

Conditions favouring the introduction and spread of diseases were mainly found in highland regions, where the largest concentrations of population were to be found and Spaniards settled in largest numbers. However, the maintenance of the empire depended on the shipment of goods and people such that ports, such as Portobello and Veracruz, earned early reputations for being unhealthy and within a short time were inhabited largely by non-native populations. Densely populated regions not only attracted outsiders and therefore new infections, but their nucleated settlement patterns encouraged their spread.

Among non-state societies opportunities for the introduction and spread were more limited. Often outside contacts were restricted to a few missionaries, soldiers or slave raiders, while the small size and dispersed settlement pattern often limited their spread. Although diseases were not dependent on contact with Spaniards, but could run ahead of the invaders through native population chains, as seems to have been the case in Central Andes,[44] the ability of diseases to spread in areas of low population density was limited, since the shortage of new susceptibles to infect meant that 'fade outs' were common.[45] Population density *per se* was not the only factor determining the ability of a disease to spread, but also the precise character and location of settlements, as well the nature and intensity of social contacts between them.[46] Hostile relations would have generally discouraged their spread, even though occasionally infections might be transmitted during a brief raid, while friendly relations manifest in

---

[44] Newson (1992), pp. 88–92.
[45] Cliff and Haggett (1988), pp. 245–46; Haggett (1994), pp. 10–11; Neel (1977), p. 170.
[46] Ramenofsky (1990), pp. 37, 41–42.

trade, social gatherings and visiting the sick, would have aided their transmission.

Endemicity

Population size and distribution also determine in part the ability of diseases to become endemic. Here it is important to note a difference between chronic and acute infections. Chronic diseases do not kill their hosts or provoke immune responses that result in the death of the disease organisms. As a consequence they may persist for long periods being maintained in human or non-human hosts. Since their survival is not dependent on the presence of a large number of susceptibles, they can be found in small populations.[47] For example, chickenpox viruses can survive in populations of less than one thousand, and even in isolated family units.[48] Acute infections, on the other hand, such as measles and smallpox, are generally spread by face to face contact and are characterised by short periods of infection. Since they normally confer lifelong immunity on survivors and are only infectious for short periods, generally less than two weeks, they only become endemic where human populations are of sufficient size to generate enough susceptibles to maintain the disease indefinitely. The ability of populations to do this depends in part on population size, but also on the birth rate.

In a classic paper, Bartlett (1960) calculated that for measles to become endemic, 7,000 susceptibles would need to be generated from an urban population of between 250,000–300,000; Black (1966: 210), using evidence from island communities, suggested a threshold of over 500,000. Since smallpox spreads less rapidly than measles, the population threshold required for it to become endemic has been estimated at 200,000.[49] Below these thresholds and where the population is small and dispersed, the shortage of new susceptibles to infect results in frequent "fade outs". In areas of low population density therefore acute infections fail to become endemic and future outbreaks are dependent on diseases being re-introduced. Hence small communities may remain disease-free for long periods, but since they

---

[47] Black (1975), pp. 515–18, (1980), pp. 45–49; Cockburn (1971), p. 50; Fenner (1970), pp. 48–68; Garruto (1981), pp. 560–64; McKeown (1988), pp. 38, 49.
[48] Fenner (1970), pp. 58, 64.
[49] Fenner *et al.* (1988), p. 118.

are unable to develop immunities to acute infections, when they are introduced they continue to be associated with high mortality among adults as well as children. Although endemic diseases that take a regular toll of infants and children might result in a larger number of deaths than infrequent epidemics accompanied by high mortality,[50] the overall demographic impact of the latter might be higher because they are generally accompanied by adult losses which may undermine the economic and social functioning of the group, rendering it unable to achieve demographic recovery.[51]

Clear differences emerge between state and non-state societies in their ability to sustain infections and thereby develop immunities to them. State societies probably suffered the heaviest losses from epidemics in the early colonial period due to the ease with which diseases could be introduced and spread, but in most cases sufficient numbers remained to enable acute infections to become endemic and for populations to develop immunities to them. Among non-state societies, on the other hand, individual communities might suffer high mortality, but the overall impact of an epidemic would be moderated since not all communities would have been affected. However, the reduced population made it even more difficult for diseases to become endemic, so that when they were re-introduced from outside they continued to cause high mortality among all age groups, that in the longer term might hold population growth. Whether or not this can partially account for the low population density in the Philippines in pre-Spanish times, it seems clear that despite trading contacts with Asia the Filipinos had been unable to acquire immunity to Old World diseases because of the low population density and its dispersion through thousands of islands (Newson, 1999).

Birth Rate

The ability of acute infections to become endemic is dependent not only on population size and distribution, but on a range of other factors, including the birth rate, migration and on levels of immunity.[52] The birth rate has often been regarded as central to under-

---

[50] McKeown (1976), p. 69,
[51] McGrath (1991), p. 417; McNeill (1979), p. 96; Whitmore (1992), p. 482.
[52] Cohen (1989), p. 49.

standing endemicity[53] and the ability of societies to recover from epidemics.[54] In non-contracepting societies the birth rate is largely determined by social practices such as age at marriage, breast-feeding, child spacing and sexual taboos.[55]

In pre-Columbian times state societies generally promoted population growth. Among the Incas premarital sexual intercourse was encouraged and state participation in the arrangement of marriages suggests a concern for population expansion.[56] Concern for the unborn child and infants is reflected in the apparent absence of abortion and infanticide and restrictions on female labour in pregnancy and until infants reached one-year old, while the fact that women were generally married by their twenties suggests that their reproductive capacities were maximised. Certain rituals among the Aztec, such as the flower wars (*guerras floridas*) which culminated with the annual sacrifice of over fifteen thousand captives,[57] effectively reduced the population, but birth control does not appear to have been practised. Indeed women who died in childbirth were deified and children were regarded as gifts from the gods and as such were cherished and indulged.[58] Like the Inca, Aztec women appear to have married around age fifteen and men a few years later.[59]

Colonial rule similarly supported population expansion for ideological and practical reasons. Even though the Church officially frowned on the marriage of minors, unofficially early marriage was encouraged to prevent immoral behaviour, to expand the labour force and to maximise tribute income. It might also fall in response to demographic crises.[60] For whatever reason, marriage age in the early colonial period often declined. For example, in the 1560s Bishop Landa noted that Indians were marrying at twelve and thirteen years, whereas previously they had married at twenty.[61] Even though marriage age may have increased later in the colonial period it remained

---

[53] Anderson and May (1979), p. 366; Black (1966), pp. 207–211.
[54] Thornton, Miller and Warren (1991), pp. 30–39.
[55] Marcy (1981), pp. 309–23.
[56] Newson (1995), p. 141; Rabell and Assasourian (1977), pp. 35, 37; Silverblatt (1987), pp. 90, 101–102.
[57] Cook (1946a).
[58] Clendinnen (1991), pp. 174–92; Conrad and Demarest (1990), pp. 171–72.
[59] McCaa (1994), p. 14.
[60] Gutierrez (1991), p. 274.
[61] Cited in Cook and Borah (1974, Vol. 2), pp. 51–52.

low. My own research on western Honduras in the early eighteenth century revealed that 13 per cent of women between ten and fourteen were married as were 78 per cent of those between fifteen and nineteen.[62] Overall marriage age in colonial Spanish America was considerably lower than in Europe or North America[63] and was not an impediment to population increase.

Christian marriage also heralded a change from polygamous to monogamous unions which, perhaps contrary to what might be expected, generally has a positive affect on the birth rate.[64] In pre-Columbian times polygyny was not widely practised and tended to be restricted to elites. In the early colonial period polygyny seems to have persisted and in some cases may even have increased, perhaps in response to imbalanced sex ratios created by higher levels of male absenteeism or mortality in conflict and forced labour, and as it no longer became the exclusive privilege of elites.[65] However, as the Church gradually exerted its influence over native beliefs monogamy became the dominant form of marriage.

Probably a more significant influence on birth rates in state societies was the crumbling of any traditional barriers to marriage as kinship ties were broken as a result of wars, population displacements and epidemics. In the early colonial period social relations appear to have been very fluid with few restrictions on marriage or re-marriage so that the pool of potential marriage partners was maximised with consequent benefits to fertility.

Operating against these positive influences on marriage and the birth rate were the negative impacts of labour systems, migration and physiological and psychological reactions to stress brought on by colonial rule[66] that undermined social relations and depressed fertility rates. Colonial systems of forced labour that operated in state societies often required the prolonged absence of workers leading to reductions in the frequency of sexual intercourse and marriage breakdown.[67] This was generally true of forced labour employed in mining since minerals had to be mined where they were found and

---

[62] Newson (1986), p. 231.
[63] Marcy (1981), pp. 309–10.
[64] Hern (1992), pp. 53–64, (1994), pp. 127, 137; Krzywicki (1934), pp. 201–202.
[65] Cline (1993), pp. 473–76, 479–80; McCaa (1994), pp. 16, 22–23; Wachtel (1977), p. 91.
[66] Sánchez-Albórnoz (1990), p. 201.
[67] Menken (1979), pp. 114–15.

workers often had to travel long distances from their communities. Even more significant in this case, and probably more widely, was fugitivism to escape such labour drafts which similarly weakened family ties and depressed fertility levels.[68] Populations appear to have survived to a greater degree in regions where the periods of employment outside the community were relatively short or indeed where workers could return home at night. This was the case in Ecuador where many of the textile factories were actually located in native communities.[69] It might also be expected that social relations would be maintained to a higher degree where workers were temporarily employed on local haciendas, though, as will be noted below, this form of labour sometimes had other adverse effects on subsistence production. In general family structures were maintained to a greater degree in more isolated regions which lacked intense Spanish settlement, mines or large scale commercial agricultural enterprises.[70]

Birth intervals were extended not only due to the prolonged separation of spouses or instability in marriage, but also by physiological and psychological responses to the changed circumstances of colonial rule. Unconscious stress-induced amenorrhea, which was probably most prevalent in the early conquest period, would have reduced conception. While the Church sought to discourage abortion and infanticide, some early colonial observers suggested that in the early colonial period they increased due to parents being unable to support their offspring or not wishing them to endure the hardships they had experienced.[71] While birth control practices may have contributed to reduced fertility, probably the breakdown in social relations was more significant. What seems clear is that despite the advantages of low marriage age, in the early colonial period families were generally smaller than those that had prevailed, either before conquest or later in the colonial period, and that they were failing to reproduce themselves. González and Mellafe (1965: 68–69) note that in Huánuco family size had fallen to 2.5 persons in 1560 from a pre-Columbian norm of six, and Borah (1951: 42) similarly notes that in the mid-sixteenth century families in Mexico only averaged

[68] Bakewell (1984), pp. 111–13, Cole (1985), p. 27.
[69] Newson (1995), p. 225.
[70] González and Mellafe (1965), p. 68.
[71] Sánchez-Albórnoz (1974), pp. 54–56; Wachtel (1977), pp. 93–94.

3.2 persons whereas by the end of the seventeenth century this had risen to five.

The populations of non-state societies were below the thresholds necessary for most acute infections to become endemic, so that even where the birth rate remained high they were unable to generate sufficient children to sustain them in endemic form. However, in most cases the birth rate fell. Population losses from epidemics or conflict resulting from attempts at missionization or to control hostile groups, often resulted in adult deaths that not only resulted in an immediate reduction in reproductive capacity, but disrupted reproduction until new unions were formed or a new reproductive group emerged.[72] In small communities the formation of new unions was often more difficult due to the small size of marriage pools, often marked differences in sex ratios and the existence of cultural restrictions on marriage and re-marriage.[73] In order to ensure biological survival, groups might have had to modify their population policies and social practices, such as marriage rules.[74] It is noteworthy that many surviving indigenous societies are exogamous and in the past may have been prepared to absorb or be absorbed by outsiders.[75]

The imposition of Christian forms of marriage on those gathered in the missions should in theory have had beneficial effects on the birth rate. As already noted, monogamy generally contributes to higher fertility than polygamy and the suppression of abortion and infanticide should also have contributed to population growth. However, the punishment of these practices including the failure of women to produce children on the suspicion that they were practising abortion were largely counterproductive since they increased levels of stress and demoralisation.[76] Other aspects of the missionisation process also contributed to lower birth rates. In many cases communities and individual families were broken up as Indians were brought into the missions by force and as those gathered in the missions often took the opportunity to flee. Adding to processes of social fragmentation which broke marital ties and disrupted reproduction, was the resentment of mission life, which involved the suppression of their own

---

[72] Malvido (1982), pp. 185–86.
[73] Early and Peters (1990), pp. 137, 140; Kunitz (1994), p. 9.
[74] Johnston et al. (1969), p. 33; Wagley (1951), pp. 95–104.
[75] Dobyns (1983), pp. 306, 310–11; McGrath, (1991), p. 414; Milner (1980), p. 47; Thornton (1986), pp. 128–29.
[76] Block (1994), p. 126; Jackson (1994), p. 126; Sweet (1995), pp. 25–26.

social practices and beliefs and the imposition of a regimented routine, which resulted in abstinence from sexual intercourse, abortion, infanticide or stress-induced amenorrhea.[77] A Jesuit missionary in the province of Mainas in Ecuador in the seventeenth century reported that previously fertile women when brought into the missions "like wild birds when captured or caged become sterile".[78] The birth rate was also held back by the shortage of women in the missions.[79] Reasons for this imbalance in the sex ratios of missions are not clear but could relate to female infanticide, despite missionary efforts to suppress it, higher levels of disease mortality among pregnant women, the absence of adequate maternity care, or inadequacies in recording. Finally, even where children were born, the expansion of mission populations was hindered by high infant and child mortality that derived from the overcrowded and insanitary conditions that often prevailed, especially in the dormitory-like accommodation in which Indians were housed.[80] Whatever the causes, most mission populations were sustained not by the birth rate, but by the addition of new converts.[81] While the low birth rates in the missions limited the growth of the pool of susceptibles, the inexorable desire to win more converts continuously replenished mission populations and effectively established sedentary settlements as nodes in a network of communications that extended from regions where diseases had become endemic.

Immunity

The pool of susceptibles was affected not only by population size and the birth rate, but also by levels of immunity. Most immunity is acquired through constant exposure to diseases either because they have become endemic, or, less likely, in situations where there are very intense contacts with a distant region where the disease is sustained in endemic form. In such circumstances those who are more resistant reproduce and those who are not die in childhood. Historical

---

[77] Block (1994), pp. 81–82; Jackson (1994), pp. 137–39, 161; Rausch (1984), p. 72.
[78] Figueroa (1904), p. 23.
[79] Block (1994), p. 81; Cook (1940), p. 17; Jackson (1994), pp. 126, 161.
[80] Jackson (1994), pp. 131–35, 161; Sweet (1995), p. 13.
[81] Cook (1940), pp. 16–19; Sweet (1995), p. 13.

experience suggests that at least a century of constant exposure is required for a disease to become endemic.[82]

Immunity may also be acquired through racial mixing. Unions between Indians and Europeans and Africans produced offspring who had some immunity to Old World diseases. African populations provided some immunity to smallpox and malaria, and Spaniards to smallpox, measles and other childhood diseases. Levels of racial mixing varied widely according to the intensity of contact between the races and their relative numbers. The growth of the mestizo population was most precocious in Mexico which in the early colonial period suffered some of the highest levels of Indian depopulation and Spanish immigration, whereas it was slower in the Andean region where both were lower.[83] In both regions racial mixing was highest in the towns and mining areas where commercial activities drew immigrants from a wide range of racial backgrounds. Due to less frequent contacts with outsiders, racial mixing was generally less common in non-state societies, at least until depopulation undermined their viability as independent groups.[84] Early exceptions were those nomadic groups which proved difficult to control, such as in northern Mexico and southern Chile, where slavery prevailed and captives were often sold in the towns where isolated from their communities they were rapidly absorbed into the expanding population of mixed races.[85] By the beginning of the nineteenth century the mixed races in Spanish America accounted for about 30 per cent of the total population and the percentage was even higher in some regions.[86] Hence although racial mixing probably had little impact on levels of immunity in the early colonial period over time its significance almost certainly increased thereby contributing to decreasing levels of disease mortality.

Nutrition

Nutrition is considered to play a major role in disease susceptibility.[87] However, the direct relationship between malnutrition and infec-

---

[82] Alchon (1991), p. 58; Jannetta (1987), pp. 19–21; De Bevoise (1995), p. 98.
[83] Bakewell (1997), p. 164.
[84] Sánchez-Albórnoz (1974), pp. 135–36.
[85] Góngora (1975), pp. 130–31; Jara (1961), pp. 163–66; Zavala (1967), p. 81.
[86] Rosenblat (1954), p. opp. p. 36.
[87] McKeown (1988), pp. 52–55.

tion is difficult to substantiate since malnourished individuals are also likely to experience poor living conditions, such as crowded accommodation and inadequate sanitation, that also favour the spread of disease. Furthermore, malnutrition does not always result in increased susceptibility for in some cases deficiencies in protein or particular vitamins and minerals may actually provide some resistance to infection.[88] For example, many disease organisms need iron to thrive, so that short-term iron deficiency may assist the body to fight infection. It is also important to note that the link between disease susceptibility and malnutrition is stronger for some diseases than for others.[89] In the case of measles and most respiratory and intestinal infections levels of morbidity and mortality appear to increase with poor nutrition, whereas smallpox, plague, yellow fever and malaria seem to be relatively unaffected.[90] Even where nutritional status might normally affect disease susceptibility, it is probably insignificant in the case of particularly virulent strains and among non-immune populations. However, where micro-organisms become endemic, malnutrition may exert a greater influence on disease mortality, particularly infant and child mortality,[91] and class and gender differences may become more significant. Hence Klein (1975: 207–208) has suggested that larger families in Chulumani and Pacajes in Upper Peru in 1786 might be related to better access to land, and therefore food, that enabled families to maintain children past infancy.

Inasmuch as disease susceptibility is related to nutritional status, it is important to note that the latter depends not only on food supplies and diets, but also on energy requirements.[92] Greater food intakes are required to ensure adequate nutrition in colder environments and where individuals are involved in arduous labour or are constantly fighting infection. Hence, all other things being equal, those who lived in crowded conditions in the highlands and were employed in arduous tasks such as mining or porterage are more likely to have been malnourished. Due to the complexity of the processes at work it is difficult to make broad generalisations about

---

[88] Cohen (1989), p. 167.
[89] Cohen (1989), p. 167; Livi-Bacci (1991), pp. 35–39; McKeown (1988), pp. 52–53; Rotberg and Rabb (1983), pp. 305–308.
[90] McKeown (1988), p. 52.
[91] Harpending, Draper and Pennington (1990), pp. 257–58.
[92] Rotberg and Rabb (1983), pp. 305–308; Walter and Schofield (1989), pp. 17–21.

nutritional levels in pre-Columbian or colonial times for they would have varied widely with environmental and social conditions.

In colonial times nutritional status depended not only on environmental conditions and the productivity of pre-contact agricultural systems, but also on the changes they experienced under colonial rule. It is clear that in pre-Columbian times some groups struggled to survive and often suffered food shortages and famines, while others enjoyed a varied and substantial diet. Carbon stable isotope analysis of skeletal remains promises to shed considerable light on nutritional status in the past, but so far its application has been limited. A current project on Health and Nutrition in the Western Hemisphere directed by Richard Steckel and Jerome Rose which examines all major skeletal collections from the Western Hemisphere indicates that the groups in Mesoamerica and the American Southwest had more severe health problems, including malnutrition, than those in Ecuador or coastal Chile. In the first two areas there is a higher incidence of porotic hyperostosis and cribra orbitalia indicative of iron-deficiency anaemia, which in the Americas is often related to a heavy dependence on the consumption of maize. Enamel hypoplasia, which is related to systemic stress that among other things can be caused by nutritional imbalances, is also more prevalent in the first two areas.[93] Evidence from Aztec codices and early colonial accounts from Mexico also indicates a pre-Columbian history of quite severe famines;[94] most likely there were other less notable periods of shortage. Even within one region nutritional status would have varied widely with local environmental and social conditions. For example, the skeletal evidence from pre-Columbian Ecuador reveals a higher incidence of iron deficiency anaemia and enamel defects among groups on the south coast, who were heavily dependent on the cultivation of maize, than among those who lived on the north coast or in the highlands where diets were more varied.[95] Not only might nutritional status be differentiated by geography, but also by social class. Carbon stable isotope analysis of skeletons from shaft tombs at La Florida in the Quito Basin indicates greater dependence on maize among the nobility.[96]

---

[93] Larsen (1994), p. 117.
[94] Cook (1946b), pp. 331–35; Hernández Rodríguez (1982), pp. 146–48; Hassig (1981).
[95] Ubelaker and Newson (in press). ???????
[96] Ubelaker, Katzenberg and Doyon (1995).

These variable patterns of nutrition changed to differing degrees in the colonial period according to the level of demographic collapse and the demands that the Spanish made on native lands, labour and production. Although these factors varied widely a general debate exists as to whether diets declined or improved in colonial times. Some have argued that diets did not decline and may even have improved since their protein content increased with the introduction of livestock, notably cattle and chickens, while they maintain that the rations provided for workers, being based on European levels of consumption, were generally adequate.[97] While these propositions can probably be substantiated in some areas, for example, the fertile Quito Basin, food supplies must have varied widely according to different ecological and social conditions.

There is insufficient space here to explore the complex processes of change to subsistence patterns under colonial rule. They were related largely to the Spanish alienation of Indian lands, the reduction in labour inputs occasioned either by depopulation or external demands for labour, and by the need to produce goods for tribute payments or trade. The extent to which subsistence systems were transformed has generally been related to the intensity of Spanish settlement and the types of commercial enterprises they established. While this observation has some validity, the character of pre-existing subsistence systems was also significant. Non-state societies, while generally coming into less intense contact with Europeans, often experienced more profound changes to their subsistence activities that resulted in poorer diets.

Loss of land has been deemed by some to be the most critical in understanding levels of depopulation in the wake of European contact.[98] since it resulted in poverty, crowding and malnutrition thereby increasing respiratory and intestinal infections and precipitating social breakdown that raised mortality rates. Similarly, but from the opposite end of the spectrum, Phelan (1959: 105–20) argues, though without specifying the precise link between agricultural production and depopulation, that the limited alienation of land and the restricted development of livestock raising in the Philippines compared to Mexico was partially responsible for the lower level of decline in the

---

[97] Cook and Borah (1979), pp. 174–76; Super (1988), pp. 28–32, 38, 63, 69–70, 87–88.
[98] Jacobs (1976), pp. 284–85; Kunitz (1994), pp. 7, 51.

islands. In the Spanish empire the alienation of native lands was generally more protracted since the Spanish, influenced by Roman Law, recognised Indian rights to land[99] and in any case they initially found more immediate sources of profit in plunder, tribute and mining. However, as land became vacant through depopulation and resettlement and the growth of internal markets provided added stimulus to agricultural production, land gradually passed into Spanish hands. It has been commonly noted that the alienation of Indian lands occurred most frequently in areas that could produce crops that were in high demand either in Europe or in local urban markets. Particularly disruptive in the lowlands were the production of sugar and cacao that also generated high demands for labour, whereas in the highlands the establishment of commercial maize and cereal production created similar demands.[100] It is sometimes argued that livestock raising was less disruptive to Indian subsistence systems since it often took place on grasslands that had not been used intensively in pre-Columbian times due to the absence of domesticated animals to raise and the lack of adequate tools to effect their cultivation. In other cases, such as the Gulf Coast of Mexico, livestock raising expanded onto cultivated lands that had been abandoned due to population decline.[101] Nevertheless, in some areas, livestock brought considerable environmental damage and destruction to native crops, and deprived communities of access to game and other wild food resources that might maintain dietary variety.[102]

Loss of land has to be viewed in the context of declining populations. Smaller communities required less land and this would have enabled the concentration of activities on the most fertile lands, thereby increasing productivity. Since epidemic mortality by striking the young, old and infirm disproportionately would have reduced the dependency ratio, initially the per capita surplus available may have increased.[103] However, not all surplus was directed at subsistence for often a significant proportion of production was channelled to meet tribute demands and other exactions. Furthermore, the benefits from increased production may have been only short term

---

[99] Elliott (1990), pp. 52–23.
[100] MacLeod (1983), pp. 196–202; Prem (1992), pp. 457–58.
[101] Whitmore and Turner (1992), p. 417.
[102] Gibson (1964), pp. 278, 280; Melville (1994), pp. 148–49.
[103] Hassig (1985), pp. 181–84; Whitmore (1992), p. 479.

since the dependency ratio would subsequently have risen as the survivors of epidemics aged and bore children. The age structure of populations in influencing patterns of food production and consumption might therefore be important in determining diets and nutritional levels.

Subsistence production was also affected by declining labour inputs due to depopulation and external demands for labour. Many intensive forms of production, such as irrigation, terracing and raised fields could not be maintained with reduced labour inputs[104] and low-yielding crops fell out of cultivation as interest focused on fewer more productive crops and those demanded as tribute. Although labour was often withdrawn from hunting, partly due to more restricted access to hunting grounds, any decline in protein availability was probably more than compensated for by the adoption of chickens and livestock.[105]

There were wide variations in the extent to which labour inputs into sub-sistence activities declined. There were major differences in levels of depopulation in the early colonial period[106] and external demands for labour varied enormously according to the number of workers required, the length and timing of their employment and distances between their workplace and residence. Subsistence production could be maintained more easily where Indians resided in their communities and worked in nearby haciendas, but in such circumstances labour demands were often at a peak when Indians needed to sow or harvest own crops in their own communities. Although mining generally required them to work at distant locations, often workers could not be employed during critical periods in the agricultural calendar, so that paradoxically such forms of employment might be more complementary to subsistence production. Furthermore, absent workers were supposedly supported by rations provided by employers, whereas those who remained in their communities continued to be a burden on subsistence production. Often, however, rations for miners were inadequate and wages were insufficient to purchase food, which in mining towns was generally expensive and in short supply, so that miners, who were generally malnourished, remained a burden on their home communities while contributing

---

[104] Keith (1976), p. 49; Denevan (1992), pp. 373, 378.
[105] Gade (1992), pp. 467–68; Licate (1981), pp. 114–15.
[106] Newson (1993), pp. 252–53.

little to subsistence production.[107] Although documentary sources make
frequent reference to the inability of forced labourers to attend to
their own subsistence needs, computer simulations of the impact of
labour shortfalls on subsistence production suggest that drafts would
have to be of considerable magnitude to have a demographic effect.[108]
Such would seem to be the case in the Philippines where heavy
demands for labour and food supplies provoked by wars with the
Dutch have been viewed as *the* major cause of depopulation in the
early seventeenth century.[109]

Even though the diets of miners may have been inadequate, particularly given the arduous work they were required to perform, it
is not certain that all those who lived in the towns and were dependent on their employers or the market for food were similarly malnourished. In Spanish America towns were essential to the functioning
and maintenance of the empire so that laws and institutions, such
as the *pósito*, a public granary, and *alhóndiga*, to oversee the sale of
grain were introduced to ensure regular, cheap supplies of food for
the towns.[110] Unlike non-state societies where such forms of storage
and redistribution were largely absent, these might prove critical in
times of temporary shortage or crisis, though access to food supplies
would have varied between social groups according to class, race,
gender and age.[111] One advantage of permanent employment in
Spanish households or haciendas was that workers were assured of
food. For this reasons times of crises often saw a migration to centres of Spanish employment.[112]

For the most part non-state societies came into less intense contact with Spaniards, but their subsistence systems were more vulnerable to the changes brought by colonial rule. The economies of
non-state societies, which were generally based on shifting cultivation and the exploitation of wild food resources, were often highly
adapted to specific environments. Even without the direct contact
with Europeans, epidemics resulting in high adult mortality would

---

[107] Bakewell (1984), pp. 104–132; Cole (1985), pp. 25, 28, 31–32; Super (1988),
p. 60.
[108] Whitmore (1992), p. 482.
[109] Phelan (1959), p. 100.
[110] Hassig (1985), pp. 241–246; Super (1988), pp. 10, 39–50.
[111] Wrigley (1969), p. 102.
[112] Farris (1982), pp. 203–204; Hassig (1985), p. 246.

have threatened the survival of many groups. Falling numbers might result in decreased production, weaken reciprocal social obligations, and cause a shift in emphasis on different activities, sometimes closing off subsistence options altogether and rendering communities more vulnerable in the face of environmental perturbations.[113] Balée (1992: 49–51) notes that in general agriculture becomes increasingly implausible with groups of under fifty persons. Food production prospects depend on whether subsistence strategies or co-operative activities could remain viable with reduced populations. In small societies the loss of only a small number of people with special skills, such as hunting, might be a serious threat to food supplies, particularly in regions of marked seasonality or where groups are dependent on a limited range of resources.[114] The vulnerability of these groups is often enhanced further by the limited surpluses they produce and their lack of familiarity with methods of food storage.

In most cases the missionisation of non-state groups threatened their nutritional status even further, although here again the economic viability of missions varied with environmental circumstances and pre-existing subsistence patterns. The missionary orders attempted to "civilise" these groups by congregating them into permanent settlements and instructing them in agricultural techniques, while suppressing the exploitation of wild food resources as "barbaric" and offering opportunities for fugitivism. Anxious to ensure their economic viability, the missionaries generally introduced metal tools, new crops and livestock and often introduced or extended irrigation systems. The fate of missions varied. Food shortages appear to have been particularly common in areas inhabited by nomadic or semi-nomadic groups where the soil was too poor or wild food resources too meagre to support permanent settlements. Hence, food shortages were common in the Franciscan missions of California[115] and in some missions in the Upper Amazon[116] and Colombian Llanos.[117] Even in areas where food supplies remained adequate, there is some evidence

---

[113] Larson *et al.* (1994), p. 276.
[114] Colson (1979), p. 23; Dobyns (1983), pp. 16, 332; Hill (1989), p. 12; Levine and LaBauve (1997), pp. 97–99; Krech III (1978), p. 717; McGrath (1991), pp. 407–19; Wolfe (1982), p. 111.
[115] Aschmann (1959), p. 209; Cook (1943), p. 55; Sweet (1995), pp. 31–36.
[116] Newson (1995), pp. 320–21.
[117] Rausch (1984), pp. 72, 74.

that they lacked variety and were deficient in iron.[118] The missions
appear to have been most successful economically where agriculture
was well established prior to missionisation and where changes to
subsistence patterns were less fundamental. These included the Jesuit
missions among the sedentary farming communities of northwest New
Spain[119] and of the Llanos de Mojos, Bolivia,[120] as well as the missionary parishes of the Philippines.[121]

Responses to Epidemic Crises

Levels of disease mortality were not only influenced by the virulence
of the pathogen and levels of immunity, but also by the ability of
societies to respond effectively to the crises that epidemics precipitated. The ability of the society to make an effective response depended
on whether or not it had the resources or management structures
to ensure that basic needs and medical care were provided, and on
a correct interpretation of the cause of the disease and how, if possible, it might be contained. Broad differences emerge between state
and non-state societies, and between those who came under Spanish
administration and those who remained outside.

In many pre-Columbian societies sickness and death were attributed to supernatural causes. Sickness was often seen to derive from
disharmony with nature, society and the gods that could be restored
through herbal remedies, rituals or offerings in which sorcerers or
shamans played central roles.[122] In pre-Columbian times native medical systems were in many cases reasonably competent in treating
disease and aiding recovery, but, where they were not suppressed as
pagan practices, they were generally ineffective in combating the
acute infections imported from the Old World. The failure of traditional healers and remedies to cope with these diseases, particularly when Spaniards appeared unaffected, served to undermine native

---

[118] Larsen *et al.* (1990), pp. 413–17, 422, (1994), pp. 125, 135; Sweet (1995), pp.
15–16; Walker *et al.* (1989), pp. 353–55, 361.
[119] Deeds (1995), pp. 89–90; Reff (1991), pp. 266–67; Ruhl (1991), p. 571.
[120] Block (1994), pp. 56–57.
[121] Phelan (1959), pp. 108–110.
[122] Alchon (1991), pp. 25–29; Newman (1976), pp. 670–71; Orellana (1987), pp.
27–52.

beliefs and induce fatalistic attitudes towards death that probably raised mortality rates.

Mortality rates associated with epidemics may have been moderated where societies came under Spanish administration for Spaniards unaffected by the diseases were able to organise practical responses to crises and provide nursing care that aided recovery. In some cases public health measures, such as quarantining, preventing the passage of people or goods or cleaning the streets may have reduced the spread of some diseases,[123] though their efficacy would have depended on their appropriateness to the epidemic concerned. Quarantining might effectively isolate diseases spread by face-to-face contact, such as smallpox and measles, but would have little effect on reducing the incidence of a disease spread by a vector, such as malaria or typhus, where changes to environmental conditions would be more appropriate.[124] Since the causes of most acute infections have been isolated only in the last two hundred years, in most cases the ability of the colonial authorities to contain or moderate their impact was probably limited. Similarly the medical treatments introduced by the Spanish were probably of little intrinsic value or advance on those employed in pre-Columbian times. However, the Christian obligation to care for the sick resulted in the establishment of hospitals, priestly visitations and in the establishment of *cofradías* which often provided moral support that enabled victims' own biological responses to overcome the disease and thereby reduce mortality levels.[125] Evidence from historically more recent epidemics among non-immune populations indicates the importance of medical care in aiding recovery.[126] For example, in a smallpox epidemic among the Hopi in 1898–1899 the crude death rate among those who received care was only 6 per cent whereas of those who declined it 74 per cent died.[127]

Nursing care may include the provision of basic needs such as food and water which state societies were generally better placed to deliver. Not only did they produce larger surpluses that were often

---

[123] Alchon (1991), pp. 62–63; Alchon (1992), p. 181; Casanueva (1992), pp. 191–92.
[124] McGrath (1991), pp. 410–17.
[125] Carmichael (1983), pp. 59–60; Crosby (1976), p. 294; McCaa (1995), pp. 420–22.
[126] Frost (1990), p. 435; Wolfe (1982), p. 116.
[127] Frost (1990), p. 437.

stored for use in times of shortage, but they also had leaders and political structures that facilitated the distribution of food and the mobilisation of labour to ensure food production was maintained. Pre-Columbian storage systems existed among the Aztec and Inca,[128] some of which, at least at the local level, are likely to have continued into colonial times. In addition, it has already been noted that the Spanish developed food storage and distribution systems to ensure that the towns were well provisioned. Despite the advantages of food surpluses and the existence of storage and distribution systems, the social inequality that characterised state societies meant that not everyone had equal access to these supplies in times of crisis.

Non-state societies were generally less well placed to cope with epidemic crises. Food supplies were often threatened by the lack of storage techniques and by adult mortality which would not only have reduced labour inputs but led to a loss of historical knowledge of coping strategies. Furthermore, where leaders are not the victims of epidemics, they generally lack the authority to organise practical responses to epidemic crises that might aid survival.[129] The well known study by Neel and others (1970: 427) of the impact of a measles epidemic that afflicted the Yanomama in the 1960s recorded that village life collapsed completely leaving only a few members capable of providing food and water or tending the sick, and with the concern for well-being seldom extending beyond the immediate family. These observations were echoed by those involved in providing medical care during the Alaskan epidemic of 1900,[130] and the lack of community support has similarly been noted among non-state societies experiencing food shortages.[131]

Not only might mortality rates be raised by the collapse of support mechanisms, but an epidemic might raise mortality rates indirectly in other ways. A common response to sickness is flight which might carry an infection to hitherto uninfected groups.[132] When smallpox broke out in the Jesuit mission of Santiago de la Laguna in the Amazon headwaters in 1680, its inhabitants fled downriver in seventy-five canoes carrying the disease to distant communities.[133] In

---

[128] D'Altroy and Earle (1992), pp. 41–45; Hassig (1981), pp. 172, 174, 177.
[129] Colson (1979), pp. 25–26; Stannard (1991), p. 531.
[130] Wolfe (1982), pp. 110–11, 116.
[131] Colson (1979), p. 25.
[132] Frost (1990), pp. 436; McGrath (1991), pp. 410; Wolfe (1982), p. 109.
[133] Newson (1995), p. 313.

other cases sickness and death might be attributed to sorcery that required revenge, so that epidemics were often accompanied by enhanced levels of mortality resulting from intertribal warfare.[134] The establishment of missions may have marginally reduced disease mortality attributable to these causes. The missions commonly had food stores to overcome crises and the missionaries, largely untouched by the epidemics, were able to care for the sick and provide them with food and water, while they also sought to suppress intertribal warfare.[135] In many cases, however, the practical help provided may have been insufficient to overcome the "loss of the will to survive" that often afflicted mission populations.

Conclusion

The aim of this essay has been to stress the significance of specific environmental and social contexts for understanding the introduction, spread and impact of acute infections that accompanied Spanish expansion overseas. However, it is worth noting some broad geographical and temporal differences in their impact that derive in part from differences in the pattern of infection. In the early colonial period state societies suffered the heaviest disease mortality for it was here that the Spaniards settled in largest numbers introducing a wide range of infections whose spread was facilitated by their dense populations. These societies also bore the brunt of conquest with wars and depopulation causing major political, economic and social upheavals that heightened disease mortality despite the efforts of the colonial authorities to ensure adequate food supplies and medical care. Nevertheless, despite heavy population losses, sufficient numbers remained for diseases to become endemic and for Indians to develop immunities to them, so that in the longer term the impact of acute infections was moderated. Initially this process was retarded by the relatively low birth rate, but over time this increased and in many areas populations developed immunities through racial mixing. The nutritional status of individuals probably had little influence on

---

[134] Early and Peters (1990), p. 80; Ferguson (1990), pp. 241–42; Hill (1989), pp. 12–13; Newson (1995), p. 318.
[135] Caraman (1976), pp. 119, 144; Deeds (1995), p. 93; Rausch (1984), pp. 68, 74; Reff (1991), pp. 260–63, 278; Newson (1995), pp. 313, 318.

mortality rates associated with the first wave of epidemics, but as they became endemic it probably affected levels of infant and child mortality and thereby the degree of demographic recovery that was achieved. Hence, there were significant differences in the extent and timing of population increases that were experienced in most former state and chiefdom societies.

In areas where the population was small and dispersed the opportunities for the introduction of diseases were fewer and their spread was more difficult. The result was that not every community would have been hit by every epidemic so that the *overall* impact of a single epidemic would have been less than in state societies, but insufficient numbers remained for acute infections to become endemic. As a consequence, when they were reintroduced they continued to cause high mortality that affected adults as well as children, which had particularly adverse effects on the birth rate and food production. The impact of each epidemic would have been heightened by the lack the strong leadership needed to foster a 'will to survive' and mobilize community efforts to cope with disaster and also by inappropriate responses to crises. Thus while overall disease mortality might be moderated, though this would depend on the frequency of reinfection, the indirect impact of epidemics might raise mortality rates to levels greater than those suffered by state societies and threaten any demographic recovery.

These broad differences in the pattern of infection may *partially* account for the continued decline of tribal peoples in lowland areas of Latin America during the colonial period, while most former state societies suffered high levels of depopulation in the early colonial period but were later characterised by a degree of demographic recovery, the timing of which varied from region to region.[136] It began in Mexico in the 1620s, occurred a few decades later in Central America, but was not experienced in the Central Andes until the middle of the eighteenth century. Although it may be hypothesized that such differences in demographic trends may be related to differences in the pattern of infection, it is difficult to generalize about differences in their aggregate effects for clearly the impact of epidemics, particularly on small populations, would depend, among other things, on the frequency of re-infection. Demographic trends

---

[136] Newson (1985), pp. 43–45; (1993), p. 253; Sánchez-Albórnoz (1984), pp. 28–29.

in the colonial Philippines do not conform to that hypothesised for non-state societies, but appear to be similar to that for highland regions of Spanish America with a decline in the early seventeenth century being followed by a marked recovery in the eighteenth and nineteenth centuries. This trend has generally been attributed to changing political and economic conditions rather than to changes in the impact of disease.[137] This topic needs further investigation, but since this paper has focused on the impact of acute infections, it serves to emphasise that differences in disease mortality alone cannot wholly explain demographic trends, which also reflect changes in fertility as well as the direct impact of other factors on mortality levels, such as wars, losses on expeditions, ill treatment and food shortages. These factors may not only affect demographic trends directly, but through interacting with biological processes also influence patterns of infection and mortality.

The aim of this paper has been to argue that it is now time to move beyond crude generalisations about the impact of Old World diseases and to recognise that disease mortality varied widely according to particular environmental and social circumstances, perhaps even more so in the seventeenth century as acute infections became endemic in many regions. As such, it is misguided to envisage a single pandemic as carrying off say 30 per cent of the population in every region that it infected, however tempting this may be in the absence of adequate information. Not only would epidemics have had a variable impact, but their significance relative to others factors implicated in any decline would also have varied. This is not to argue against generalising about the impact of Old World diseases, but to suggest that their validity depends on a full appreciation of the complexity of the processes at work.

Bibliography

Alchon, S.A. 1991 *Native Society and Disease in Colonial Ecuador.* Cambridge University Press, Cambridge.
——— 1992 Disease, Population and Public Health in Eighteenth-Century Quito. In *"Secret Judgments of God:" Old World Disease in Colonial Spanish America,* edited by N.D. Cook and W.G. Lovell, pp. 159–82. University of Oklahoma Press, Norman.

---

[137] Reid (1987); Owen (1987b), pp. 51–57.

Allison, A.C. 1982 Coevolution Between Hosts and Infectious Disease Agents and its Effects on Virulence. In *Population Biology of Infectious Diseases*, edited by R.M. Anderson and R.M. May, pp. 245–267. Springer-Verlag, Heidelberg and New York.

Altman, I. and J.M. Lockhart 1976 *Provinces of Early Mexico*. University of California Press, Berkeley and Los Angeles.

Anderson, R.M. and R.M. May 1979 Population Biology of Infectious Diseases: Part I, *Nature* 280: 361–67.

———— 1991. *Infectious Diseases of Humans: Dynamics and Control*. Oxford University Press, Oxford.

Appleby, A.B. 1980 The Disappearance of Plague: A Continuing Puzzle. *Economic History Review* 33 (2): 161–73.

Aschmann, H. 1959 *The Central Desert of Baja California*. Ibero-Americana 42. University of California Press, Berkeley and Los Angeles.

Ayala Mora, T. 1957 Epidemiología de la malaria en el Ecuador y su evaluación en la campaña de eradicación. *Revista Ecuatoriana de Higiene y Medicina Tropical* (Guayaquil) 14 (4): 29–86.

Bakewell, P. 1984 *Miners of the Red Mountain: Indian Labor in Potosí, 1545–1650*. University of New Mexcio Press, Albuquerque.

———— 1997 *A History of Latin America*. Blackwell, Oxford.

Balée, W. 1992 People of the Fallow: A Historical Ecology of Foraging in Lowland South America. In *Conservation of Neotropical Forests: Working from Traditional Resource Use*, edited by K.H. Redford and C. Padoch, pp. 35–57. Columbia University Press, New York.

Bartlett, M.S. 1957 Measles Periodicity and Community Size. *Journal of the Royal Statistical Society, Series A* 120: 48–70.

Black, F.L. 1966 Measles Endemicity in Insular Populations: Critical Community Size and its Evolutionary Implications. *Journal of Theoretical Biology* 11: 207–211.

———— 1975 Infectious Diseases in Primitive Societies. *Science* 187: 515–18.

———— 1990 Infectious Disease and Evolution of Human Populations: The Example of South American Forest Tribes. *Disease in Populations in Transition: Anthropological and Epidemiological Perspectives*, edited by A.C. Swedlund and G.J. Armelagos, pp. 57–74. Bergin and Garvey, New York.

———— 1992 Why Did They Die? *Science* 258: 1739–40.

Block, D. 1994 *Mission Culture on the Upper Amazon: Native Tradition, Jesuit Enterprise, and Secular Policy in Moxos, 1660–1880*. University of Nebraska, Lincoln and London.

Borah, W. 1951 *New Spain's Century of Depression*. Ibero-Americana 35. University of California, Berkeley and Los Angeles.

———— 1964 America as Model: The Demographic Impact of European Expansion on the Non-European World. *Actas y Memorias, 35⁰ Congreso Internacional de Americanistas*, Vol. 3, pp. 379–87.

———— 1992 The Historical Demography of Aboriginal and Colonial America: An Attempt at Perspective. In *Native Population of the Americas in 1492*, edited by W.M. Denevan, pp. 13–41. University of Wisconsin Press, Madison.

Borah, W. and Cook, S.F. 1969. Conquest and Population: A Demographic Approach to Mexican History. *Proceedings of the American Philosophical Society* 113 (2): 177–83.

———— 1963 *The Aboriginal Population of Central Mexico on the Eve of Spanish Conquest*. Ibero-Americana 45. University of California Press, Berkeley and Los Angeles.

Butlin, N.G. 1983 *Our Original Aggression*. George Allen and Unwin, Sydney.

Caraman, P. 1976 *The Lost Paradise: The Jesuit Republic in South America*. The Seabury Press: New York.

Carmack, R.M. 1991 The Spanish Conquest of Central America: Comparative Cases from Guatemala and Costa Rica. In *Columbian Consequences*, Vol. 3, edited by D.H. Thomas, pp. 389–410. Smithsonian Institution Press, Washington and London.

Carmichael, A.G. 1983 Infection, Hidden Hunger and History. In *Hunger and History*, edited by R.I. Rotberg and T.K. Rabb, pp. 51–66. Cambridge University Press, Cambridge.

Casanueva, F. 1992 Smallpox in Late Eighteenth Century Chile. In *"Secret Judgments of God:" Old World Disease in Colonial Spanish America*, edited by N.D. Cook and W.G. Lovell, pp. 183–212. University of Oklahoma Press, Norman.

Clendinnen, I. 1991 *The Aztecs: An Interpretation*. Cambridge University Press, Cambridge.

Cliff, A. and Haggett, P. 1988 *Atlas of Disease Distributions*. Blackwell, Oxford.

Cline, S. 1993 The Spiritual Conquest Re-examined: Baptism and Christian Marriage in Early Sixteenth-Century Mexico. *Hispanic American Historical Review* 73 (3): 452–80.

Cockburn, A.T. 1971 Infectious Diseases in Ancient Populations. *Current Anthropology* 12: 45–62.

Cohen, M.N. 1989 *Health and the Rise of Civilization*. Yale University Press, New Haven and London.

Cole, J. 1985 *The Potosí Mita, 1573–1700*. Stanford University Press, Stanford.

Colson, E. 1979 In Good Years and in Bad: Food Strategies of Self-Reliant Societies. *Journal of Anthropological Research* 35: 18–28.

Conrad, G.W. and A.A. Demarest 1984 *Religion and Empire: The Dynamics of Aztec and Inca Expansionism*. Cambridge University Press, Cambridge.

Cook, N.D. 1980 *Demographic Collapse: Indian Peru, 1520–1620*. Cambridge University Press, Cambridge.

———— 1998 *Born to Die: Disease and New World Conquests, 1492–1650*. Cambridge University Press, Cambridge.

Cook, S.F. 1940 *Population Trends among the California Mission Indians*. Ibero-Americana 17. University of California, Berkeley and Los Angeles.

———— 1946a Human Sacrifice and Warfare as Factors in the Demography of Pre-colonial Mexico. *Human Biology* 18: 81–102.

———— 1946b The Incidence and Significance of Disease among the Aztec and Related Tribes. *Hispanic American Historical Review* 26: 320–35.

Cook, S.F. and W. Borah 1971–1979 *Essays in Population History* 3 Vols. University of California Press, Berkeley and Los Angeles.

Cooper, D.B. and K.F. Kiple. 1993 Yellow Fever. In *The Cambridge World History of Human Disease*, edited K.F. Kiple, pp. 1100–1107. Cambridge University Press, Cambridge.

Corpuz, O.D. 1988 *The Roots of the Filipino Nation* Vol. 1. AKLAHI Foundation, Quezon City.

Crosby, A.W. 1976 Virgin Soil Epidemics as a Factor in the Aboriginal Depopulation in America. *William and Mary Quarterly* 3rd Ser. 33 (2): 289–99.

———— 1992 Hawaiian Depopulation as a Model for the Amerindian Experience. In *Epidemics and Ideas: Essays on the Historical Perception of Pestilence*, edited by T. Ranger and P. Slack, pp. 175–202. Cambridge University Press, Cambridge.

D'Altroy T.N. and T.K. Earle 1992 Staple Finance, Wealth Finance and Storage in the Inka Political Economy. In *Inka Storage Systems*, edited by T.V. LeVine, pp. 31–61. University of Oklahoma Press, Norman.

De Bevoise, K. 1995 *Agents of the Apocalypse: Epidemic Disease in the Colonial Philippines*. Princeton University Press, Princeton.

De Boer, W. 1981 Buffer Zones in the Cultural Ecology of Aboriginal Amazonia: An Ethnohistorical Approach. *American Antiquity* 46: 364–77.

Deeds, S.M. 1995 Indigenous Responses to Mission Settlement in Nueva Vizcaya. In *The New Latin American Mission History*, edited by E. Langer and R.H. Jackson, pp. 77–108. University of Nebraska Press, Lincoln and London.

Denevan, W.M. (Ed.) 1992a *Native Population of the Americas in 1492*. University of Wisconsin Press, Madison.

——— 1992b The Pristine Myth: The Landscape of the Americas in 1492. *Annals of the Association of American Geographers* 82 (3) 369–85.

Diamond, J. 1998. *Guns, Germs and Steel*. Vintage, London.

Dobyns, H.F. 1966 Estimating Aboriginal American Population: An Appraisal of Techniques with a New Hemispheric Estimate. *Current Anthropology* 7: 395–416.

——— 1983 *Their Number Become Thinned: Native American Population Dynamics in Eastern North America*. University of Tennessee Press, Knoxville.

Doeppers, D. 1968 Hispanic Influences on Demographic Patterns in the Central Plain of Luzon, 1565–1780. *University of Manila Journal of East Asiatic Studies* 12: 11–96.

Dunn, F.L. 1965 On the Antiquity of Malaria in the Western Hemisphere. *Human Biology* 37: 385–93.

——— 1993 Malaria. In *The Cambridge World History of Human Disease*, edited K.F. Kiple, pp. 855–63. Cambridge University Press, Cambridge.

Early, J.D. and J.F. Peters 1990 *The Population Dynamics of the Mucajai Yanomama*. Academic Press, New York.

Elliott, J.H. 1990 The Seizure of Overseas Territories by the European Powers. In *The European Discovery of the World and its Economic Effects on Pre-Industrial Society*, edited by H. Pohl, pp. 43–61. Franz Steirner Verlag, Stuttgart.

Ewald, P.W. 1994. *Evolution of Infectious Disease*. Oxford University Press, Oxford.

Farris, N.M. 1984 *Maya Society Under Colonial Rule: The Collective Enterprise of Survival*. Princeton University Press, Princeton.

Fenner, F.L. 1970 The Effects of Changing Social Organisation on the Infectious Diseases of Man. *The Impact of Civilisation on the Biology of Man*, edited by S. Boyden, pp. 48–76. Australian National University Press, Canberra.

——— 1980 Sociocultural Change and Environmental Diseases. In *Changing Disease Patterns and Human Behaviour*, edited by N.F. Stanley and R.A. Joske, pp. 7–26 Academic Press, London and New York.

——— 1982 Transmission Cycles and Broad Patterns of Observed Epidemiological Behaviour in Human and Other Animals. In *Population Biology of Infectious Diseases*, edited by R.M. Anderson and R.M. May, pp. 103–119. Springer-Verlag, Heidelberg and New York.

Fenner, F.L., Henderson, D.A., Arita, I., Jezek, Z. and Ladnyi, I.D. 1988 *Smallpox and its Eradication*. WHO, Geneva.

Ferguson, R.B. 1990 Blood of the Leviathan: Western Contact and Warfare in Amazonia. *American Ethnologist* 17: 237–57.

Figueroa, F. de 1904 Relación de las misiones de la Compañía de Jesús en el país de los Maynas. V. Suárez, Madrid.

Friedlander, J. 1969 Malaria and Demography in the Lowlands of Mexico: An Ethno-Historical Approach. In *Forms of Symbolic Action*, edited by R.F. Spencer, pp. 217–33. American Ethnological Society, Seattle and London.

Frost, R.H. 1990 The Pueblo Indian Smallpox Epidemic in New Mexico, 1898–1899. *Bulletin of the History of Medicine* 64: 417–45.

Gade, D.W. 1992 Landscape, System, and Identity in the Post-Conquest Andes, *Annals of the Association of American Geographers* 82 (3): 460–77.

Ganson, B. 1989 The Evuevi of Paraguay: Adaptive Strategies and Responses to colonialism, 1528–1811. *The Americas* 45 (4): 461–88.

Garruto, R.M. 1981 Disease Patterns of Isolated Groups. In *Biocultural Aspects of Disease*, edited by H. Rothschild, pp. 560–64. Academic Press, New York.

Gibson, C. 1964 *The Aztecs Under Spanish Rule*. Stanford University Press, Stanford.

Góngora, M. 1975 *Studies in the Colonial History of Spanish America*. Cambridge University Press, Cambridge.

González, E.R. and R. Mellafe 1965 La función de la familia en la historia social hispanoamericana colonial. *Anuario del Instituto de Investigaciones Históricas* 8: 57–71.

Grieshaber, E.P. 1979 Hacienda-Indian Community Relations and Indian Acculturation, *Latin American Research Review* 14 (3): 107–28.

Guttierez, R.A. 1991 *When Jesus Came the Corn Mothers Went Away: Marriage, Sexuality and Power in New Mexico, 1500–1846*. Stanford University Press, Stanford.

Haggett, P. 1994 Prediction and Predictability in Geographic Systems. *Transactions of the Institute of British Geographers NS* 19: 6–20.

Harpending, H.C., P. Draper and R. Pennington 1990 Cultural Evolution, Parental Care and Mortality. In *Disease in Populations in Transition: Anthropological and Epidemiological Perspectives*, edited by A.C. Swedlund and G.J. Armelagos, pp. 251–65. Bergin and Garvey, New York.

Hassig, R. 1981 The Famine of One Rabbit; Ecological Causes and Social Consequences of a Pre-Columbian Calamity. *Journal of Anthropological Research* 37 (2): 171–81.

———— 1985 *Trade, Tribute and Transportation: The Sixteenth-Century Political Economy of the Valley of Mexico*. University of Oklahoma Press; Norman.

Henige, D.H. 1978. On the Contact Population of Hispaniola: History as Higher Mathematics. *Hispanic American Historical Review* 58: 217–37.

———— 1993 Counting the Encounter: The Pernicious Appeal of Verisimilitude. *Colonial Latin American Historical Review* 3: 325–61.

———— 1998 Numbers from Nowhere: The American Indian Contact Population Debate. University of Olklahoma Press, Norman, Olklahoma.

Hern, W.M. 1992 Polygyny and Fertility Among the Shipibo of the Peruvian Amazon. *Population Studies* 46 (1): 53–64.

———— 1994 Health and Demography of Native Amazonians: Historical Perspective and Current Status. *Amazonian Indians from Prehistory to the Present: Anthropological Perspectives*, edited by A. Roosevelt, pp. 123–49 University of Arizona Press, Tucson and London.

Hernández Rodríguez, R. 1982. Epidemias y calamidades en el México prehispánico. In *Ensayos sobre la historia de las epidemias en México* Vol. 1, edited by E. Florescano and E. Malvido, pp. 139–56. Instituto Mexicano del Seguro Social, Mexico City.

Hill, J.D. 1989 Ritual Production of Environmental History among the Arawakan Wakuénai of Venezuela. *Human Ecology* 17 (1): 1–25.

Jackson, R.H. 1994 *Indian Population Decline: The Missions of Northwestern New Spain, 1687–1840*. University of New Mexico Press, Albuquerque.

Jacobs, W.R. 1974 The Tip of the Iceberg: Pre-Columbian Indian Demography and Some Implications for Revisionism. *William and Mary Quarterly* 3rd Ser. 31: 123–32.

Jannetta, A.B. 1987 *Epidemics and Mortality in Early Modern Japan*. Princeton University Press, Princeton, N.J.

Jara, A. 1961 *Guerre et Société au Chili*. Institut des Hautes Études de l'Amérique Latine. Paris.

Johnston, F.E., K.M. Kensinger, R.L. Jantz, and G.F. Walker 1969 The Population Structure of the Peruvian Cashinahua: Demographic, Genetic and Cultural Relationships. *Human Biology* 41: 29–41.

Keith, R.G. 1976 *Conquest and Agrarian Change: The Emergence of the Hacienda System on the Peruvian Coast*. Harvard University Press, Cambridge, Mass.

Kiple, K. 1984. *The Caribbean Slave: A Biological History*. Cambridge University Press, Cambridge.

Klein, H. 1975. Hacienda and Free Community in the Eighteenth Century in Alto Perú. *Journal of Latin American Studies* 7: 221–48.

Kondrashin, A.V. 1986 Malaria in Southeast Asia. *Southeast Asian Journal of Tropical Medicine and Public Health* 17 (4): 642–55.

Krech III, S. 1978 Disease, Starvation and Northern Athapaskan Social Organization. *American Ethnologist* 5: 710–32.

Kroeger, A., H. Heyna, G. Pawelig and E. Ileckova 1977 La salúd y la alimentación entre los indígenas Schuaras del Ecuador. *Revista Ecuatoriana de Higiene y Medicina Tropical* (Guayaquil) 30 (2): 119–67.

Krzywicki, L. 1934 *Primitive Society and its Vital Statistics*. Macmillan and Co., London

Kunitz, S.J. 1994 *Disease and Social Diversity: The European Impact on the Health of Non-Europeans*. Oxford University Press, Oxford.

Larsen, C.S. 1994. In the Wake of Columbus: Native Population Biology in the Post Contact Americas. *Yearbook of Physical Anthropology* 37: 109–54.

Larsen, C.S., M.J. Schoeninger, D.L. Hutchinson, K.F. Russell and C.B. Ruff 1990 Beyond Demographic Collapse: Biological Adaptation and Change in the Native Populations of La Florida. In *Columbian Consequences*, Vol. 2, edited by D.H. Thomas, pp. 409–28. Smithsonian Institution Press, Washington.

Levin, B.R., A.C. Allison, H.J. Bremermann, L.L. Cavalli-Sforza, S.A. Levin, R.M. May and H.R. Thieme 1982 Evolution of Parasites and Hosts. In *Population Biology of Infectious Diseases*, edited by R.M. Anderson and R.M. May, pp. 213–43. Springer-Verlag, Heidelberg and New York.

Levine, F. and A. LaBauve 1996 Examining the Complexity of Historic Population Decline: A Case Study of Pecos Pueblo, New Mexico. *Ethnohistory* 44 (1): 75–12.

Licate, J.A. 1981 Creation of a Mexican Landscape: Territorial Organization and Settlement in the Eastern Puebla Basin, 1520–1605. Department of Geography Research Papers 201. University of Chicago Press, Chicago.

Livi-Bacci, M. 1991 *Population and Nutrition: An Essay on European Demographic History*. Cambridge University Press, Cambridge.

Lockhart, J. 1991 Trunk Lines and Feeder Routes: The Spanish Reaction to American Resources. In *Transatlantic Encounters: Europeans and Indians in the Sixteenth Century*, edited by K.J. Andrien and R. Adorno, pp. 90–120. University of California Press, Berkeley and Los Angeles.

MacLeod, M.J. 1982 Ethnic Relations and Indian Society in the Province of Guatemala ca. 1620–ca. 1800. In *Spaniards and Indians in Southern Mesoamerica: Essays on the History of Ethnic Relations*, edited by M.J. MacLeod and R. Wasserstrom, pp. 189–214. University of Nebraska Press, Lincoln and London.

Malvido, E. 1982 Efectos de las epidemias y hambrunas en la población colonial de México (1519–1810). In *Ensayos sobre la historia de las epidemias en México* Vol. 1, edited by E. Florescano and E. Malvido, pp. 179–97. Instituto Mexicano del Seguro Social, Mexico City.

Marcy, P.T. 1981 Factors Affecting the Fecundity and Fertility of Historical Populations. *Journal of Family History* 6: 309–26.

McArthur, N. 1967 *Island Populations of the Pacific*. Australian National University Press, Canberra.

McCaa, R. 1994 Marriageways in Mexico and Spain, 1500–1900. *Continuity and Change* 9 (1): 11–43.

McGrath, J.W. 1991 Biological Impact of Social Disruption Resulting from Epidemic Disease. *American Journal of Physical Anthropology* 84: 407–19.

McKeown, T. 1976 *The Modern Rise of Population*. Edward Arnold, London.

——— 1988 *The Origins of Human Disease*. Basil Blackwell, Oxford.

McNeill, W.M. 1976 *Plagues and Peoples*. Oxford University Press, Oxford.

——— 1979 Historical Patterns of Migration. *Current Anthropology* 20 (1): 95–98.

Meinig, D.W. 1986 *The Shaping of America Vol. 1 Atlantic America 1492–1800*. Yale University Press, New Haven.

Melville, E.G.K. 1994 *A Plague of Sheep: Environmental Consequence of the Conquest of Mexico*. Cambridge University Press, Cambridge.

——— 1997. Global Developments and Latin American Environments. In *Ecology and Empire: Environmental History of Settler Societies*, edited by T. Griffiths and L. Robin, pp. 185–98. Keele University Press, Edinburgh.

Menken, J. 1979 Seasonal Migration and Seasonal Variation on Fecundability: Effects on Birth Rates and Birth Intervals. *Demography* 16: 103–19.

Milner, G.R. 1980 Epidemic Disease in the Postcontact Southeast. *Mid-Continental Journal of Archaeology* 5 (1): 39–56.

Myers, T.P. 1976 Defended Territories and No-man's-lands. *American Anthropologist* 78: 354–55.

Neel, J.V. 1977 Health and Disease in Unacculturated Amerindian Populations. In *Health and Disease in Tribal Societies*, CIBA Foundation Symposium 49, pp. 155–68. Elsevier, Amsterdam.

——— W.R. Centerwall, N.A. Chagnon and H.L. Casey 1970 Notes on the Effects of Measles and Measles Vaccine in a Virgin-soil Population of South American Indians. *American Journal of Epidemiology* 91: 418–29.

Newman, M.T. 1976 Aboriginal New World Epidemiology and Medical Care, and the Impact of Old World Disease Imports. *Journal of Physical Anthropology* 45; 667–72.

Newson, L.A. 1985 Indian Population Patterns in Colonial Spanish America. *Latin American Research Review* 20 (3) 41–74.

——— 1986 *The Cost of Conquest: Indian Decline in Honduras under Spanish Rule*. Westview Press, Boulder, Col.

——— 1992 Old World Epidemics in Early Colonial Ecuador. In *"Secret Judgments of God:" Old World Disease in Colonial Spanish America*, edited by N.D. Cook and W.G. Lovell, pp. 84–112. University of Oklahoma Press, Norman.

——— 1993a The Demographic Collapse of Native Peoples of the Americas, 1492–1650. *Proceedings of the British Academy* 81: 247–88.

——— 1993b Highland-Lowland Contrasts in the Impact of Old World Diseases in Early Colonial Ecuador. *Social Science and Medicine* 36 (9): 1187–95.

——— 1995 *Life and Death in Early Colonial Ecuador*. Norman: University of Oklahoma Press.

——— 1999 Disease and Immunity in the Pre-Spanish Philippines. *Social Science and Medicine* 48: 1833–1850.

Orellana, S.L. 1987 *Indian Medicine in Highland Guatemala*. University of New Mexico Press, Albuquerque.

Osterhammell, J. 1997. *Colonialism: A Theoretical Overview*. Markus Wiener, Princeton and Ian Randle, Kingston.

Owen, N.G. (Ed.) 1987a *Death and Disease in Southeast Asia: Explorations in Social, Medical and Demographic History*. Oxford University Press, Oxford.

——— 1987b The Paradox of Nineteenth-Century Population Growth in Southeast Asia: Evidence from Java and the Philippines. *Journal of Southeast Asian Studies* 18 (1): 45–57.

Parker, G. (Ed.) 1995 *The Cambridge Illustrated History of Warfare: The Triumph of the West*. BCA, London.

Patch, R.W. 1994. Imperial Politics and Local Economy in Central America 1670–1770. *Past and Present* 143: 77–107.

Phelan, J.L. 1959 *The Hispanization of the Philippines: Spanish Aims and Filipino Responses 1565–1700*. University of Wisconsin, Madison.

Pimental, D. 1968 Population Regulation and Genetic Feedback. *Science* 159: 1432–37.

Pineo, R.F. 1990 Misery and Death in the Pearl of the Pacific: Health Care in Guayaquil, Ecuador 1870–1925. *Hispanic American Historical Review* 70 (4): 609–37.

Powell, P.W. 1975 *Soldiers, Indians and Silver: North America's First Frontier War.* Center for Latin American Studies, Arizona State University, Tempe.

Prem, H.J. 1992 Spanish Colonization and Indian Property in Central Mexico, 1521–1620. *Annals of the Association of American Geographers* 82 (3): 444–460.

Rabell, C.A. and Assaodurian, C.S. 1977 Self-Regulating Mechanisms of the Population in a Pre-Columbian Society: The Case of the Inca Empire. In *International Population Conference* (Mexico, 1977) 3: 25–42. Deronaux, Liège.

Ramenofsky, A.F. 1987 *Vectors of Death*: University of New Mexico, Albuqerque,
——— 1990 Loss of Innocence: Explanations of Differential Persistence in the Sixteenth-century Southeast. In *Columbian Consequences*, Vol. 2, edited by D.H. Thomas, pp. 31–48. Smithsonian Institution Press, Washington.

Rausch, J.M. 1984 *A Tropical Plains Frontier: The Llanos of Colombia, 1531–1831.* University of New Mexico Press, Albuquerque.

Reff, D.T. 1991 *Disease, Depopulation and Culture Change in Northwestern New Spain, 1518–1764.* University of Utah Press, Salt Lake City.

Reid, A. 1987. Low Population Growth and Its Causes in Pre-Colonial Southeast Asia. In *Death and Disease in Southeast Asia: Explorations in Social. Medical and Demographic History*, edited by N. Owen, pp. 33–47. Oxford University Press, Oxford.
——— 1988 *Southeast Asia in the Age of Commerce 1450–1680 Vol. I: The Lands Below the Winds*, pp. 57–58. Yale University Press, New Haven and London.

Roberts, L. 1989 Disease and Death in the New World, *Science* 246, 1245–47.

Rotberg, R.I., and T.K. Rabb (Eds.) 1983 *Hunger and History.* Cambridge University Press, Cambridge.

Ruhl, D.L. 1990 Spanish Mission Paleoethnobotany and Culture Change: A Survey of the Archaeobotanical Data and some Speculations on Aboriginal and Spanish Agrarian Interactions in La Florida. In *Columbian Consequences*, Vol. 2, edited by D.H. Thomas, pp. 555–80. Smithsonian Institution Press, Washington.

Rullu, J. 1991 Population of the French Overseas Territories in the Pacific, Past, Present and Projected. *The Journal of Pacific History* 26 (2), 169–186.

Sánchez-Albórnoz, N. 1974 *The Population of Latin America: A History.* University of California Press, Berkeley.
——— 1984 The Population of Colonial Spanish America. In *The Cambridge History of Latin America* Vol. 2, edited by L. Bethell, pp. 3–35. Cambridge University Press, Cambridge.
——— 1990 Demographic Change in America and Africa Induced by European Expansion, 1500–1800. In *The European Discovery of the World and its Economic Effects on Pre-Industrial Society*, edited by H. Pohl, pp. 195–206. Franz Steirner Verlag, Stuttgart.

Schurz, W.L. 1959 *The Manila Galleon.* E.P. Dutton and Co., New York.

Service, E.R. 1955 Indian-European Relations in Colonial Latin America. *American Anthropologist* 57: 411–25.

Shea, D.E. 1992 A Defense of Small Population Estimates for the Central Andes in 1520. In *The Native Population of the Americas in 1492* (2nd ed.), edited by W.M. Denevan, pp. 157–80. University of Wisconsin Press, Madison.

Silverblatt, I. 1987 *Moon, Sun and Witches: Gender Ideologies and Class in Inca and Colonial Peru.* Princeton University Press, Princeton.

Slack, P. 1981 The Disappearance of Plague: An Alternative View. *Economic History Review* 34 (3): 469–76.

Smith, C.T. 1970 Depopulation of the Central Andes in the Sixteenth Century. *Current Anthropology* 11: 453–64.

Somolinos d'Ardois, G. 1982 La viruela en la Nueva España. In *Ensayos sobre la historia de las epidemias en México*, Vol. 1, edited by E. Florescano and E. Malvido, pp. 237–49. Instituto Mexicano del Seguro Social, Mexico City.

Stannard, D.E. 1989 *Before the Horror: The Population of Hawai'i on the Eve of Western Contact*. University of Hawai'i, Honolulu.

―――― 1991 The Consequences of Contact: Toward an Interdisciplinary Theory of Native Responses to Biological and Cultural Invasion. In *Columbian Consequences*, Vol. 3, edited by D.H. Thomas, pp. 519–39. Smithsonian Institution Press, Washington.

Super, J. 1988 *Food, Conquest and Colonization in Sixteenth-Century Spanish America*. University of New Mexico Press, Albuquerque.

Svanborg-Eden, C. and B.R. Levin 1990 Infectious Disease and Natural Selection in Human Populations: A Critical Re-examination. In *Disease in Populations in Transition: Anthropological and Epidemiological Perspectives*, edited by A.C. Swedlund and G.J. Armelagos, pp. 31–46. Bergin and Garvey, New York.

Sweet, D. 1995 The Ibero-American Frontier Mission in Native American History. In *The New Latin American Mission History*, edited by E. Langer and R.H. Jackson, pp. 1–48. University of Nebraska, Lincoln and London.

Taylor, W.B. 1972 *Landlord and Peasant in Colonial Oaxaca*. Stanford University Press, Stanford.

Thornton, R.T. Miller and J. Warren 1991 American Indian Population Recovery Following Smallpox Epidemics. *American Anthropologist* 93 (3): 28–45.

Thornton, R. 1986 History, Structure and Survival: A Comparison of the Yuki (Ukom-no'm) and Tolowa (Hush) Indians of Northern California. *Ethnology* 25: 119–30.

Ubelaker, D.H. and Newson, L.A. Patterns of Health and Nutrition in Prehistoric and Historic Ecuador. In *The Backbone of History: Health and Nutrition in the Western Hemisphere*, Vol. 1, edited by R.H. Steckel and J.C. Rose. Cambridge University Press, Cambridge.

Ubelaker, D.H., Katzenberg, M.A. and Doyon, L.G. 1995. Status and Diet in Precontact Highland Ecuador, *American Journal of Physical Anthropology* 97: 403–411.

Upham, S. 1986 Smallpox and Climate in the American Southwest. *American Anthropologist* 88: 115–28.

Wachtel, N. 1977 *The Vision of the Vanquished. The Spanish Conquest of Peru Through Indian Eyes*. Harvester Press, Hassocks.

Wagley, C. 1951 Cultural Influences on a Population. *Revista do Museu Paulista* 5: 95–104.

Walker, P.L., P. Lambert and M.J. DeNiro 1989 The Effects of European Contact on the Health of Alta California Indians. In *Columbian Consequences*, Vol. 1, edited by D.H. Thomas, pp. 349–64. Smithsonian Institution Press, Washington.

Walter, J., and R. Schofield 1989 Famine, Disease and Crisis Mortality in Early Modern Society. *Famine, Disease and the Social Order in Early Modern Society*, edited by J. Walter and R. Schofield, pp. 1–73. Cambridge University Press, Cambridge.

Watson, R.B. and R. Hewitt 1941 Topographical and Related Factors in the Epidemiology of Malaria in North America, Central America and the West Indies. In *A Symposium on Human Malaria with Special Reference to North America and the Caribbean Region*, edited by F.R. Moulton, pp. 135–47. American Association for the Advancement of Science, Publication 15. Washington, DC.

Whitmore, T.M. 1991 A Simulation of the Sixteenth-century Population Collapse in the Basin of Mexico. *Annals of the Association of American Geographers* 81 (3): 464–87.

Whitmore, T.M. and Turner, B. 1992 Landscapes of Cultivation in Mesoamerica on the Eve of Spanish Conquest, *Annals of the Association of American Geographers* 82 (3): 402–425.

Wolfe, R.J. 1982 Alaska's Great Sickness, 1900: An Epidemic of Measles and Influenza in a Virgin Soil Population. *Proceedings of the American Philosophical Society* 126 (2): 91–121.

Zavala, S.A. 1967 *Los esclavos indios en Nueva España*. El Colegio Nacional, Mexico City.

Zulueta, J. de 1956 Malaria in Sarawak and Brunei. *Bulletin of the World Health Organization* 15: 651–71.

7. THE IBERIAN ADVANTAGE

Lawrence A. Clayton

"A la espada y al compás, Mas, y mas, y mas, y mas"[1]

Every generation writes its own history, reflecting the cultural bias of the age. So, as we consider the question of why Europeans successfully spread their influence over much of the world between the fifteenth and nineteenth centuries, one has to read the great masters of the past. In this genre, Carlo M. Cipolla, John H. Parry, and Charles R. Boxer stand out, for example, as the master historical craftsmen of their age. The telling of the story, the reenactment of the great episodes, the scholarship, the erudition, and the wonderful strength of their narrative are hard to surpass. More contemporary historians, such as Geoffrey Parker, also took their sights on the fascinating question: "just how did the West, initially so small and so deficient in most natural resources, become able to compensate for what it lacked through superior military and naval power?"[2] Even natural scientists, such as the physiologist Jared Diamond, have cast the net out to answer the question, "why did wealth and power become distributed as they now are, rather than in some other way?" Or, as Diamond colorfully framed the question by his New Guinea friend Yali, "Why is it that you white people developed so much cargo and brought it to New Guinea, but we black people had little cargo of our own?"[3]

In our summary of the elements that historians of the past identified as prominent in what we have styled the "Iberian Advantage," perhaps the most prominent is religious conviction. Religious passion

---

[1] From frontispiece of Bernardo de Vargas Machuca, *Milicia y descripción de las Indias* (Madrid, 1599), showing "a Spanish captain, Vargas Machuca, whose description of the Indies of 1599, showed him in the frontispiece with one hand on his sword, and the other holding a pair of compasses on top of a globe. Beneath was the inscription" quoted above. From J.H. Eliot, *The Old World and the New, 1492–1650* (Cambridge: Cambridge University Press, 1996 [1970]), p. 53.

[2] Geoffrey Parker, *The Military Revolution: Military Innovation and the Rise of the West, 1500–1800* (Cambridge: Cambridge University Press, 1988), p. 4.

[3] Jared Diamond, *Guns, Germs, and Steel: The Fates of Human Societies* (New York: W.W. Norton & Co., 1997), pp. 15, 14.

and evangelical obsession marked the age. The Spanish Reconquest of the Iberian peninsula for Christianity reached a crescendo in the late fifteenth century, while the "crusading spirit" of a Prince Henry the Navigator "set the Portuguese upon a career of overseas expansion" in the first half of the century.[4] Religious enthusiasm and the goad to proselytize and convert thus carried them like a swelling wave beyond the confines of Europe into the waters around Africa, to Asia, and finally to the Americas.

But religious zealots and passion drove other people as well, none more successfully than the Muslim culture competing with Christians across the Mediterranean and southern European world in the fifteenth and sixteenth centuries. The Ottoman Turks were as passionate and committed as the warriors of Prince Henry and the knights of Queen Isabella of Castile and King Ferdinand of Aragon. Besides, many have commented along the lines of Cipolla who observed that "religion supplied the pretext and gold the motive."[5]

Beyond the crusading spirit, there was "courage, discipline, and organising ability" that endowed European maritime culture with special strengths.[6] But the voyages of the Chinese eunuch Zheng He in the early fifteenth century were themselves immensely successful examples of organizing ability, discipline, and, we have to opine, courage as well.

Zheng He led at least seven major maritime and naval expeditions for the Mings from China into the Indian Ocean. The first one in 1405 sailed as far as Sri Lanka and numbered 62 ships and over 27,000 men! He reached as far as the Persian Gulf and the east coast of Africa in the early fifteenth century, making contact and trading in ports from Hormuz to Mozambique. That the Chinese did not follow up on these fantastic maritime endeavors is the subject of some debate, but that they possessed an extremely well organized and focused presence at sea is beyond doubt.[7]

---

[4] J.H. Parry, *The Establishment of the European Hegemony: 1415–1715: Trade and Exploration in the Age of the Renaissance* (New York: Harper Torchbook, 1961 [1949]), p. 13.

[5] Carlo M. Cipolla, *Guns, Sails and Empires: Technological Innovation and the Early Phases of European Expansion, 1400–1700* (n.p.: Minerva Press, 1965), p. 136.

[6] Parry, *Establishment*, p. 13.

[7] See Louise Levathes, *When China Ruled the Seas: The Treasure Fleet of the Dragon Throne, 1405–1433* (New York: Oxford Univ. Press, 1994).

So, if the establishment of European dominance was not attributable in the main to religious passion, organization, or discipline, then what can we ascribe it to? What about technology?

In the realm of technological advancements, or, put another way, technological superiority, Parry wrote that "one of the most obvious characteristics of European civilisation is its preoccupation with technical problems and its mastery of a wide range of mechanical devices."[8] Were Europeans simply better tinkers? This is hardly the stuff of voyages of epic proportions and conquests that changed the course of history. Reading on, Parry notes that "technical skill and the ability to turn theoretical knowledge to practical material ends have been major factors in the extension of European influence round the world . . . the scientific knowledge of the time, whether the result of genuine discovery or of the revival of classical knowledge, was turned very quickly to practical account." Here, I believe, we are getting warmer.

Carlo Cipolla made the connection between technological innovation and expansion even more direct. "Exchanging oarsmen for sails and warriors for guns meant essentially the exchange of human energy for inanimate power. By turning wholeheartedly to the gun-carrying sailing ship the Atlantic peoples broke down the bottleneck inherent in the use of human energy and harnessed, to their advantage, far larger quantities of power."[9]

Roger C. Smith, a late twentieth century student of the subject, was as equally clear as the earlier masters. "Ships and guns were the most important tools of technology that made possible the Iberian nautical revolution."[10] I have titled this essay the "Iberian Advantage" since I'm not sure if the technological advances qualify as a true revolution, in the same way the invention of the printing press "revolutionized" the dissemination of knowledge in the fifteenth century, or the computer did the late twentieth century. Semantics aside, the road to understanding the Iberian advantage combines many elements, none more important than the technological element.

Having expressed this bias, now let us consider two principal areas: one, the discrete elements that made up this technological advantage,

---

[8] Parry, *Establishment*, p. 13.

[9] Carlo M. Cipolla, *Guns, Sails, and Empires: Technological Innovation and the Early Phases of European Expansion, 1400–1700* (New York: Pantheon Books, 1965), p. 81.

[10] Roger C. Smith, *Vanguard of Empire: Ships of Exploration in the Age of Columbus* (New York: Oxford Univ. Press, 1993), p. 208.

and two, the cultural matrix which proved a fertile bed for the flowering of the advantage.

The technological elements are multitudinous, but relatively easily identified and analyzed. They include not only ships and guns, but charts and maps, navigational instruments, prior (ancient) knowledge and new investigations. The cultural matrix subsumes the warring worlds of Christendom and Islam, the rise of Protestantism, the equally powerful mercantile drive for commerce and worldly gain, the personal desire of adventure, and, perhaps the hardest to define, but one of the most telling, the psychology of the individual mariner-explorers of the age.

At the beginning of the rise of the European dominance between the fifteenth and nineteenth centuries stand the mariners who sailed for Portugal and Spain. Actually, they were not all Spaniards or Portuguese, but, rather, quite an eclectic bunch. Perhaps the greatest of them all—Christopher Columbus—was Genoese-born, and, like Columbus, it was not unusual for natives of one country to sail in the service of another. Sebastian Cabot, an Italian, laid English claims to the New World in 1497–98 for Henry VII of England, while Ferdinand Magellan, a Portuguese, made, arguably, the greatest voyage in the history of mankind between 1519–1520 in the service of the Spanish. Some of the most important cosmographers and mapmakers were Italians and Germans, and a number were even drawn from the ranks of the ancients. To wit, Ptolemy's *Geography*, a map of the world which first drew in lines of latitude and longitude and made a reasonable estimate of the size of the globe, was produced in the second century AD by a Hellenized Alexandrian. Lost for centuries, it was reproduced in Europe around 1410 and gave European mariners a standard view of the world from antiquity.

As we move to a consideration of the technological advances of the period, it turns out that European mariners, shipbuilders, geographers, cosmographers, and mapmakers were not so much creators and innovators, but magnificent adapters. They took pieces—of knowledge, such as Ptolemy's *Geography* and Pierre d'Ailly's *Imago Mundi*, of shipbuilding practices, of esoteric inventions such as of gunpowder by the Chinese—and adapted them to their needs. More of the needs in the moment. First to the tools.

At the very core of the Iberian advantage that developed in the fifteenth and sixteenth centuries was the simple ability to get back to where you sailed from. Any fool can put out to sea, and with a fair wind and some luck, go a long way, perhaps even fetch up on an island, a far shore, a distant haven, but, more than likely, simply disappear in the trackless seas that make up more than two-thirds of the surface of the earth. The trick was to know how to return home. And to do that one needed to know how to navigate.

The word "know" keeps cropping up in our consideration. Implied is "knowledge," and the expanding knowledge of the seas and how to navigate them marked one important element in the Iberian advantage. Sparing the details, we know that Europeans of the fifteenth century had learned how to find their latitude by observations of certain celestial bodies, such as the North Star—Polaris—, and sun, for instance. By employing instruments such as the astrolabe (an Arab invention), cross-staff, and quadrant, themselves, they measured the angle between the horizon and the celestial body. After "shooting" the North Star which occupied a relatively steady position over the polar region, they could then deduce their latitude, measured in degrees north of the Equator. This simple calculation was okay if one were in the northern hemisphere where Polaris could be observed.

If, on the other hand, one sailed across the equatorial region into the Southern Hemisphere, as did the Portuguese in the second half of the fifteenth century while probing down the African coast, then the North Star gradually disappeared. This was a problem, but the solution gives us some insight into one area of the Iberian advantage—the ability to experiment successfully, to innovate, to move beyond the frontier of known knowledge and "push the envelop" of experience, in the jargon of the Space Age.

Many, such as Amerigo Vespucci, attempted to identify the "southern Pole Star." On a voyage south of the Equator along the coast of South America in 1499, Vespucci was keenly "desirous of being the author who should identify the pole star of the other hemisphere." Always with a personal touch, Vespucci wrote that "I lost many a night's sleep in contemplation of the motion of the stars around the South Pole . . . but I was unable to succeed . . . [and] did not observe any star which had less than ten degrees of motion around the pole."[11]

Here is a good example of the Iberian advantage. Vespucci, on this particular voyage in the service of Portugal, was *competing* to find

---

[11] J.H. Parry, ed., *The European Reconnaissance: Selected Documents* (New York: Harper & Row, 1968), pp. 177–178.

the solution to reliable navigation in the southern hemisphere. Other Portuguese navigators and pilots were also being encouraged by the Portuguese Crown to *discover* and *apply* the solution. It came around 1500, or at the very moment that Vespucci was afloat in the equatorial oceans. Portuguese mariners had discovered the Southern Cross earlier in their voyages down the coast of Africa, and by 1506 Pedro Anes was teaching fellow pilots how to sail by that constellation.[12]

The other form of celestial navigation developed by the Portuguese was by taking solar observations. However, if the sun was being shot, then tables of declination had to be first consulted to determine where one expected to find the sun in the skies on any given day of the year. These tables were first produced in the 1480s by Portuguese astronomers for practical navigation. Pilots, such as Columbus, knew how to find their latitude with some degree of reliability, a knowledge that was constantly being encouraged by both Portuguese and Spanish sovereigns.

In 1508, for example, the Spanish crown established the office of pilot major in Seville. First held by Amerigo Vespucci, and then other distinguished and successful pilots such as Sebastian Cabot, the pilots major essentially ran a school for pilots, debriefing ones returning from voyages, keeping a master chart (the *padrón real*), and effectively keeping the edge on the Iberian advantage. One of the great masters of naval and maritime history, Samuel Eliot Morison, observed that "Portugal, but no other country, had a similar system for regulating voyages," and Morison added, "Englishmen such as Richard Hakluyt openly admired the Spanish regulations for training pilots."[13] Bailey W. Diffie, a long-time student of the Portuguese empire, was even more emphatic: "On the high seas, where it counted, the Portuguese led—and northern Europe lagged."[14]

Determining longitude was more difficult, for, to do so, one needed a very accurate timepiece, or chronometer. A suitable one was not developed until the eighteenth century. One could determine longitude by some complicated mathematical formulas and very precise celestial observations that could only be done on land. At sea or on

---

[12] Bailey W. Diffie and George D. Winius, *Foundations of the Portuguese Empire, 1415–1580* (Minneapolis: University of Minnesota Press, 1977), p. 141.
[13] Samuel Eliot Morison, *The European Discovery of America: The Southern Voyages, AD 1492–1616* (New York: Oxford University Press, 1974), p. 475.
[14] Diffie and Winius, *Foundations*, p. 143.

strange shores, the precise figuring of longitude was impossible. So, for longitude, mariners employed a host of devices and their own experienced observations as they traveled over the seas to estimate how far and in what direction they had traveled after leaving a place—such as their home port—whose coordinates—latitude and longitude—they were certain of.

Apart from celestial navigation, pilots employed numerous other devices and methods to navigate. Most of these come under the term dead reckoning, which basically drew upon various instruments and charts to plot one's course. Experienced mariners such as Columbus were masters of the craft. To summarize this phase of navigation is not fair, for it involved an eclectic mixture of semi-precise, almost scientific measures combined with man's intuitive sixth sense that sometimes seemed more in touch with the divine than the mere practice of a craft.

Of the various instruments, perhaps the compass was the most important. Its invention has variously been ascribed to the Chinese and Arab maritime cultures of the East, but, more than likely, it came from the Vikings, working its way down to the Italians of the twelfth or thirteenth centuries, and from the Mediterranean thence into the Iberian area.[15] The principle was certainly known in the Middle Ages—that an iron needle magnetized with a lodestone and floated in water or some other liquid would tend to point north. It was adapted and refined for use at sea by attaching the needle to a pivot or pin, swung on gimbals so it could move freely to compensate for the motion of the sea, and put into a box or binnacle to protect it from the weather. It became a reliable element in the Iberian advantage. Pilots learned to adjust to the quirks of the compass which was often deflected from pointing to true north by the magnetic fields of the earth. Compass variation—still compensated for in modern ships and aircraft—could vary as many as ten or fifteen degrees or more, making navigation in strange waters a dicey business.

To help keep track of the business of sailing with greater and greater reliability, Iberians borrowed from the Mediterranean practice of making very detailed coastal charts, called *portolani*, to record courses and distances between known points. These charts were quite

---

[15] Heinrich Winter, "Who invented the compass," *Mariner's Mirror*, 23:95–102 (1937), cited in Diffie and Winius, *Foundations*, pp. 124–125, fn. # 2.

accurate and reliable for most short hauls between ports, headlands, and other recognizable geographic features. Portuguese and Spanish pilots, and those others sailing in the Iberian service, delivered specific and detailed reports of their voyages that were then committed to charts for future reference. As early as 1352, the King of Aragon required all ships to carry two maritime charts.[16] This may seem like an incidental detail in analyzing the Iberian advantage, but is not. It formed part of a coherent, deliberate effort to expand the boundaries of geographical knowledge (we will deal with various motivations below) that *consciously* pushed the frontier beyond the known. Or, as a famous epigraph from Spain of the late sixteenth century summed it up. "A la espada y al compas, y mas, y mas, y mas."[17] Or, "With the sword and the compass, and more, and more, and more."

Rounding out the pilot's instruments were devices to measure the passage of time and distances, as well as at least one very necessary technique for piloting close into shore, especially along strange and new lands. Computing distances sailed was a function of speed and time. How fast did we go in the last half-hour, in the last ten minutes, in the last three minutes? A chip log was in use by the early sixteenth century. A simple device, one tied knots in a line and allowed that line to stream out in the wake as one timed it. The result was so many knots per hour, or nautical miles per hour, a measure of speed still used at sea and in aviation today. Fifteenth century navigators however, such as the immensely experienced Columbus, did not have "chip" logs and basically had to estimate their speed and distance. Currents, strong winds, and tacking, for example, complicated the solution. This is when a sailor's sixth sense kicked in, when experience combined with a feel for the sea to produce a reliable guestimate on course and distance made good that day, that week, that month.

Finally, the lead line proved an indispensable tool. It is a simple device. A lead weight is attached to a line and heaved overboard as ships approached shallow waters. The line was marked in some fashion, such as in fathoms (about six feet), to show depth. The changes in depth were then sung out by the leadsman to the pilot

---

[16] Diffie and Winius, *Foundations*, p. 131.
[17] Quoted in J.H. Eliot, *The Old World and the New, 1492–1650* (Cambridge: Cambridge University Press, 1996 [1970]), p. 53.

and navigator who relied on changes in depth to indicate channels, shoals, and shallow waters the ship might be nearing.

Among the technological advances of the age, one stands out from all the others in the literature of the subject, and everyone tends to agree: there occurred a remarkably fast innovation in ship design and construction that enabled Iberian mariners—and by extension those other Europeans who followed, such as the English, Dutch, and French—to establish a mastery at sea. From Africa to the Malacca Straits, to China, to the Americas, European ships overpowered their competitors—native maritime cultures—and set up a maritime and naval supremacy that pushed Europe to dominate much of the world.

Concomitant with ship design was the adaptation of the gun to naval warfare, a transition so important that Parker noted it constituted a "revolution in naval warfare . . . in early modern Europe which . . . opened the way to the exercise of European hegemony over most of the world's oceans for much of the modern period."[18]

The history of ship design and evolution is an immensely varied subject, complicated by the many terms and languages employed, the parallel evolution of ship types in some instances, the various claims of different nationalities that sometimes obscure fact from nationalist myth. For our purposes, the principal breakthroughs came in the fourteenth and fifteenth centuries when Iberians, for all practical purposes, adapted existing ships and sails to produce two vessels, the caravel and the *nao*, or ship, that carried the explorers far beyond the confines of European and Mediterranean waters.

By way of background, seagoing vessels had evolved into two general types, the long ship and the round ship. The longship, a descendant of both Mediterranean and Scandinavian forerunners, was propelled most often by oars, was quite maneuverable, and was employed for the most part as a warship. Generically termed "longship," in Spanish literature it appears most often as a *galera*. *Galeras* and variations of the type formed the backbone of the Christian fleet that defeated the Turks at Lepanto on 7 October 1571.

The round ships in the Iberian fleets were relative newcomers compared with the *galeras* which traced their lineage to the ancient Phoenicians and Vikings. The roundship, or *nao*, sometimes called *navío* by the Spanish, was driven solely by sails, tended to be quite broad in relation to its length, rode fairly deeply in the water, and,

---

[18] Parker, *Military Revolution*, p. 83.

compared to the *galeras*, maneuvered sluggishly in adverse conditions. It was preferred by merchants who could ship large amounts of cargo at a low operating cost, since the crews necessary to man these vessels were a fraction of the sailors and soldiers a *galera* required. The galleys that fought at Lepanto each carried almost 400 men, prompting one observer to note that "when every man is at his post, only heads can be seen from prow to stern."[19] The origin of the roundship were probably Mediterranean, although the Arabian maritime culture of the Indian Ocean also produced vessels with similar characteristics.

The breakthrough for the eventual supremacy of the roundship over the longship came some time in the late Middle Ages. Until then, square sails, set on one or two masts, had been the common means of propulsion. With a following or quarterly wind the vessels moved a decent clip and answered the helm reasonably well. However, winds forward of the beam left these wide, deep merchantmen with little alternative but to wait patiently for fairer breezes and better days. The solution to the problem was the adoption of probably an Arabic invention, the lateen sail, which was added to the after or mizzenmast. The lateen sail had long been in use in the Mediterranean and its evolution is associated with that area, just as the square sail is thought to have evolved in Northern Europe.

The lateen sail, roughly triangular, could be worked into a variety of positions to catch the wind coming from virtually any direction except dead on. The Portuguese were the first successfully to utilize lateen-rigged caravels that carried explorers slowly down the African coast in the fifteenth century, discovering and colonizing some of the Atlantic island chains as well, such as the Azores and Madeiras. But the lateen-rigged caravels also had some disadvantages. They were hard to come about when tacking and their awkwardness in this respect limited their size, and thus the power they provided. Thus, when lateen sails were combined with square sails, a configuration was achieved which combined power—square sails—with maneuverability—lateen sails. Here terms get confusing, for we have various descriptions—carrack, full-rigged ship, *nao, navío*, galleon—all which represent various stages in the improvement in this new ship design that came about in the fifteenth century.

---

[19] Parker, *Military Revolution*, p. 89.

Other improvements in hull construction further facilitated the Iberian advantage. Sometime around 1000 AD ". . . instead of putting together the external skin of the ship first . . . shipbuilders put up the internal ribs and then tacked the hull planking to the external framework."[20] This method of ship construction allowed for a number of clear advantages: larger ships; more flexible hull designs and shapes; and it was less demanding in shipwrights' time and skills.

This experimentation in hull design and sail configurations was a dynamic process, combining the various traditions to produce the caravels, carracks, and galleons of the age of exploration. All the while this phase of technological improvement was occurring in hull and sails, Iberians and other Europeans were also experimenting with what proved to be a most lethal combination and, indeed, perhaps a "revolution" in naval warfare, by adapting guns on ships.

The Chinese invented gunpowder (around the ninth century AD) and probably were the first to manufacture metal-barreled canon in the thirteenth century. By the middle of the fourteenth century the Chinese under the Ming dynasty were putting artillery on ships. And they were effective. A Portuguese flotilla in 1522 was defeated off Tunmen, and the Europeans were imprisoned and then executed.[21]

The Chinese presence at sea, indeed, from about the tenth through the fourteenth centuries, was impressive. Hundreds of ships, both naval and merchant, projected naval power and made money for the Chinese. They experimented and designed new types of ships such as paddlewheel boats, galleys, rams, and outriggers, spurred on by cash rewards from the government.[22] By the ". . . early fifteenth century, the great Ming navy consisted of 3,500 vessels: 2700 of them were warships at the dozens of coastal patrol stations up and down the coast, 400 were warships based at Xinjiangkou near Nanjing, and 400 were armed transport vessels for grain."[23] Let us remember for a moment that Columbus's expedition, at the end of the century, consisted of three rather small, albeit sturdy, craft.

---

[20] Robert Gardiner and Richard W. Unger, eds., (*Cogs, Caravels and Galleons, The Sailing Ship 1000–1650*) (London: Conway Maritime Press, 1994), Richard Unger, "Introduction," p. 8.

[21] Parker, *Military Revolution*, p. 83.

[22] Jung-Pang Lo, "The emergence of China as a sea power during the late Sung and early Yuan periods," *The Far Eastern Quarterly*, Vol. 14, No. 4 (Aug., 1955), 489–503.

[23] Louise Levathes, *When China Ruled the Seas: The Treasure Fleet of the Dragon Throne*,

Then, somewhat inexplicably, the Chinese failed to develop their early lead in naval architecture and artillery, or take advantage of a dominant presence at sea. They continued to rely on a host of other strategies, on land and at sea, that precluded, it would seem, radical improvements in their artillery. Why did the Chinese not pursue this technological edge which, when combined with a display of massive organization at sea manifested in the Zheng He voyages of the early fourteenth century, endowed them with the ability to project power and commerce at sea?[24]

In fact, the Chinese gutted the magnificent fleets of the Mings that had taken the eunuch Zheng He on his voyages of exploration, trade, and empire into the Indian Ocean in the early fourteenth century. By mid-century, only half of the fleets existed. Imperial edicts in 1500 and 1525 forbade the building of oceangoing ships. As Louise Levathes wrote, "in less than a hundred years, the greatest navy the world had ever known had ordered itself into extinction. Why?"[25] Why indeed? In the answer we get some new insight in the Iberian advantage.

Here we start to shade off a bit into the second theme of this essay, the cultural context of the Iberian advantage. In this instance, let us look at it negatively for a moment. Rather than why the Iberians/Europeans took off technologically with guns, why did the Chinese not do so?

Parker cogently stated the case: "But [for the Chinese] to possess guns is one thing; to use them effectively quite another." The basic argument made by Parker was that the Chinese had been unable to use guns at sea effectively to repel Japanese pirates in the sixteenth century. Instead, the Chinese relied on tried and true ways,

---

1405–1433 (New York: Oxford University Press, 1994), p. 174. My thanks to colleague, Ronald R. Robel, Chinese historian at the University of Alabama, for directing me to this book and Jung-Pang Lo's article.

[24] Jung-Pang Lo, "The emergence of China as a sea power during the Late Sung and Early Yuan Periods," in, republished from *The Far Eastern Quarterly*, Vol. 14, No. 4 (Aug., 1955), 489–503, in which he describes Chinese naval forces during the early Ming period (or the late thirteenth and early fourteenth centuries): "At its maximum strength during the reign of Yung-lo, it consisted of a central fleet of four hundred ships stationed at Nanking, a coastal defense fleet of twenty-eight hundred ships to ward off raids by the *wako* from Japan, a maritime transport fleet of three thousand ships, and, the pride of the Ming navy, a fleet of over two hundred and fifty "treasure ships" (*pao-ch'uan*), each with a capacity of five hundred men." p. 292.

[25] Levathes, *When China*, p. 175.

massing troops and overwhelming their rivals with bows, lances, and swords. Cannon were judged too unreliable, too difficult to supply, too cumbersome, too inaccurate, and too often prone to explode when fired. So, not significantly being able to improve their warfare with guns, in the case of ship-borne artillery, "the Chinese deliberately rejected it."[26] Here we have a clear case of an advantage not taken. It proved more expedient to be traditional, than to bear the cost of experimentation. Cipolla judged the Chinese decision in the larger context of culture. So does Louise Levathes in her pioneering study of the Zheng He voyages of the early fourteenth century.

In Cipolla's argument, the Imperial Court "was heavily influenced by the fact that Chinese rulers had always been apprehensive of foreign influence, for they realized that the idea of the 'barbarians' being superior to Peking would be political dynamite." Here we move beyond cannons, and their efficacy against Japanese pirates, although that manifestation of a larger cultural context is important. Cipolla argued that the gentry and scholar-officials of China were against *innovation*. While there *were* examples of Chinese who promoted the adaptation of new guns and their manufacture, ". . . the efforts of a few were not enough to compensate for the immobile conservatism of the many."[27]

This profoundly conservative caste to society immobilized the Chinese on the technological front. Cultural pride and traditional tastes, scholar-bureaucrats with little desire to engage in commerce and practical science, all contributed to the crisis. "In the past the Chinese had never had to give up their cultural pride: the foreign rulers always adopted the Chinese civilization. Hence there was nothing in their history to guide them through their modern crisis."[28]

Levathes tends to attribute the precipitous decline of the Chinese navy, and concomitantly, technological improvements, to the dynamics of internal politics as well, although all of this predated the Japanese pirate threat of the sixteenth century. "Part of the answer has to do with court politics and the heightened tension between the eunuchs and the Confucian advisers to the emperor in the mid-fifteenth century. Seafaring and overseas trade were the traditional domain of eunuchs, and in striking down those enterprises the

---

[26] Parker, *Military Revolution*, pp. 83–84.
[27] Cipolla, *Guns, Sails*, pp. 118, 119.
[28] Cipolla, *Guns, Sails*, p. 120.

Confucians were eliminating a primary source of their rivals' power and income."[29] Increasing threats from the Monguls on the northern and western borders of China also took attention away from the sea, but the principal elements in China's withdrawal from the sea appear to be internal.

Coincidentally, the Iberian advantage too was fueled by internal changes in Europe which, on the other hand, *favored* change, adaptation, experimentation, and expansion. The comparison between the European cultural disposition to promote change, and the Chinese resistance to change was noted by Father Louis Le Comte (1655–1728), a French traveler and Jesuit. The Chinese did not want to "make use of new instruments and leave their old ones without an especial order from the Emperor to that effect. They are more fond of the most defective piece of antiquity than of the most perfect of the modern, differing much in that from us (Europeans) who are in love with nothing but what is new."[30]

Cipolla's argument may, however, have been far too impressionistic and anecdotal, although we reproduce one paragraph that is fun to read as a summary of his thesis.

> Nothing, I think, can better serve than the following delightful episode to illustrate the prevailing Chinese aura of patrician detachment and amateurish style. When in 1626 Yuan Ch'ung-huan had to defend Ning-yuan against the attacking Manchus and eventually decided to resort to "foreign guns," the general direction of artillery operations was put in the hands of his Fukienese cook who, incidentally, put up a very good show.

> If a Fukienese cook was good enough as captain-major of artillery against the "barbarians" who were pressing against China from the steppes, much more was needed to fight against the "barbarians" who were coming from the sea. But the scholar-officials of the Celestial Empire did not have much more at their disposal.[31]

Contrast the above view with Parker's: ". . . the peoples of East Asia, by contrast [to the Muslim world] were able to keep the West at bay throughout the early modern period because, as it were, they already knew the rules of the game. Firearms, fortresses, standing armies and warships had long been part of the military tradition of

---

[29] Levathes, *When China*, p. 175.
[30] Cipolla, *Guns, Sails*, pp. 120, 121, quoting from L. Le Comte, *Empire of China* (London, 1737), p. 68.
[31] Cipolla, *Guns, Sails*, pp. 121, 122.

China, Korea, and Japan."[32] So, were the scholar-bureaucrats casting cannons instead of composing poems? The answer lies in a much
wider, and detailed, consideration of the military revolution that was
taking place across the world, and far beyond the confines of this
essay. However, we do note that Parker contends that "the distinctive 'world order' of both China and Japan endured intact until the
Industrial nations of the West deployed steamships, steel artillery,
and sepoys against them in the mid-nineteenth century. They did
not fall before the military revolution."[33]

As we consider the rise of European superiority at sea in the
fifteenth and sixteenth centuries, we need to maintain some perspective. It was not an unqualified, meteoric rise, marked by shell-
shocked Muslims in the Indian Ocean and Chinese junks drifting to
oblivion as Iberian, and later Dutch and English, warships and traders
swept the oceans of their competitors. There were setbacks. But there
was the near inexorable rise of Iberian superiority at sea, and the
ease with which the Spanish conquered much of the Americas.
Although disease played as much, if not a greater role, than technology in that part of the world, the role of cannon and technology employed are worth considering in some detail.

It has been fashionable now for some time to emphasize weapons,
and specifically, guns, as preeminent factors in the rise of the European
dominance, and not without some just cause.[34] A sampling of the
literature is clearly unambiguous on this subject. "Non-European
countries never succeeded in filling the vast technological gap [refer-
ring to guns and artillery] that separated them from Europe. On
the contrary, in the course of time the gap grew conspicuously larger."
". . . Between 1450 and 1650, the emergence of the heavily armed
[with artillery] sailing ship transformed the situation." And, ". . . one
of the most important technological innovations during the fifteenth
century was the introduction of artillery at sea."[35]

While the literature on guns and ships is large, and still growing,
we can abstract it for the purposes of this essay.[36] Beginning with

---

[32] Parker, *Military Revolution*, p. 136.

[33] Parker, *Military Revolution*, p. 145.

[34] William McNeil, article in *Journal of World History*, 9:2 (1998), pp. 00–00.

[35] The quotes are from Cipolla, *Guns, Ships*, p. 129; Parker, *Military Revolution*,
p. 89, Smith, *Vanguard of Empire*, p. 148, in the same order they appear in the text.

[36] For a wonderfully illustrated example of the literature, see Peter Padfield, *Guns
at Sea* (New York: St. Martin's Press, 1974).

small, breech-loading, cast or wrought iron guns, and capable of firing about a 4-pound shot, seagoing cannons evolved in the fifteenth and sixteenth centuries into effective weapons. As early as the 1430s, Portuguese caravels carried small guns, some mounted on swivels for aiming, most of them delivering missiles as diverse as stone, iron, and lead projectiles. The names of the various guns are myriad, representing not only an industry or art in rapid transition, but national variances.

One of the earliest technological breakthroughs came with the introduction of the muzzle-loading bronze cannons in the fifteenth century. Here we have to pause in an essay that is not technical, but devoted in some ways to the technological improvements in ships and guns that drove the Iberian advantage. Breech-loaded cannons, or those loaded by opening them at the breech end, were cheaper and easier to fabricate, but had some intrinsic weaknesses: they were prone to bursting the barrel or blowing the breechblock out and could only be built for relatively small charges of powder. Muzzle-loading bronze cannon, on the other hand, possessed increased strength because of the fabrication process (casting them in a single piece) and could deliver a much heavier projectile over a longer distance. Bronze muzzle-loaders were, however, expensive to build and demanded a much higher degree of technical skill. As a result, the usual Iberian ship of exploration was equipped often with a combination of muzzle- and breech-loaders, of different calibers and types.

On Vasco da Gama's first voyage into the Indian Ocean, for example, each of his larger ships carried about twenty bombards, or breech-loading cannon, and an unknown number of smaller guns.[37] "It is clear that Portuguese voyages of exploration were heavily laden with firepower."[38] In da Gama's second voyage to the Indian Ocean in 1502, even more guns bristled from his decks. How effective were da Gama's guns in the Indian Ocean? Before we consider that central question, we need to back off a bit and consider a couple of other elements, equally important in determining the Iberian advantage.

Principally among these was that of the implication of the invention and use of gunpowder and cannons in the overall nature of warfare. I do not believe Roger Smith overstated the case when he

---

[37] This section on guns drawn from Smith, *Vanguard of Empire*, pp. 154ff., Padfield, *Guns at Sea*, pp. 25ff., Parker, *Military Revolution*, pp. 89ff.

[38] Smith, *Vanguard of Empire*, p. 157.

wrote, ". . . mastery of controlled explosions represented a major forward leap in the evolution of human technology from the dawn of
the discovery of fire toward our own nuclear age . . . [and]explosive
devices adapted for shipboard use quickly altered the complexion of
naval warfare."[39] Or, put another way, the power to wage war at
sea was dramatically transformed by the addition of artillery at sea.
Instead of arrows, swords, ramming, and whatever else could be
thrown and thrust at an enemy, now one had the possibility of doing
the damage *more efficiently* and by *standing off* from one's opponent.

Where warfare at sea had not advanced much in thousands of
years—basically it had involved closing with the enemy and engag-
ing in hand to hand combat—now the ship was transformed from
a *carrier* to a weapon itself. When writing of how Mediterranean merchantmen—roundships with small crews—might more effectively
defend themselves in the fifteenth century against the pirates often
infesting that sea, Peter Padfield envisioned the following scene:

> What better defence than a row of quick-firing, breech-loading pieces
> mounted on swivels to command any direction the pirates might choose
> for their boarding tactics? For gunpowder, to a far greater extent than
> the crossbow, *replaced human energy* [emphasis added]. Once the row of
> guns were loaded, *one man* with a lighted match could set them off
> one after the other, and another man could follow him knocking out
> the wedges which held the chamber in position, removing the cham-
> ber and replacing it with another previously-filled chamber after insert-
> ing a ball or bag of old nails in the barrel. Two men could keep up
> a hail of fire for a short time, a few more would be sufficient to repel
> boarders not similarly equipped.[40]

But what if you wished to increase both efficiency and the *efficacy* of
your artillery at sea? One answer was bigger and more powerful
guns. But where to put them? Certainly not high up in the castles
fore and aft, or even arrayed in numbers on the main deck, for all
that weight that high up on a ship's superstructure created dangerous instability. "Starting (according to tradition) around 1500 in the
port of Brest in Brittany, and quickly spreading all over Atlantic
Europe, hinged gun-ports were cut into the sides of the larger ships,
making it possible to deploy artillery along their entire length on
several levels."[41] Now larger and more powerful cannons could be

---

[39] Smith, *Vanguard of Empire*, p. 149.
[40] Padfield, *Guns at Sea*, p. 20.
[41] Parker, *Military Revolution*, p. 90.

fired that produced a *lethal* impact on enemy hulls and rigging. While the technology continued to be refined in the sixteenth century, reaching a high tide of sorts for the English, for example, with the defeat of the Spanish Armada in 1588, the basic ingredients for the Iberian advantage at sea were in place by 1500.

In that year, one other element of the new naval warfare was mentioned in the instructions that King Manuel of Portugal gave to Pedro Cabral as he prepared for the second Portuguese expedition to India. If he met Muslim ships, "'you are not to come to close quarters with them if you can avoid it, but you are to compel them with our artillery alone to strike sail . . .' so that '. . . this war may be waged with greater safety, and . . . less loss may result to the people of your ships.'"[42]

Da Gama's second voyage to India in 1501 and 1502 proved the worth of the growing Iberian advantage. Calicut, the site of the first Portuguese station in India, had already been bombarded by Pedro Cabral after the Muslims had harassed the Portuguese. Da Gama's ships were even more heavily armed than Cabral's. The gauntlet was thrown down.

The Arabs put together a fleet of over 70 ocean-going dhows, accompanied by scores of smaller craft.[43] They would soon rid themselves of these Portuguese invaders. The Arab fleet carried some crude guns, perhaps mortars, some even made of wood, but they were undergunned when compared to the Portuguese. Arab tactics, very traditional in naval warfare up to then, were to close quarters, board, and defeat their foes in hand-to-hand fighting. Da Gama sailed to meet the challenge, reiterating the orders given to Cabral. "Don't close. Keep your distance. Use your artillery."

The ensuing battle off the Malabar coast in 1502 is a classic, one of ". . . the decisive battles of the world."[44] It is hard to describe a naval battle of such dimensions, involving thousands of men, hundreds of ships, and maneuvers and tactics that covered hours and many square miles at sea. However, Peter Padfield's description of the battle is excellent; one section follows:

> After much cheering and dinning of gongs and other instruments by
> the Arabs, the fight was opened when the Portuguese caravels, sailing

[42] Parker, *Military Revolution*, p. 94; Padfield, *Guns at Sea*, p. 25.
[43] The following account from Padfield, *Guns at Sea*, pp. 25–28.
[44] Padfield, *Guns at Sea*, p. 27.

in line ahead well to the windward of the enemy, came abreast of
Cojambar's [Arab admiral] leading rank or bunch. Each then dis-
charged its two heavy pieces on that side of the flagship. "With this
first discharge our [Portuguese] men made such good work that they
brought down the mast of the [Arab] flagship, which fell over and
stove in the ship and killed many Moors; and another shot hit it full
and passed through near the poop, which it shattered much . . ." The
caravel gunners reloaded their pieces as rapidly as they could, using
"bags of powder which they had ready for this purpose made to measure so that they could load again very speedily." From this continuing cannonade by the caravels three large dhows were stove in low
down and sank, and many of the others seem to have been driven
into confusion, colliding with each other and bunching up so that the
Portuguese ships which had now arrived at the scene [da Gama with
the main body] simply brailed up their sails and 'fired into the thick'
and "it was not possible to miss."[45]

The battle continued through the afternoon, the Portuguese battering the Arabs at a range which prevented the Arabs from closing
and grappling. When the Muslims did manage to close the range
enough, they loosened hails of arrows, but the Portuguese gunners
simply ducked down, reloaded, and continued to blast away. In the
end, as darkness fell, the sea was spread with "Arab wreckage and
drowning men and bodies . . . what remained of Cojambar's once
great fleet fled the slaughter under cover of darkness. Da Gama lost
not a single ship."[46]

The Iberian advantage, in hull design and construction, sail
configuration, navigation, and gunnery, hit full stride with this tremendous victory by a relatively small Portuguese fleet operating alone,
thousands of miles away from the security of hearth and home. There
were reverses in the many naval battles ahead of the Portuguese in
the sixteenth century as they strung their trading posts and commercial power across the Indian Ocean, thence down the Malacca
Straits and into the lands and archipelagos of the famed Spice Islands
of the South China Sea and Pacific Ocean. Geoffrey Parker, in his
book *The Military Revolution* recounts many of the Portuguese reverses
at the hands of a Muslim sea power that kept the Portuguese from
establishing unquestioned control of the sea. But, Parker has to admit

---

[45] Padfield, *Guns at Sea*, pp. 26–27.
[46] Padfield, *Guns at Sea*, p. 27.

that ". . . usually, it is true, the Europeans won, but at a terrible cost . . ."[47] But, they won.

We have devoted much to the technological improvements in ships and guns that enabled the Iberians to take the advantage in the fifteenth and sixteenth centuries. But, in a way, we have deftly skirted around the question of "why," tending rather to focus on the "how." Or, as some would phrase it, on the "proximate" or immediate causes, rather than the "ultimate" or distant causes. That St. Thomas Aquinas, one of the great thinkers in history, wrote that all ultimate causes emanate from God probably would only muddle the analysis at this stage. However, if we WERE to follow the philosophical and theological implications of the question, "why the Europeans?" then it may lead to a far different conclusion than one concerned with mere technology. That endeavor we leave for another time. In this final section, we will try to come to terms with the "why" in its simplest, secular meaning.

Aside from technology, what were some of the other ingredients in the successful expansion of Europe? We think timing, or, more exactly, the *sustained momentum* across time was probably as, if not *more*, important than any other single ingredient in the European expansion; these elements include the traditional ones of technology and religious fervor, for example, and some identified by contemporary scholarship which include geography, botany, zoology, archaeology, and epidemiology popularized by students of the environmental school of causation such as Jared Diamond.[48] However, before timing, there exist several other elements that need to be identified.

Among the traditional elements was the peculiar development of national or state capitalism in Portugal in the fourteenth and fifteenth centuries.[49] This meant that, in effect, the Crown both participated directly in entrepreneurial exploration as a ". . . giant mercantile corporation . . .," and directly stimulated activities as a ". . . colonial franchiser which entrusted the management of its assets to others

---

[47] Parker, *Military Revolution*, p. 105.

[48] See Diamond's book, *Guns, Germs, and Steel*, especially p. 405, for the environmental explanation; and also others such as Alfred Crosby, *The Columbian Exchange: Biological and Cultural Consequences of 1492* (Westport, Conn.: Greenwood Press, 1972) and William McNeill, *Plagues and Peoples* (Garden City, N.Y.: Doubleday, 1976).

[49] This theme developed fully in Diffie and Winius, *Foundations of the Portuguese Empire*, especially Chapter 18, "Institutions of Trade and Government," pp. 301ff.

and allowed them the greatest share of the profits. . . ."[50] This was made possible by a long period of domestic political stability in the fifteenth and sixteenth centuries that set the stage for the Portuguese push into the world's oceans and markets.[51]

Diffie and Winius wrote of this advantage in terms that bear repetition:

> The state capitalism of the Portuguese was one of the most unusual experiments of early modern Europe . . . never before or since has one of them [Western governments] become the entrepreneur of an entire imperial undertaking and thrown its whole resources into the creation of profits from a trading monopoly on its overseas discoveries. This was facilitated through the use of a pattern that emerged from earlier medieval practice, was perfected in the course of African trading, and ultimately came to be applied on a vast scale to the Indian Ocean.[52]

For reasons unique to their national development, ". . . neither the Spanish nor the French, constantly at war with one another, could have attempted it during the first half of the sixteenth century, nor could the early Tudors, who lacked the capital, let alone the commercial experience or the navigational experience."[53] Beyond the mercantile and entrepreneurial skills of the Portuguese—from the monarchs on down through the bankers and investors from Genoa who provided much needed capital during this period—there existed a spiritual edge to the Iberian advantage that has to be reckoned with. In their book on Columbus and his times, Carla Rahn Phillips and William D. Phillips basically summarized in several sentences the context of the Iberian advantage.

"His [Columbus's] scheme had the potential to tie together and accomplish the dreams that European merchants, monarchs, missionaries, and mystics had held since the end of the Crusades. An established sea route to Asia would surely produce great riches, and it might also lead to an alliance with the Grand Khan against the Muslims and an unprecedented opportunity to spread the Christian message."[54] Or, as summarized even more succinctly by Louis B.

---

[50] Diffie and Winius, *Foundations*, p. 301.
[51] My thanks to my colleague Prof. John Beeler, naval historian at the University of Alabama, who brought this element of the Iberian advantage to my attention.
[52] Diffie and Winius, *Foundations*, p. 312.
[53] Diffie and Winius, *Foundations*, p. 312.
[54] William D. Phillips, Jr. and Carla Rahn Phillips, *The Worlds of Christopher Columbus* (Cambridge: Cambridge University Press, 192), p. 124.

Wright, the motivations and desires were encapsulated in the phrase, for gold, glory, and the gospel, although not necessarily in that order.[55]

The religious component of the Iberian advantage is one of the most compelling elements in the complex equation of motivation. Many European Christians of the Middle Ages expected the Second Coming of Christ and therefore they needed first to spread the Word to the world. "Go ye therefore and teach all nations . . ." Matthew 28:19,20 "Go ye into all the world, and preach the Gospel to every creature . . ." Mark 16:15. Intensely evangelical orders founded in the period, principally the Franciscans and the Dominicans, were devoted to, among other ends, a strong missionary effort to fulfill Scripture and thus prepare for the Second Coming. This effort took on special meaning in the Americas after the discovery, but the pros-elytizing spirit in Christianity was very much in evidence from the earliest history of the Church. After all, the Apostle Paul's mission was to the Gentiles, moving the message of Jesus Christ rapidly beyond the confines of the Chosen People, the Jews, to encompass—effectively—the world.

Of no less importance was the growing hostility between the Muslims and Christianity. The Crusades of the eleventh and twelfth centuries brought the Holy Lands temporarily into the hands of Christian warriors, but by the end of the thirteenth century, all the crusading efforts had been extinguished by the Muslims. The desire to recapture the Holy Lands was never too far from the surface of Iberian navigators and explorers. Columbus reminded Ferdinand and Isabella in the prologue to the diary of his first voyage that he urged them "'. . . to spend all the profits of this my enterprise on the con-quest of Jerusalem.'"[56]

One of the most fundamental elements in the complex of reli-gious motives was the ongoing Reconquest of the Iberian peninsula itself. The Reconquest of Moorish Spain for Christianity began around 1000 AD and, after nearly five centuries of intermittent warfare, was about to conclude at the end of the fifteenth century with the his-toric victory of Ferdinand and Isabella over the last Moorish king-dom of Granada. Earlier in the century, Prince Henry the Navigator

---

[55] Wright, Louis B. *Gold, Glory, and the Gospel; the Adventurous Lives and Times of the Renaissance Explorers* (New York, Atheneum, 1970).
[56] Phillips and Phillips, *Worlds of Christopher Columbus*, p. 124.

took part in the Portuguese capture of the North African city of Ceuta in 1415. The spring by the Portuguese across to Africa was not a decision lightly taken, nor one simply driven by religion. It was a business and strategic decision, one to help secure the safety of the southern Portuguese coast from raids, to provide security for Italian galleys enroute to England and Flanders and for Portuguese trade to the Mediterranean, to establish a base in the Mediterranean to attack Muslim commerce, and, a bit more difficult to document, to give King Joao's knights and warriors, and especially his three energetic sons, Duarte, Pedro, and Henry, a chance "to win their spurs of knighthood on the battlefield."[57] Underlying the very businesslike nature of the decision to attack and seize Ceuta was the act as a "a holy and honorable thing."[58]

Here we have manifested an important element in the Iberian advantage—the commercial or mercantile motive grafted very easily onto the religious dimension of the Reconquest. Trade between Portugal and Africa had been in existence for years, the gold, sugar, leather, textiles, and cereals of Northwest Africa being exchanged for copper, arms, wood, lacquer and other European products. The Portuguese advance into Africa through the capture of Ceuta represented a commercial venture as much as a religious quest. As in the Reconquest of the Iberian peninsula itself, there was not only fame and honor to be achieved in a defeat of the Moors, but it was a lucrative enterprise, marked not only by the taking of booty and prisoners (to be ransomed for handsome amounts depending upon their rank), but also by the establishment of new commercial and strategic outposts.

At the center of these activities was Prince Henry, dubbed "the Navigator" by succeeding generations, but, who, in reality, was not much of a sailor or navigator.[59] What he did do, however, was to ambitiously promote his own economic interests and the interests of Portugal which included setting himself up in North Africa, conquering Granada from the Muslims, exploring and trading along the

[57] Bailey W. Diffie and George D. Winius, *Foundations of the Portuguese Empire, 1415–1580* (Minneapolis: University of Minnesota Press, 1977), pp. 49, 53.

[58] Diffie and Winius, *Foundations*, p. 51.

[59] Diffie and Winius, *Foundations*, p. 121, demythologize Henry, who they said was not a man of scientific learning, nor did he surround himself or seek much advice from men of cosmographical and navigational skills, nor did he maintain a "school" at Sagres.

African coast, and badgering the King and Pope ceaselessly, and successfully, for concessions and favors related to his interests. He helped acquire for Portugal the Madeiras, the Azores, and the Cape Verde Islands, went after the Canaries (which ultimately fell to Castile), and, finally, but perhaps most important, he was the governor and administrator of the Order of Christ.

The Order of Christ had been set up in 1319, charged with defending Christians from Muslim attack in Portugal, and prosecuting the war against them in their own territory.[60] Prince Henry took his Christianity seriously, and it dovetailed neatly into his commercial side. To wage war on Muslims was just, honorable, holy, AND profitable. So was the encouragement of the seaborne exploration of Africa.

The stage was thus set in the fifteenth century for the full flowering of the Iberian advantage. By mid-century when Constantinople fell to the Turkish Ottomans (1453), the orientation of European trade was already shifting from the Mediterranean to the Atlantic, with Portugal leading the way down the African coast and into the Atlantic islands. The trade in African slaves was growing, and profitable, as Portuguese explorers pushed down west Africa. Trade between Portugal and Africa become even more lucrative. Horses, saddles, stirrups, cloth, caps, hats, saffron, wine, wheat, salt, lead, iron, steel, copper, and brass all moved south and east from Portugal to be traded for African slaves, gold, animal skins, gum arabic, civet, cotton, malagueta pepper, cobal, parrots, and even camels![61] It remained for the visionary Columbus to challenge the Portuguese crawl down around Africa on their way to Asia by proposing to sail directly West to reach the East.

Columbus's voyages (1492–1502) of course led to the Spanish conquest of the Americas, and the wealth of the Indies fueled the meteoric rise of Spain in the sixteenth century. The Iberian advantage was given an immense boost by the wealth generated from Portuguese commerce as it expanded into Asia, and the Spanish conquest as it spread across the rich empires of the Aztec and Inca.

In the world of aviation propulsion, there are ways to boost power for short periods of time that enhance speed. The penalty for switching on the afterburners in jet aircraft, however, is a tremendous

---

[60] Diffie and Winius, *Foundations*, p. 26.
[61] Phillips and Phillips, *Worlds of Columbus*, p. 55.

drain on resources, in this case fuel. But when the afterburners kick in, the rush of power and speed is dramatic. The conquest of the Indies and the early expansion in and dominance of the Muslim/Arabic trade routes in Asia provided the afterburner kick for the Iberians. The basic elements of the advantage were already in place: ship and sail design, navigational improvements, guns and the refashioning of the ship as a weapons platform, the commercial and religious motivation, the cultural disposition to promote change and invention.

The Iberian advantage set up the platform for other Europeans, principally the English, Dutch, and French, to launch their own imperial endeavors. Here we return to timing as the central, perhaps the ultimate, or primary, cause of the European rise to prominence. It was not enough simply to possess the ability to extend their power at sea, such as the Chinese did so successfully in the early fourteenth century, nor to adopt technology, such as advanced guns, as the Japanese did in the fifteenth century.[62] In each case, the Chinese and Japanese abandoned spectacular successes that could have successfully replicated the European seaborne expansion.

Borrowing one final phrase from the air and space age, we might say the Iberians had the "right stuff" in the fifteenth century. The Chinese were certainly able to make things happen in the world of exploration, maritime endeavor, and naval warfare. But the coincidence of timing, technology, and political and economic culture that drove the Iberians to success were not sustained subsequent to the brilliant Chinese accomplishments of the age of Zheng He. In the case of the Spanish and Portuguese, however, it not only all came together, but the initiative was seized by successors to the Iberians, especially of course the Dutch, English and French. Each possessed a maritime culture that easily matched the Iberian one. As one European innovator reached the top of his orbit, another one followed, like the stages of a rocket, each building on the preceding one. And like the rockets that take man into space, the ships propelled the Europeans into the world, to Africa, to Asia, to the Americas, and ultimately even to the frozen Polar regions. Without the sustained advancement at sea by the Iberians and their later Northern European competitors, there would have been no rise of the European hegemony.

---

[62] See Noel Perrin, *Giving Up the Gun: Japan's Reversion to the Sword, 1543–1879* (Boston: D.R. Godine, 1979).

8. "BLACK WITH CANOES".
ABORIGINAL RESISTANCE AND THE CANOE: DIPLOMACY, TRADE AND WARFARE IN THE MEETING GROUNDS OF NORTHEASTERN NORTH AMERICA, 1600–1821

David McNab, Bruce W. Hodgins and Dale S. Standen

Introduction

Aboriginal oral traditions in northeastern North America recall through their stories the significance of the canoe in Canada's history. Early in the twentieth century the hereditary Chief Peterwegeschick recalled that, in the 1820's, the citizens of the Bkejwanong First Nation (also known as the Walpole Island First Nation) participated in extensive trade, among other places, at Detroit and that his father "went there to trade when he was very small. He told me [Chief Peterwegeschick] that the St. Clair was often black with canoes in their journeying to the trading post at Detroit".[1] The canoe, especially its birchbark variety was, for at least five centuries, the most important Amerindian[2] device of technology; it was an essential part of their knowledge which was bequeathed to the European newcomers. The canoe, in war and diplomacy, along with trade, was the principal means by which Aboriginal autonomy and sovereignty were long secured. (See Figure 8.1)

A "Celestial Craft of Souls":
The Significance of the Canoe in Aboriginal Oral Traditions

The English word "canoe" is derived from the Arawak (Tainos) word for "boat." In the fifteenth century the Spanish appropriated the

---

[1] Nin.Da.Waab,Jig. Files, Sarnia *Canadian-Observer*, Saturday, July 18, 1925, p. 14.
[2] The terms "Anishinabe", "Aboriginal" and "Amerindian" will be used in this paper synonymously to refer to "Aboriginal people" who are defined in Canada's written Constitution (1982) as "Indians, Inuit and Metis". Today they are often referred to as First Nations, Aboriginal Peoples, or First Peoples.

Arawak word and it became "canoa." The term was used at the time of Christopher Columbus's voyages to the Caribbean as meaning a hollowed-out log used by "uncivilized Nations" as a boat which is propelled by paddles through the water.[3] The Ojibwa word for "canoe" is "Chiimaan(an)" (boat(s)). Indeed the major water transportation from the southern Ontario mainland to Manitoulin Island and the north country is by the modern ferry aptly named the Che-Che-maun, or big canoe (also Che-mun, boats).

The history of Aboriginal people comes from the oral traditions.[4] Without "pen and ink," First Nations remember and understand and have recorded their internal and external landscapes using their oral traditions and their stories. These stories were, of course, also recorded, but not by pen and ink in European languages; rather in wampum belts, in pictographs on stone and in birchbark scrolls.[5] Central to these stories are those of creation. Their focus is on water as an integral part of the four natural elements of earth, water, air, and fire. The canoe links these elements. For Aboriginal people the canoe is spiritual in its origin. Resting horizontally across a plane of water and with a paddle held vertically, the canoe represents the four sacred directions. As such, it is a holistic representation or symbol of life and the human journey through the mortal world to the world of the spirits.[6]

In yet another dimension, the canoe still is, as Blake Debassige has shown, a veritable "celestial craft of souls."[7] It is a metaphor

---

[3] Liz Wylie, *In the Wilds, Canoeing and Canadian Art* (Kleinburg, Ontario: McMichael Canadian Art Collection, 1998), p. 8.

[4] Basil Johnston, *Ojibwa Ceremonies* (Toronto: McClelland and Stewart, 1982), pp. 155–75; *The Manitous, The Spiritual World of the Ojibway* (Toronto: Key Porter Books, 1995). Johnson understood the significance of this oral tradition when he observed, in 1768, that ". . . whosoever has any affairs to transact with Indians must know their forms and in some measure comply with them, and to our Ignorance, negligence and Hauteur in these points we must attribute the little esteem they have for us." *The Papers of Sir William Johnson*, Prepared for publication by Milton W. Hamilton, Vol. VI (Albany: The University of the State of New York, 1928), Letter, Johnson to Henry Moore, September 20, 1768, Fort Stanwix, 400. On Iroquoian oral tradition see Mary A. Druke, "Iroquois treaties, common forms, varying interpretations", in Francis Jennings (ed.), *The History and Culture of Iroquois Diplomacy: An Interdisciplinary Guide to the Treaties of the Six Nations and Their League* (Syracuse: Syracuse University Press, 1985), pp. 85–98, 90.

[5] Peter S. Schmalz, *The Ojibwa of Southern Ontario* (Toronto: University of Toronto Press, 1991), p. 15.

[6] Edward Benton-Banai, *The Mishomis Book, The Voice of the Ojibway* (Saint Paul, Minnesota, Red School House, July, 1988), pp. 1–2.

[7] Wylie, *In the Wilds*, p. 27.

FIGURES

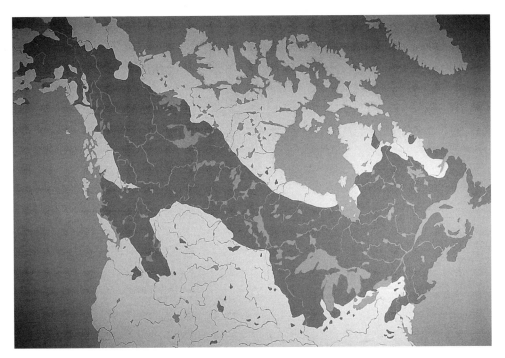

Figure 8.1. A map of the birchbark country. The authors would like to thank the Frost Centre for Canadian Studies and Native Studies, Trent University, for the use of this map.

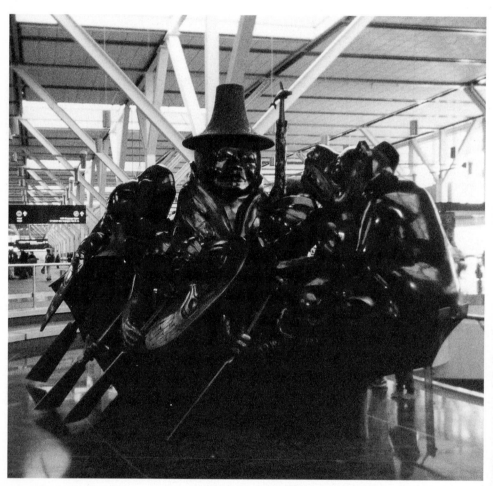

Figure 8.2. The jade canoe: a sculpture by Bill Reid entitled "The Spirit of Haida Gwaii". See fn. 14.

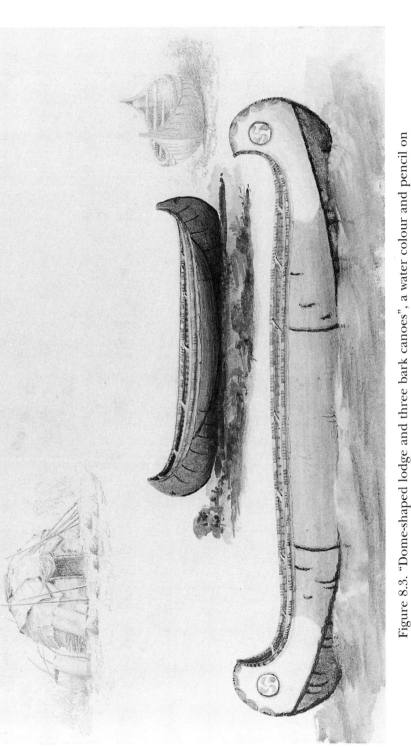

Figure 8.3. "Dome-shaped lodge and three bark canoes", a water colour and pencil on paper drawing by Paul Kane. The authors would like to thank Mr Ken Lister of the Royal Ontario Museum, Toronto, Canada, for his assistance in obtaining copies of the three Paul Kane pictures reproduced in this article. (ROM # 946.15.22.)

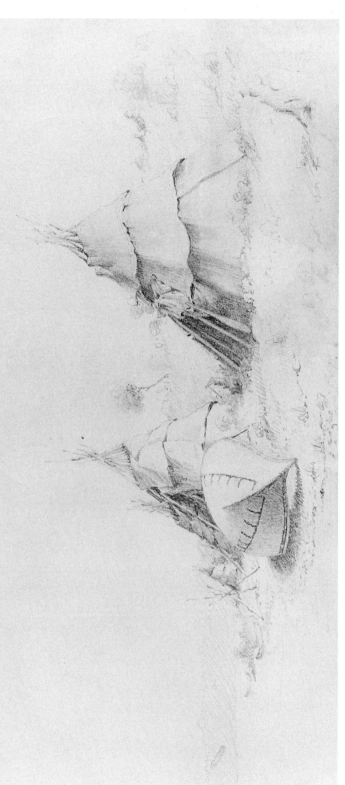

Figure 8.4. "Encampment with conical lodges and canoe", pencil on paper drawing by Paul Kane. (Royal Ontario Museum, Toronto, Canada # 946.15.37.)

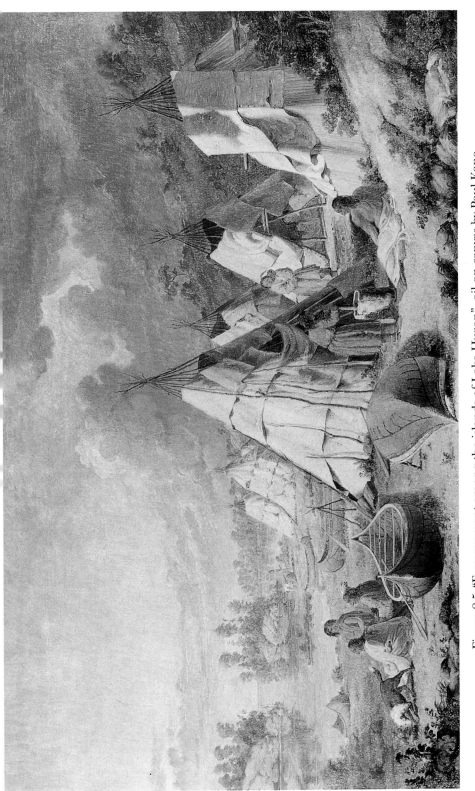

Figure 8.5. "Encampment among the islands of Lake Huron", oil on canvas by Paul Kane. (Royal Ontario Museum, Toronto, Canada # 912.1.8.)

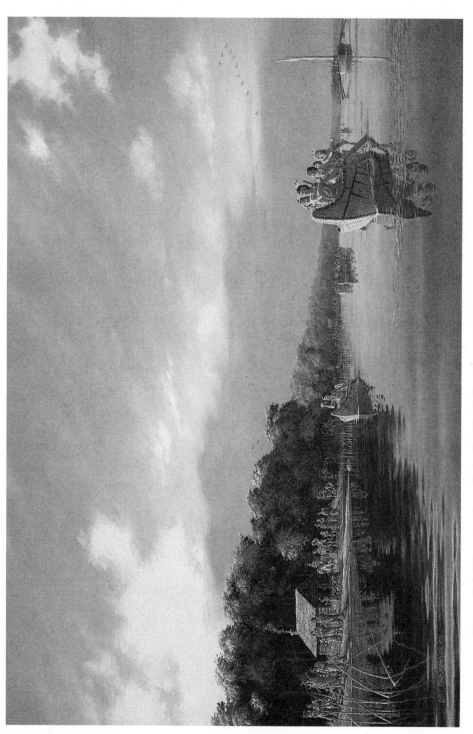

Figure 8.6. "Retreat along Lake St. Clair" October, 1813 by Peter Rindlisbacher. The authors would like to thank Peter Rindlisbacher for permission to reproduce this painting.

related to the creation of Turtle Island-North America. In this respect the canoe is depicted in many Aboriginal creation stories. To illustrate this significance, one such story from Ojibwa mythology is that of the muskrat. In this story the canoe is the huge log on which the Anishinabe, or Original Man, managed to climb after the Great Flood covered the surface of the Earth. Some of the earliest canoes on Turtle Island were, of course, hollowed-out logs.[8] And so the water, and the canoe, came before the land. The canoe provides the vehicle for reaching the four directions and provides the principle of balance connecting the four natural elements of earth, water, air and fire.[9]

The canoe is spiritual; yet it is also a practical form of Amerindian science as well as art. Amerindian technology and science are ecologically-based on knowledge of the natural and spirit worlds.[10] One of the greatest gifts which Aboriginal people brought to the Covenant Chain of Silver was the technology of the birchbark canoe. Birchbark was extremely light and plentiful in the Great Lakes watershed. Moreover, in addition to the making of canoes, the birchbark was used for fuel, the making of lodges as well as maps to guide the traveler in the canoe to her/his destination aided by the star maps at night.[11]

So valuable was this scientific invention that it was soon appropriated by the European visitors for use by missionaries, explorers, the military, professional artists, as well as fur traders.[12] The significance of the canoe in Aboriginal oral traditions and history cannot be overemphasized. It is central to the creation stories, to the cultures

---

[8] Benton Banai in *The Mishomis Book*, pp. 31–33.

[9] McNab, "Introduction", *Circles of Time*, 1999, pp. 1–19.

[10] Dickason, "Art and Amerindian worldviews", in David T. McNab (ed. for *Nin.Da.Waab.Jig.*), *Earth, Water, Air and Fire*, Studies in Canadian Ethnohistory (Waterloo: WLU Press, 1998), pp. 25–26. In this sense every Aboriginal person is at once an artist as well as a scientist.

[11] Schmalz, *Ojibwa*, p. 15.

[12] Wylie, *In the Wilds*, p. 8. This fact was well illustrated on October 15, 1754 when Anthony Henday, a Hudson's Bay Company's trader, met with the Chief of the Blackfoot Confederacy in their Territory and was told that "it was far off, & they could not live with buffalo flesh; and that they could not leave their horses &c and many other obstacles, though all might be got over if they were acquainted with a Canoe; and could eat Fish, which they never do." On the Atlantic seaboard, the Mi'kmaq were excellent at making and using canoes. Nicolas Denys, the seventeenth century French trader, described in 1680 the details of the work that went into the construction of a Mi'kmaq canoe.

providing a balance practically and spiritually as a means—an instrument—of understanding the natural world and providing a means of working within it. Olive Dickason has commented that the "connection between worldviews and art" is "so close that they can be regarded as two aspects of the same reality."[13]

This reality is also continuous and modern. It can be found in the monumental canoe sculpture by Bill Reid "The Spirit of Haida Gwaii" which stands now in front of the Canadian Embassy in Washington, D.C. James Tully has described it as follows:

> Cast in bronze, it recreates a group of thirteen human, animal and bird figures interacting with each other as they head into the unknown in a Haida canoe, under the guidance of Chief Kilstlaai. Wrapped in the skin of the mythical sea wolf and holding a speaker's staff that tells the Haida story of creation.[14]

Tully has drawn on this sculpture for his view of Canada's "strange multiplicity". However, Tully completely misrepresents Bill Reid's "The Spirit of Haida Gwaii" as well as Aboriginal people. There is nothing "strange" about Bill Reid's view of Canada. See Figure 8.2.

The canoe also has a practical everyday function. In this respect, it differs markedly from European-based works of art in which the canoe appears primarily for exotic or local colour usually with the presence of Amerindians against a backdrop of either European urban life or the "wilderness."[15] Above all else, the canoe links the four

---

[13] Dickason, "Art and Amerindian worldviews", in *Earth, Water, Air and Fire*, op. cit., p. 21.

[14] A jade replica of the Black Canoe is also in the Vancouver International Airport. See the photograph in this chapter taken by David T. McNab on January 30, 2000. David is a cousin of Bill Reid, who was a descendant of Dr. John Frederick Kennedy, David's great-great-great uncle. The political philosopher, James Tully in his 1995 book, *Strange Multiplicity, Constitutionalism in an age of diversity*, Cambridge: Cambridge University Press, 1995, makes a contribution to Canadian constitutional and federalist discussions using Bill Reid's canoe sculpture. But Tully's analysis also misses the mark for he has misinterpreted the central figure in the canoe as only a facilitator in constitutional discussions. Perhaps he does not understand the broader spiritual role of the Great Mystery or the story-teller in Aboriginal oral traditions. See pp. xi, xv, 17–34, 202–212. Tully presented his work in the first John Robert Seeley Memorial lectures at Cambridge University in 1994.

[15] Wylie, *In the Wilds*, pp. 8–9. The mid-nineteenth century works of art by Paul Kane is a case in point. They are the subject of a recent noteworthy exhibit of Paul Kane's sketches and oil paintings of which Ken Lister is the curator at the Royal Ontario Museum in Toronto. This article is illustrated, in part, from that exhibit. The authors would like to thank Ken Lister for his advice on Kane and the canoe.

elements of earth, water, air and fire. It is an integral part of Amerindian trade, warfare, diplomacy and economy since the initial encounters in northeastern North America in the fifteenth (Basques fishermen and traders) and sixteenth centuries as well as a central vehicle in Amerindian resistance to the incursions of European Empires.[16]

The Canoe as a Diplomatic Invention:
Gus Wen Tah, The Covenant Chain of Silver

The canoe is the central or focus point to the international relationship that is represented, among others, in the Two Row Wampum belt.[17] Made from wampum shells by Amerindian artists, this belt represented the main gift of Amerindian diplomacy to the European Empires. There is a specific relationship characterized in the Belt. The Belt has two rows of purple wampum on a white background. One row represents the Amerindian Nations; parallel to it is another row which symbolized the European Nations. The two rows are emblematic of two canoes being paddled down a river side by side but never meeting. This relationship was used in diplomacy and trade between Europeans and Aboriginal people, in peace negotiations after warfare. It also was subsequently embodied in the Treaty-making process which included both peace and friendship as well as arrangements regarding uses of lands and natural resources.

The Two Row Wampum embodied the Covenant Chain of Silver and what it represented in the relationship between the English imperial government and the Amerindian Nations. The latter included

---

[16] The holistic significance of the canoe as a central point in the multi-dimensional worlds of Aboriginal people of Canada can be seen in the traveling exhibition "Down from the shimmering sky masks of the Northwest Coast", curated by Peter MacNair, Robert Joseph and Bruce Grenville, December 5, 1998 to February 28, 1998 in Toronto. This exhibit opened at the Vancouver Art Gallery in the summer of 1998 and a catalogue by the same name was published by the Vancouver Art Gallery and Douglas & McIntyre. Central to this exhibit was a canoe made by Henry Hunt, a Kwakwaka'wakw artist, which holds seated masked figures in white. In this regard the canoe represents a vehicle for the transformation of souls from the mortal to the sky world.

[17] This section and subsequent sections are based largely on McNab, "'We joined hands; they were lashed together strongly', the St. Anne Island Treaty of 1796", an unpublished Historical Report prepared by David T. McNab for the Bkejwanong First Nation, dated February 14, 1996. See also "'Water is her lifeblood': The waters of Bkejwanong and the treaty-making process", in *Earth, Water, Air and Fire: Studies in Canadian Ethnohistory* (Wilfrid Laurier University Press, 1998), pp. 35–63.

the Iroquois Confederacy, the Abenaki, Malecite and Mi'kmaq Confederacies as well as the Western Confederacy of Algonquian-speaking peoples such as the Ojibwa, Ottawa (Odawa) and Potawatomi, among others. The wampum itself represented the relationship as one of Peace, Mutual Respect and Trust.[18]

The Covenant Chain was continually renewed by both the English Crown, the Haudenosaunee and the Anishinabe. Later other Amerindian Nations entered into the Covenant Chain as well.[19] For example, Sir William Johnson,[20] the Superintendent General of Indian Affairs for the Northern Department (stationed near Albany on the banks of the Mohawk River), observed its history and significance in 1748 when he met in Council with the Iroquois Confederacy:

> . . . our first Friendship Commenced at the Arrival of the first great Canoe or Vessel at Albany, at which time you were much surprized but finding what it contained pleased you much, being Things for your Purpose, . . .
>
> After this was agreed on and done you made an offer to the Governor to enter into a Bond of Friendship with him and his People which he was so pleased at that he told you he would find a strong Silver Chain which would never break, slip or Rust, to bind you and him in Brothership together, . . .[21]

The canoe was clearly a prominent symbol in the Two Row Wampum and in the Covenant Chain of Silver. For the Iroquoian and Algonkian-speaking Amerindian Nations as well as the European Nations, it continued to be an important fixture of international diplomacy, war

---

[18] Paul Williams, "The chain", L.L.M. Thesis (Osgoode Hall Law School, 1982). In the written record, the Covenant Chain dates back at least to the mid-seventeenth century to a Treaty, which was entered into on September 24, 1664, between the Haudenosaunee and the English Crown at Albany, at the forks of the Mohawk and Hudson Rivers in present-day New York state. The Treaty stated that the English Crown, replacing the relationship that the Haudenosaunee formerly had with the Dutch, which would provide "the Indian Princes" and "their subjects" with the same goods and trade "in the future" as they formerly had with the Dutch. The written documents relating to the Covenant Chain of Silver can be found in *Documents relative to the Colonial History of the State of New York*, ed. by E.B. O'Callaghan, Vol. VII (Albany: Weed, Parsons and Company, Printers, 1856); *The Papers of Sir William Johnson*, Prepared for publication by Milton W. Hamilton (Albany: The University of the State of New York, 1953).

[19] "Anishnabek News", Nipissing First Nation, May–June, 1995.

[20] Julian Gwyn, "Sir William Johnson", *Dictionary of Canadian Biography*, Volume IV (Toronto: University of Toronto Press, 1979), pp. 394–398.

[21] Hamilton, *Sir William Johnson*, p. 158; National Archives of Canada (NAC), Record Group 10, Vol. 1822, p. 35. See also Ian K. Steele, *Warpaths Invasions of North America* (New York: Oxford University Press, 1994), especially Chapter 4, pp.

and trade throughout the shifting conflicts and realignments wrought by the European incursions in the seventeenth and eighteenth centuries. Above all, the Chain showed the continuing sovereignty and independence of Aboriginal Nations in an international context. (See Figure 8.3.)

Borders of the Birchbark Country

As an invention of Aboriginal science, the canoe both created an initial golden age of Amerindian wealth through trade[22] and considerably slowed the process of European expansion into northeastern North America from the seventeenth to the mid-nineteenth centuries. It also effectively prevented the conquest of the Amerindian Nations and eventually provided one of the ways in which Aboriginal peoples have continued to survive and finally flourish once again in the late twentieth century. The birchbark canoe was the centrepiece of the relationship between the Amerindian Nations and the European empires in international matters, especially diplomacy, trade and warfare.

In terms of trade, the canoe was terribly significant. It made possible the fur trade of the northeastern and northwestern interior-including the St. Lawrence-Great Lakes basin and connecting waterways, the Saint John and adjacent river valleys to the east and the Hudson and James Bay watersheds to the north. Indeed this trade became the primary inland commercial activity in which the Europeans were involved in the seventeenth and eighteenth centuries.

59–79; Colin G. Calloway, *Crown and Calumet, British-Indian Relations, 1783–1815*, Norman: University of Oklahoma Press, 1987; *The American Revolution in Indian Country, Crisis and Diversity in Native American Communities*, Cambridge: Cambridge University Press, 1995.

[22] As late as 1835 the canoe was still in use for trade in Chicago. See Ralph C. Frese, "The Canadians and the Canadian canoe in the opening of the American Midwest", in *The Canoe and Canadian Cultures*, ed. John Jennings, Bruce W. Hodgins and Doreen Small (Toronto: Natural Heritage, 1999). Also note on the canoe and on traditional canoe travel the following: Timothy J. Kent, *Birchbark Canoes of the Fur Trade*, 2 Vols., Ossineke: MI. Silver Fox Enterprises, 1997; Kenneth G. Roberts and Philip Shackleton, *The Canoe: A History of the Craft from Panama to the Arctic* (Toronto: Macmillan, 1983); David Gidmark, *The Algonquin Birchbark Canoe* (Aylesbury: Shire Publications, 1974); Bruce W. Hodgins and Gwyneth Hoyle, *Canoeing North into the Unknown: A Record of River Travel, 1874–1974* (Toronto: Natural Heritage, 1994); Richard Pope, *Superior Illusions* (Toronto: Natural Heritage Books, 1998); Edward S. Rogers and Donald B., Smith (eds.), *Aboriginal Ontario: Historical Perspectives on the First Nations* (Toronto Dundurn Press, 1994).

Yet it was a partnership in fur in which the indigenous people long remained ascendant. Only latterly, in the late nineteenth century, did they became displaced economically.

In the international context of military alliances and geopolitics, to the French certainly and to a large degree the English, the canoe was the primary vehicle of travel and communication. The varieties of trade was a major enticement for these alliances. Canoes carried diverse freight as well as the mail from Europe via the entrepots of Quebec City, Montreal, Toronto and Detroit inland along the Great Lakes waterways for almost three hundred years until the coming of roads and railways in the mid to late nineteenth century. Council Fires were held and treaties were made along these same waterways. Representatives of Amerindian and European Nations were summoned to them by Amerindian messengers or runners traveling in fast express canoes with strings of wampum.

The canoe and the waterways (nastawgan) became synonymous. It is significant that, in the treaty-making process since the late nineteenth century and down to the present, the Anishinabe Nations did not cede or in any way relinquish their rights to the waterways, including the beds and the waters of the Great Lakes, on the northern side of the line-what we now know territorially as the modern nation-state of Canada.[23]

The territorial limits of canoe transportation must be carefully defined. For what became English-speaking American lands on the northeast coast, the canoe could only be used for parts of what became Maine-Vermont-New York, perhaps some border areas along Lake Champlain and the Mohawk-Hudson rivers. At the same time its use included all of the North Atlantic region, including Newfoundland. Apart from the very small and narrow valley of the St. Lawrence, and a very few pocket valleys in Nova Scotia and in what became New Brunswick, European agricultural and settlement land was insignificant. This remained true at least until after the end of the War of the American Revolution.[24]

---

[23] McNab, "'Water is her lifeblood'", pp. 35–63.

[24] The territoriality of First Nations was centered on the water and the trade routes and the portages which connected them. At Bkejwanong today their lands are laid out in long, narrow strips from the water into the interior of their islands. This is definitely not the influence of the French seigneurial system of land-holding since these lands were not subject to any French influence at Bkejwanong. Moreover, the lands of the Three Fires Confederacy, as at Bkejwanong, were in

Most of the violence which can be documented from the written records of Europeans relates to European desires for wealth through trade and the quarrels of European empires—the Spanish, French and English—bent of expansion in Europe, North America and beyond. Without denying Amerindian participation in this violence in the seventeenth and eighteenth centuries, it should also be put into historical context. In this respect, in its sheer magnitude, it pales in comparison to the two World Wars resulting from European warfare of the twentieth century, or earlier.

Canoes were also vitally used in both pre-and post-contact inter-tribal warfare. Even before the early eighteenth century this fighting was seldom between the "Europeans" and "Indians." Instead, at first, this forest warfare, in which the canoe and the bow and arrow were much more effective than the gun, was engaged in by one or more Amerindian groups frequently linked to the French imperial power and one or more Amerindian groups sometimes co-joined with either the Dutch (to 1664) or the English empires. In spite of their expansionist reputation, the Iroquois, especially the Mohawk and the Seneca, frequently acted alone. Rarely, if ever, did the "Indians" act just as auxiliaries or pawns; usually they were the senior partners. They were sovereign; they were active and independent participants. In the eighteenth century the French put geopolitical goals above trade matters, but the enemy was certainly not the Amerindians. The French wished to confine the Anglo-Americans to the Atlantic coast, limiting their expansionism to territory, east of the Appalachian mountains. So, as W.J. Eccles has so strongly argued,[25] Harold Innis's

---

the same form and laid out along the Detroit River downstream from Bkejwanong and Lake St. Clair. Here it appears that, although there is a later (early eighteenth century) French settlement, the form of territoriality was the same as at Bkejwanong. Perhaps this system of territoriality was also, even in evidence for the lands along the St. Lawrence River and may also have been an Amerindian scientific invention, owing their very existence to the waterways and the canoe. Is it possible that this Amerindian form of land holding, like the canoe, the snowshoe and the toboggan, may have been copied from the Amerindian village structure of land-holding in which the premium was put on access of families to water and the canoe? For southwestern Ontario it should be noted that it was only later in the late eighteenth century that the European forms of land-holding in the forms of a rectangle and a square replaced on European maps of settlement the ribbons of land laid out along the Amerindian waters linking the circular "onegaming" (portage routes) with both the many family villages, resource-rich gathering territories and the trading routes which linked them intricately.

[25] W.J. Eccles, "A belated review of Harold Adams Innis's *The Fur Trade in Canada*, in *Essays in New France* (Toronto: Oxford University Press, 1987), pp. 61–78.

assertion that the fur trade and the canoe created the outer territorial boundaries of what became national Canada, are not correct for
the early period. The thesis is certainly wrong before 1784 and probably before 1796, and perhaps before 1816–21. In this sense Canada,
which is derived from the Mohawk/Iroquoian word Kanata, meaning a country connected by a series of villages, is territorially speaking a series of meeting grounds within First Nations' territories. This
is still true today, and it remains the bedrock of the political entity
which we call Canada.[26] It was the expansionist American nation
state which took away the southern part of the birchbark canoe
country from the Amerindian Nations and the future Canada.

In the first half of the eighteenth century there was a French-
Anishinabe "empire," or more correctly termed a diplomatic alliance
system, which was predominantly Anishinabe in numbers, politics
and land ownership. This system stretched geographically in an arc
from the Gulf and the River St. Lawrence through Detroit and the
old Midwest southward to the Ohio valley and down the Mississippi
to New Orleans. The English-Americans were hemmed into the
broad Atlantic coastal strip. In the old northeast lay Acadia-Nova
Scotia, Cape Breton Island and Newfoundland. This area, now called
the four Canadian provinces of New Brunswick, Nova Scotia, Prince
Edward Island and Newfoundland, was fought over by the English
and French empires until 1763. Also, on the inside, or on the broad
face, of the arc, later to be known as upstate New York there was
the lands of the Haudenosaunee (also known as the Iroquois Confederacy also as the Five, then the Six, Nations). North and northwest was the vast Rupert's Land comprising the Cree, the Dene, the
Blackfoot Confederacy and the Metis Nation. This huge area was
as late as 1800 less than 1% English-Orkney-Highland Scot. In spite
of its Royal Charter of 1670 asserting exclusive English trading rights,
the Hudson's Bay Company did not, and never could, rule or even
claim ownership over Rupert's Land; much of this land was only
vaguely within an English sphere of influence.

The European metropoles had, of course, the population and the
military power to sustain centuries of expansion and wealth-building
which wrought great economic and cultural changes in northeastern
North America as well as to Europe itself. But, in the seventeenth
century, few in Europe could have foreseen this great transforma-

---

[26] John Jennings, "Introduction", *Canexus II*, 1999.

tion. The canoe, the fur trade, the topography and the climate slowed down this complex phenomenon in the St. Lawrence Valley and even more broadly across the northeast. Given the geography, demography and social, political and cultural structures of Amerindians at contact, there was no concerted attempt to repel the new migrants. Except for recurring French-Mohawk conflict in the seventeenth century, there was little hostility on the frontiers of contact. There was little hostility, but there was considerable condescension and indifference; often the newcomers never welcomed any viewpoint other than their own without attempting to understand the Amerindian perspectives.

The evidence shows that Amerindian groups sought from the initial encounters to use Europeans for their own social and political purposes. From this perspective, questions of European military superiority or transoceanic transportation capacity were almost irrelevant. The Amerindian realization that Europeans may not be controllable was highly localized, coming at widely different times. The timing of decimation by Eurasian pathogens, while personally major and very tragic, seemed to be to the Europeans almost irrelevant. As a result the Amerindian Nations of the Great Lakes did not show signs of feeling seriously threatened in their control of their territories until the late eighteenth century. Further north and northwest this threat came very much later.

The place of the birchbark canoe in this history needs to be considered like that of the other technologies, as a dependent variable. Everyone within the birch forest zone had access to the canoe before and after the Europeans came. And the canoes, of all diverse shapes and sizes, were also manufactured trading items. So the Anishinabe groups within the birch forest zone traded canoes with their neighbours to the south where the birch forest ended. European traders bought or likewise were caught up in this trade. The French trade would have been impossible along the interior waterways without the large-scale freight canoe as the only method of cheap transportation.[27]

The French empire of trade, involving fur and much more in return for kettles, ornamental beads, axes, guns and blankets, was

---

[27] This is true likewise of all Amerindian tools and artwork, including the snowshoe, the toboggan and the moccasin and other leather clothing which was made for the weather and climate of northeastern North America.

based on the hull of the Anishinabe birchbark canoe. But the French, like the English, did not have a monopoly over the "Indian" trade. The reality was hardly a monopoly. French traders at their western posts sometimes had a limited form of control over the French trade through a licensing system. This system kept other French traders out of the area but did not make any impact on their major competitors, the Amerindian traders and the Anglo-Americans who had an extensive supply of English goods. The only significant advantage that the French had was the willingness of the Great Lakes Anishinabe Nations to accept the trade alliance with the French, including the French posts throughout, and to tolerate for so long (until well into the eighteenth century) the French refusal, militarily, to allow English traders beyond the Ohio valley. The relationship was very complex, but if there had been no such thing as a birch tree, would the circumstances have differed greatly? It seems reasonable to imagine that Amerindians of the northern waterways would have invented some other similarly ingenious and adaptable conveyance. But the birch tree did exist. So, the birchbark canoe was very important.

On the Atlantic side of the continent the diverse Algonkian-speaking Nations (Mi'kmaq, Malecite, Algonquin, Innu) and the Iroquois Confederacy, held the birchbark canoe as a wonderful technological invention and form of art. The canoe rendered the Gulf of the St. Lawrence very much like the Mediterranean in former times. Island-hopping, the Mi'kmaq moved with relative ease around the Gulf of the St. Lawrence from New Brunswick to Nova Scotia, Cape Breton Island and Newfoundland. The Europeans simply did not have anything that could compare with the canoe for inshore travel or for inland water travel.[28]

We now use the phrase "fur trade" to include as an internal part to it the beaver, the canoe and the paddle in intercultural diplomacy. We also include a French and English opposition to far interior agrarian settlement except for the post-1800 pemmican-buffalo-based Metis culture in the Red River valley and the adjacent prairies. The culture of the Metis Nation also developed, in part, as a response to the fur trade which needed pemmican made from buffalo meat

---

[28] This was certainly true at least until the invention or local re-invention of the Hudson's Bay Company's York boat in the early nineteenth century; even the York boat was relatively clumsy compared with the birchbark canoe and had serious weight problems when it came to the necessity of portaging through much of the interior.

and used for the vital provisioning of the canoe voyages and the trading posts. And even part of the Metis Nation of the Great Lakes was built on the birchbark canoe with trade as its backbone.

While and wherever the canoe reigned supreme, Aboriginal people were not marginalized and certainly not conquered. Instead of a "partnership in fur,"[29] perhaps, given the now extensive literature on the significance of the Covenant Chain of Silver as a diplomatic device for alliances, it would be more accurate to say "an alliance in fur, peace, commerce and war." In this arrangement Amerindians were, according to European expectations, supposed to remain "Indians," meaning as "savages," somehow, in spite of their scientific utilitarian knowledge, frozen primitively in time.[30] Pioneers, farmers, and pastoralists and pathogens were usually joint, but distant, threats and so frequently were the missionaries.

The Metis and the French Canadians developed for bulk transport the large birchbark freight canoes so central to the fur trade based until 1821 on the St. Lawrence and Ottawa valleys and the Great Lakes.[31] There, the great 36-foot canots du Maitre or Montreal canoes and the 26-foot canots du Nord or North canoes, the latter used in the pays d'en haut, were made along the St. Lawrence. Many of the actual builders were either Metis or French Canadians. Until after the English conquest of New France the management and control of the trade were primarily French Canadian. Thereafter, the ownership and management of the boats and the trade were in the hands of Scottish merchants based in Montreal. Whoever were the owners they all used Amerindian science and technology. Only the size varied according to the job required in the trade. They continued to be staffed by Anishinabe, by Metis, by resident Mohawks and French Canadians.

To the north the Hudson's Bay Company's personnel residing in their posts along the Bays rarely traveled inland before the 1780's. They expected the Amerindians to paddle down in huge canoe flotillas. There is now an extensive literature on that topic, and the work of the historical geographer Arthur Ray is critical to understanding how significant was the active participation of the Amerindians,

---

[29] Daniel Francis and Toby Morantz, *Partners in Fur* (Kingston and Montreal: McGill-Queen's University Press, 1983).

[30] Dickason, *The Myth of the Savage and the Beginnings of French Colonialism in the Americas* (Edmonton: The University of Alberta Press, 1997 (1994)).

[31] Kent, *Birchbark Canoes*, pp. 37–115.

by means of the canoe, in manipulating and controlling this trade.[32] After 1777 competition from Scottish pedlars and merchants from Montreal forced the Bay traders and agents to move inland.

The canoe is to northeastern North America, and certainly to Canada, what the horse is to the United States.[33] The Amerindian canoe and its linked "Indian" trade, enhanced by the fur trade, enhanced the economic life of Aboriginal people from the fifteenth through to the twentieth century.[34] This process was markedly different from that experienced in the Thirteen Colonies or in Australia as well as the Spanish and Portuguese colonies to the south in Central and South America. The Amerindian canoe and northern ecology-topography were central to Amerindian relations with the newcomers. The canoe postponed severely the overall impact of European cultural change on the North American landscape and with it, the Amerindian Nations who lived there.

Seventeenth Century Conflicts and Realignments

The history of the canoe, the interaction with and resistance by Amerindian people to European empires has been cast primarily through the lenses of the written records left by the French and the English recorders of European history. What has loomed large from this European-based perspective, is the incidence of wars and the movements of peoples on the "Canadian frontier." This interpretation is based largely on seeing history, like the European concept of "wilderness," as if it were a blank page of white paper.[35] Recalling the history of the canoe changes this perspective radically.

---

[32] A.J. Ray, *Indians in the Fur Trade, Their Role as Hunters, Trappers and Middlemen in the Lands Southwest of Hudson Bay, 1660–1870*, Toronto: University of Toronto Press, 1974, pp. 51–60. According to James Knight at York Factory, 172 Amerindian canoes arrived in 1715, mainly paddled down the Hays River by Cree and Assiniboine; the pattern continued until about 1780.

[33] Jennings, "Introduction", *The Canoe in Canadian Cultures*, 1999.

[34] It enabled the Amerindians to continue to resist and survive and ultimately flourish again by the late twentieth century.

[35] This presentist view of history is self-serving, recalling the conquests of the landscape—in which Amerindians appear to be invisible—by European explorers and settlers. Aboriginal people and their place are minimized in numbers and in action while often ignoring the impact of disease, trade and the seasonal movements by Aboriginal people within their Territories. Whether from the perspectives of the French or the English records, the result is the same; Aboriginal people are

A more inclusive interpretation of the process of historical development would center on the Amerindian-controlled trade, trading networks rather than concentrating only on warfare and conquest in large European wars.[36] In fact, as one historian has pointed out recently, the Amerindian Nations inhabiting the St. Lawrence waterway system, the Atlantic region as well as the Hudson and James Bay areas, were not conquered.[37] Using birchbark canoes and defensive guerrilla tactics in warfare, they could win battles and wars against European land-based armies in the forests of northeastern North America and along its vast waterway systems. Long before the "man with a large hat" came, however, the Anishinabe had been trading among themselves for centuries. The trade had its origins within their society and economy.[38] This trade would not have been possible but for the birchbark canoe. The Indian trade with the French flourished throughout the Great Lakes basin and elsewhere in the northeastern part of North America.[39] Trading places were located at the confluences of the Great Lakes and rivers such as at Cape Breton Island, Halifax, St. John river valley, Wendake (Quebec City), Montreal, Allumette Island on the Ottawa river, Fort Ontario (Oswego, New York), Fort Niagara, Toronto, Detroit, Sault Ste. Marie and Michilimackinac, just to mention some of the most prominent.

The military events of the seventeenth century in northeastern North America could be characterized as one of the initial invasion north of the Great Lakes by the Iroquois Confederacy (the Onondaga, Seneca, Cayuga, Mohawk, Delaware and the Oneida). This conflict has been called the "trade or beaver wars." Initiated by a series of trading relationships which flowed from the diplomatic alliances between the Dutch and the Amerindian Nations, this warfare was between the French and the English empires.

---

seen to be like wolves or other animals in the wilderness—as nomads and beasts—and not as human beings.

[36] These still exist but have become less visible, or have gone "underground", like the potlatch for most of the twentieth century, to prevent prosecution by government authorities) Douglas L. Cole, *Captured Heritage, The Scramble for Northwest Coast Artifacts* (Vancouver: Douglas & McIntyre, 1985).

[37] Steele, *Warpaths*, pp. 246–247.

[38] Benton-Banai, *The Mishomis Book*, pp. 103–113.

[39] Nicolas Denys, *The Description and Natural History of the Coasts of North America (Acadia)*, Translated and Edited, with a Memoir of the author, collateral documents, and a reprint of the original, by William F. Ganong, Ph.D. (Toronto: The Champlain Society, 1908), pp. 448–449.

The most famous of these events occurred in 1609 one year after Quebec was founded. The French alliance, which included a force of Algonquin, Huron and Montagnais, was cemented militarily when Samuel de Champlain canoed into the very heart of the Iroquois Territory in what is now New York state and at Ticonderoga defeated the Iroquois. Champlain, using European technology—an arquebus-killed two of the Iroquois chiefs, thereby at once consolidated the French alliance with these Nations and also ignited a series of wars that lasted through the century.[40] The Iroquois became the allies of the Dutch and then the English.

Champlain understood the significance of the canoe when he wrote back to his French superiors: "With the canoe of the savages, one may travel freely and quickly throughout the country as well as up the little rivers as up the large rivers. So that by directing one's course with the help of the savages and their canoes, a man might see all that is to be seen, good or bad, within the space of a year or two." To consolidate their presence, the French sent both explorers such as Etienne Brule and priests into the northern interior of the Great Lakes. In 1615 Champlain himself traveled to Georgian Bay and joined again a major Anishinabe raid on the Iroquois south of Lake Ontario. French travels through what became known as Canada could only have been accomplished by using Anishinabe guides who were able to "read" the landscape, make birchbark maps and who possessed technology of which the canoe was of paramount importance for most of the year. In the Canadian winter, canoes were replaced on the frozen land and waterways by Anishinabe toboggans and snowshoes, both of which enabled Europeans to adapt to the new land that they had encountered.[41] Failure to use Anishinabe technology would have meant defeat for the Europeans who soon recognized the principle that the land is, as Gary G. Potts has frequently asserted, the boss. Failure to show proper respect would result in death.[42]

One of the greatest inroads that the French made in the seventeenth century was their attempt to christianize the large primarily

---

[40] Illustrations of this battle show birchbark canoes prominently on the shores of Lake Champlain while the actual fighting is taking place at the edge of the forest.
[41] Frese, "Canadian canoe", 1999.
[42] Gary Potts, "Bushman and dragonfly", *Journal of Canadian Studies*, "Refiguring Wilderness", 33(2), Summer, 1998, p. 195. This principle has not changed over the past centuries and, as a result, most non-Aboriginal Canadians live in a series of

corn-growing Huron Nation on the southern coast of Georgian Bay. By 1640 they had founded their mission at Sainte Marie among the Hurons and it was followed by the mission of Saint Peter at Manitoulin Island among the Ojibwa and Ottawa (Odawa) along the shores of Lake Huron and Georgian Bay. All of these Jesuit establishments were developed and maintained only through the use of the waterways and canoes. Even the early postal communications were accomplished by using Anishinabe modes of transport in both summer and winter, a situation that did not change until the coming of roads in the nineteenth century.

These Anishinabe-European encounters had immediate benefits in trade and diplomacy. Using birchbark canoes the French explorers and traders were able to bypass the natural barriers of Niagara and make valuable trading connections into the Ohio and the Mississippi valleys. The long-term cost of these encounters was an extremely large loss of population in Amerindian Nations through disease and warfare.

The best example was the near destruction of the Huron Nation in the mid-seventeenth century. At first weakened by disease through contact with the French and then partly exhausted by Iroquois raids and dispersed from Huronia to Christian Island, the Huron moved to a Reserve at Wendake (Village Huron, near Quebec City), and also west to an area on the shores of Lake Huron and eventually to a large Reserve (in 1790) adjacent to the Detroit River, close to what is now Windsor, Ontario. Even today at Wendake, the Huron Nation has only a very small land base and a small population of 300 citizens on-reserve and less than 200 others scattered across Canada and the United States. The Huron Nation paid an inordinately huge price for their diplomatic and trade alliance with the French empire in the early seventeenth century.

Great allied French-Anishinabe canoe voyages and canoe raids continued. There were the vast commercial expeditions by Radisson and Groseillers. Then in 1686 there was the staggering snowshoe and canoe expedition with a mixed troop of 100 persons overland from Temiscamingue on the Ottawa to James Bay where French

cities (large villages) in a ribbon within one hundred miles of the Canadian-American border. Amerindians still live north of this ribbon and are mostly in a majority in this vast geographical space.

and Amerindian forces captured and sacked several English Bay posts.[43]

Canoes played a large part in the history of the Ojibwa in the seventeenth century. The Ojibwa historian Kahgegagahbowh (George Copway) recorded that

> our nation has never been conquered; and have maintained their ground wherever they have conquered. The Sax [also variously Sacs, Sauks] tribe have tried their ingenuity, power and bravery, to drive them from the south shore of Lake Superior. The Hurons mustered their warriors against the aggressions made by the Ojibwa nation. Their war canoes were once directed against the Ojibwa nation, but they were obliged to turn back, and flee for protection, to the Shawnee nation.[44]

A major battle between the Mississauga-Ojibwa (and their French allies though the latter's military role was negligible), with the Iroquois and the English took place at the mouth of the Saugeen river on the Bruce Peninsula in the 1690's:

> . . . the combined forces gathered in two parties, one at Lake St. Clair and the other at Sault Ste. Marie, seven hundred canoes being there assembled. This latter party divided into two bands. One advanced on the enemy by way of the Ottawa valley, while the other proceeded to Penetanguishene. The Lake St. Clair division at the same time came up the east coast of Lake Huron to the mouth of the Saugeen River, where a fierce battle was fought with the Iroquois, who ultimately gave way and fled before the savage onslaught of the Ojebwa.[45]

Another battle was fought on the banks of the Thames river near Lake St. Clair, involving 400 canoes of the Three Fires Confederacy alone, against the Seneca which found that Confederacy once again the victors.[46] Peter Schmalz has described, from the oral tradition, this large battle—the battle of Skull Mound (dating from the early 1690's)—as having ". . . 400 canoes, each containing eight warriors, were involved in a two-pronged attack in the St. Clair region."

---

[43] W.A. Kenyon and J.R. Turnbull, *The Battle for James Bay 1686*, Toronto: Macmillan, 1971. For voyages by canoes during the French regime see Roberts and Shackleton, "The French period", in *The Canoe*, pp. 167–96.

[44] A. LaVonne Brown Ruoff and Donald B. Smith (eds.), *Life, Letters & Speeches, George Copway (Kahgegahbowh)*, (Lincoln and London: University of Nebraska Press, 1997), p. 90.

[45] Schmalz, *Ojibwa*, p. 22.

[46] *Ibid.*, p. 23.

This battle was followed, also in the 1690's, by further conflict using war canoes on the Otonabee River (Peterborough-Trent Valley-eastern Ontario) area. There is a vivid description of this encounter between the Mississaugas and the Iroquois from the Paudash oral tradition. From Lake Couchiching the main body in birchbark canoes

> proceeded along the portage . . . to Balsam Lake; the other party went south to Toronto. After various skirmishes the Mohawks continued their retreat down the valley of the Otonabee, and on Rice Lake. They made their first real stand at Nogojiwanong, which was the original name of the town of Peterborough, meaning the place at the end of the rapids; Katchewanock, above the present village of Lakefield, meaning the beginning of the rapids. A sharp skirmish took place here upon what is now known as Campbellford . . . After great preparation, an attack was made by the Mississaugas, both by land and water, and the Mohawks were driven after the battle, in which no less than one thousand warriors were slain, down to Rice Lake to what is now known as Roche's Point . . .[47]

These, and other Ojibwa/Mississauga victories which drove the Iroquois out of the northern side of the Great Lakes by 1700, all involved large numbers of canoes.[48]

These canoe victories occurred in spite of the superior technological firepower possessed by the Iroquois. Guerrilla tactics, aided and abetted by the mobility of the birchbark canoe, led to the realignment of power in what later became southern Ontario. The Ojibwa/Mississaugas solidified their hold on their ancient territories recovering them from the earlier Iroquois incursions. By means of the birchbark canoe the Iroquois were pushed out of what became southern Ontario, except for two small villages at Oswegatchie and St. Regis (Akwesasne).[49]

Treaties of Montreal and Albany of 1701

By the end of the seventeenth century, the Iroquois could only sue for peace with their Anishinabe and French enemies and a treaty

---

[47] *Ibid.*, p. 27.

[48] These battles also occurred "along the shore and the islands of Georgian Bay and Lake Huron" adjacent to the Bruce Peninsula, and around present-day Walkerton, Indian Hill near the Teeswater River, at Wadi-weediwon, now Owen Sound, and White Cloud Island in Colpoy Bay.

[49] Schmalz, *Ojibwa*, pp. 25–30.

was entered into at Montreal among the Five Nations and the French in 1701. By its terms, the Iroquois were no longer a military factor north of the Great Lakes.[50] One of the major results of this canoe warfare was to shift the French influence south and west and to consolidate the English empire's hold on James and Hudson Bay and the fur trade of that region. This was also a major factor in the demise of the French empire in the Seven Years Wars (1755–63), when the French tried to take over the Ohio valley from the Seneca and the encroaching Virginians.

The Treaty of Montreal of 1701 ratified peace between the French Crown and the First Nations which included both the Western or Lake Confederacy Algonkian-speakers and the Iroquois Confederacies in a tripartite format. This occurred before the Treaty of Albany of 1701 between the English Crown and the Iroquois Confederacy. The Treaty of Montreal reaffirmed the Covenant Chain of Silver and, with it, the strong diplomatic relationship between the French Crown and the Algonquian-speaking Nations of the Great Lakes.[51]

For the French this Treaty bought peace with the Iroquois Confederacy until 1746. Ojibwa and Ottawa fur traders were allowed to go to Albany to market their wares. As Schmalz has pointed out, the significance of the Montreal Treaty was profound: "In return for the Iroquois Confederacy's recognition of their occupancy of southern Ontario and for an 'open path' to Albany, the Ojibwa offered peace."[52] That same year the Treaty of Albany (between the English and the Iroquois) sought to maintain the status quo north of the Great Lakes. The intent of these Treaties was from the Amerindian

---

[50] Eccles, "Belated review", and "Sovereignty-association, 1500–1783", in *Essays*, pp. 61–78; 156–181.

[51] O'Callaghan (ed.), *Documents*, IX, pp. 722–725; Steele, *Warpaths*, pp. 148–149. On page 149, Steele has an illustration of a wampum belt from the McCord Museum of Canadian History in Montreal which is "said to represent a clause from the 'Great Peace' between the Five Nations and the French, 1701". Professor Steele describes the Treaties, as follows: ". . . Preliminaries of a peace with New France and a virtual Five Nation capitulation to the western tribes were negotiated in the summer of 1700, as was a renewal of the covenant chain with the English. The famous Montreal meeting of July 1701 brought some thirteen hundred representatives of thirty-one tribes allied with the French, together with the French and the Five Nations to ratify the 'Great Peace'."

[52] "The Five Nations, in their enfeebled state, had no alternative and they accepted. In these negotiations, the Ojibwa and the English won, and the French and the Iroquois lost." Schmalz, *Ojibwa*, p. 31.

Nations' perspective primarily one of peace and friendship, recognizing that it was necessary to have stability, peace and good trading relations. For the French empire this objective also included their attempts to keep all of their trade away from Albany. The Amerindian trade was by this time too lucrative in both fish and furs to have it disrupted by incessant warfare which was continually being provoked by European imperial rivalries. European alliances with Amerindian Nations also intensified the state and fundamental character of war. They also highlighted the significance of the birchbark canoe in that trade.

The longer term consequences of these Treaties were also of significance. Perhaps for the first time, but not the last, the French won recognition by the Iroquois Confederacy and the Lakes Confederacy as mediators in the international disputes between the Amerindian Nations and the European empires. Even though the Iroquois Confederacy still resisted the Algonquin traders at Albany, some were permitted to trade there. The Iroquois Confederacy attempted to maintain their middleman position in the trade. This economic buffer for the French was a relief and helped to maintain the status quo in the Great Lakes, as perceived by the French empire of trade. But the French still had a dilemma requiring some hostility by the Iroquois Confederacy towards the Lakes Confederacy and to accomplish this objective the French encouraged distrust surreptitiously, in spite of their official imperial role as mediators, so that their position would be maintained and imperial aims secured. Until 1715 there was a critical problem for the French as a result of the depressed markets for pelts, especially beaver, in France. The Lakes Confederacy of Nations went more to the Iroquois to sell their furs, a development partially offset by hostilities of the War of the Spanish Succession which helped to maintain the French alliance system with the Lakes Confederacy at war with the English empire.

The Treaty of Utrecht of 1713 and its Aftermath

The War of the Spanish Succession (1702–1713) pitted the French against the English empires in northeastern North America and it affected again the relations with the Amerindian Nations. In the end there were no winners and losers in this encounter—at least in North America, as the Treaty of Utrecht illustrated.

Signed at Utrecht in Holland by the representatives of the French and the English Empires, this Treaty was made to end a European war. The King of France, Louis XIV, himself was directly involved in the negotiations. But it had important repercussions for North America and for the northern Amerindian Nations in particular—the Cree, Mi'kmaq, Malecite and the other Algonkian-speaking peoples of northeastern North America.[53] The key point was that trade, including the natural resources of fish and fur in the Atlantic area and in James and Hudson Bay, and with it the birchbark canoe, remained paramount. Both trades were dependent on water transport and canoes. It also recognized the status quo antebellum of the large strategic waterways which were vital for trading purposes. Utrecht was not an Indian Treaty, and Amerindian Nations were not notified or consulted about it.[54]

After 1715 the pelt market also revived for the French traders. In order to ensure that the Treaty of Utrecht clause permitting English access to the west would remain a dead letter, the French began again to expand their network of trade/garrisoned posts in the Great Lakes theater and beyond, inciting the Nations to raid and pillage any English traders they found there. These actions led to confrontations with the English governors of New York, who in the 1720's tried to challenge the French hold on the west, but in the end did not succeed. More effective in eroding French influence in the west were independent Amerindian movements in the Ohio valley in the 1730's.[55]

Further north and northwest the Cree Nation's relationship to the fur trade of the Hudson's Bay Company remained unchanged. The

---

[53] Dale Miquelon, *New France 1701–1744 "A Supplement to Europe"*, The Canadian Centenary Series, Volume 4 (Toronto: McClelland and Stewart, 1987), pp. 51–52.

[54] McNab, "Fragments of time: The Mi'kmaq nation and Ktaqamkuk, 'The place of fog'", unpublished Historical Report prepared for the Federation of Newfoundland Indians, dated April 16, 1996. One major result was that part of the Mi'kmaq Nation's territory—Ktaqamkuk (which included Newfoundland and Cape Breton Island)—was cut in two. The English Crown proceeded to justify its take-over of the Island of Newfoundland since 1713 by denying that Ktaqamkuk existed and that the Mi'kmaq Nation had no Aboriginal rights or title. The Mi'kmaq seemingly "became" fragments of European history. However, they remained in their Territory residing on Cape Breton Island and Newfoundland and continued their resource activities and trade using their canoes and other means of Amerindian knowledge and technology to resist and indeed to survive to this day.

[55] For an analysis of the impact of trade in the aftermath of Utrecht and the economic tension between French post commanders and merchants, discussed below,

large threat of the French empire either north overland through the continent or by means of the northern Arctic routes was gone. The dominant Cree role both as middlemen and trappers in that trade continued well beyond the eighteenth century and even after the Company established its inland posts. Here the canoe reigned supreme as the major source of water transport for more than two centuries. The fur trade there was still important in 1972.

But Utrecht was not to be the last time the French and the English Crowns would attempt to carve up northeastern North America to the detriment of the interests of the Amerindian Nations. The European empires remained at the edges of the four primary waterway approaches to northeastern North America while the Amerindian Nations controlled the interior. These approaches included the Arctic Ocean into Hudson and James Bay, the eastern Atlantic seaboard of the Thirteen colonies into the Hudson and Mohawk rivers, the Gulf of the St. Lawrence into the St. Lawrence River and the Great Lakes waterway system into the interior.

The Atlantic Region After Utrecht

In spite of the Treaty of Utrecht the Mi'kmaq were still attacking English ships on the coastal seas. Two years after Utrecht was signed the Mi'kmaq found out from the English officers about Utrecht. In response, they protested to the French governor at Louisbourg who replied that Louis XIV "... knew full well that the lands on which he tread, you possess them for all time. The King of France, your Father, never had the intention of taking them from you, but had ceded only his rights to the English Crown." The Mi'kmaq trade was disrupted with the French empire. The Mi'kmaq fishery became debased.[56] Yet the Mi'kmaq Nation still continued to resist the attacks of the English empire by pursuing both peace and war.

---

see S. Dale Standen, "'Personnes sans caractère': Private merchants, post commanders and the regulation of the Western fur trade, 1720–1745" in *De France en Nouvelle-France Société Fondatrice et Société Nouvelle*, sous la direction de Hubert Watelet avec la collaboration de Cornelius J. Jaenen (Ottawa: Acten Press, 1994), pp. 265–295. For trade and canoe conflict in the Petit Nord (northern Ontario and Quebec) see Elaine Allan Mitchell, *Fort Timiskaming and the Fur Trade* (Toronto: University of Toronto Press, 1977).

[56] Dickason, *Canada's First Nations*, pp. 133–36.

Mi'kmaq forces on the waters of the Gulf of the St. Lawrence continued to raid English ships until the Treaty of Boston was entered into on December 15, 1725 (ratified in 1728) between the English Crown and the Abenaki, Malecite and Mi'kmaq Nations.[57] It ended a long war of a decade between the English and the Mi'kmaq, and other Amerindian Nations, against the English Empire.[58] Its terms included, in part, that ". . . the Indians shall not molest any of His Majestie's Subjects or their dependants [dependents] in their settlements already (made) or lawfully to be made, or in the carrying on their trade (traffick) and other affairs within said Province." It also promised compensation to the white settlers if there were any more raids on white ships or settlements by the Mi'kmaq.[59] From the Mi'kmaq perspective the treaty was soon thrown into disrepute[60] by the behaviour of the English officials who did not act "in an honourable manner and refrain from having any further designs upon their territories and their assets."[61] As a result, the Hopson Treaty of 1752, rather than the Treaty of Boston of 1725 has been seen as the central Treaty between the English Crown and the Mi'kmaq Nation.[62]

France fought another world war with the English Empire—the War of the Austrian Succession (1744–48). Louisbourg was taken for the first time in 1745 by the American colonial forces and all of Cape Breton had also fallen. The war was ended by the Treaty of Aix-la-Chapelle by which the status quo ant bellum was once more maintained in northeastern North America. The French Empire regained Louisbourg and Cape Breton Island. Article 4 stated that the Mi'kmaq citizens ". . . shall not be hindered from, but have free liberty of hunting and Fishing as usual and that if they shall think a Truck house needful at the River Chibenaccadie, or any other

---

[57] Canada, *Indian Treaties and Surrenders*, Volume 2 (Ottawa: Queen's Printer, 1891; Reprinted by Fifth House Publishers, Saskatoon, 1992), pp. 198–204. The Treaty was ratified at Annapolis Royal in Nova Scotia on September 24, 1728.

[58] L.F.S. Upton *Micmacs and Colonists, Indian-White relations in the maritimes, 1713–1867* (Vancouver: University of British Columbia Press, 1979), pp. 40–43.

[59] Canada, *Indian Treaties*, Volume 2, pp. 198–204.

[60] Dickason, *Canada's First Nations*, pp. 133–36; Daniel N. Paul, *We Were Not the Savages, A Micmac Perspective on the Collision of European and Aboriginal Civilization* (Halifax: Nimbus Publishing, 1993), pp. 76–85.

[61] Dickason, *Canada's First Nations*, pp. 133–36.

[62] Adrian Tanner and Sakej Henderson, "Aboriginal land claims in the Atlantic Provinces", in Ken Coates (ed.), *Aboriginal Land Claims in Canada, A Regional Perspective*, (Toronto: Copp Clark Pitman, 1992), pp. 132–133.

place of their resort". This article is similar to the Treaties under the Covenant Chain.[63] By this means the independence of the Amerindian trade in the North Atlantic was retained.

Beginning in 1748–49, the English began to consolidate their foothold in the Mi'kmaq Territory in the Atlantic region by building a naval fortress in Halifax to counterbalance Louisbourg. Building on Mi'kmaq lands evoked a vigorous response from the Mi'kmaq who, on September 23, 1749, once again, effectively through their actions, declared war on the English Empire.[64] Lord Cornwallis, the English governor called a meeting of his council and issued the following proclamation on October 2, 1749:

> ... The Micmacs have of late in a most treacherous manner taken 20 of His Majesty's Subjects prisoners at Canso, and carried off a sloop belonging to Boston, and a boat from this Settlement and at Chinecto basely and under the pretence of friendship and commerce. Attempted to seize two English sloops and murder their crews and actually killed several, and on Saturday the 30th of September [1749], a body of these savages fell upon some men cutting wood and without arms near the saw mill and barbarously killed four and carried one away.
>
> ... [we] do hereby authorize and command all Officers Civil and Military, and all His Majesty's Subjects or others to annoy, distress, take or destroy the Savage commonly called Micmac, wherever they are found, and all as such as aiding and assisting them, ... do promise a reward of ten Guineas for every Indian Micmac taken or killed, to be paid upon producing such Savage taken or his scalp (as is the custom in America) if killed to the Officer Commanding at Halifax, Annapolis Royal, or Minas.[65]

Cornwallis followed this act of attempted extermination, including those in Newfoundland, by attempting to reaffirm the Treaty of 1725, but it too failed. After becoming governor of Nova Scotia in 1752, Hopson negotiated a Treaty with the Mi'kmaq Nation. Immediately before the Treaty, Cornwallis's "Mi'kmaq scalping proclamation" was repealed. A brief interlude of peace was the immediate result of the Hopson Treaty.[66]

---

[63] G.F.G. Stanley, *New France, The Last Phase, 1744–1760*, The Canadian Centenary Series, Volume 5 (Toronto: McClelland and Stewart, 1968), pp. 15–32.

[64] Paul, *We Were Not the Savages*, pp. 107–108.

[65] Public Record Office (PRO), Colonial Office records, C.O. 217/9/118. A copy is available on microfilm in the Provincial Archives of Nova Scotia in Halifax. See, for an interpretation, Paul, *We Were Not the Savages*, pp. 99–114.

[66] The Treaty is named after Peregrine Thomas Hopson, (?–1759), who was a

The Mi'kmaq Nation played a prominent role in the Seven Years War. Once again, however, the French offered but little assistance. In the defence, for example, of Louisbourg in 1758 the Mi'kmaq were at "Fresh Water Cove."[67] In fact, the Mi'kmaq style of naval warfare was more effective than that employed by the English Empire.[68] Olive Dickason has summarized the Mi'kmaq role in these complex military operations:

> As the final round of the North American colonial wars got under way, the Mi'kmaq pitched into the fray on land and sea, asserting their right to make war or peace as they willed and reaffirming their sovereignty over Megumaage. Between 1713 and 1760, Louisbourg correspondence refers to well over 100 captures of vessels by Amerindians. The Amerindians liked to cruise in their captured ships before abandoning them, forcing their prisoners to serve as crew. At that time they had no use for ships of that size, just as they had no use for artillery.[69]

In the long term, with little or no assistance from the French Navy, the Mi'kmaq Nation could not, by itself, match the naval firepower of the English Royal Navy. Louisbourg fell early in the Seven Years War and with it their military alliance with the French Empire. But the Mi'kmaq Nation was never conquered.[70]

The Fox War (1710-1738)

Not all of the Great Lakes Nations acquiesced in the quest of the French for a pan-national network of alliances and trade partnerships. The most obdurate resistance from an Algonquian speaking

---

British "military officer, governor of Louisbourg, Cape Breton Island, and Nova Scotia". See Wendy Cameron, "Peregrine Thomas Hopson", *Dictionary of Canadian Biography*, Volume III (Toronto: University of Toronto Press, 1974), pp. 294–295.

[67] Richard Brown, *A history of the Island of Cape Breton with some account of the discovery and settlement of Canada, Nova Scotia, and Newfoundland* (London: Sampson Low, Son, and Marston, 1869; Belleville, Ontario, Mika Publishing Company, Canadiana Reprint Series No. 72, 1979), p. 297.

[68] A.G. Doughty (ed.), *An Historical Journal of the Campaigns in North America For the Years 1757, 1758, 1759, and 1760 by Captain John Knox*, VIII, 3 Volumes, Volume II (Toronto: The Champlain Society, 1914–1916), pp. 279–280. Captain John Knox in his *An Historical Journal of the Campaigns in North America For the Years 1757, 1758, 1759, and 1760...* recorded these events on November 24, 1758.

[69] Dickason, *Canada's First Nations*, p. 159.

[70] Brown, *Cape Breton*, p. 177.

people came from the Mesquakie, called the Fox by the French, Outagami by the Ojibwa. There were simmering hostilities and blood-feuds among many of the nations that inhabited the Great Lakes and Laurentian Shield, but the Mesquakie stand out in their pro-clivity to offend and quarrel with others. Little is known of them before 1667 when the French Jesuit Father Claude Allouez first encountered them at a mission he established on Chequamegon Bay on the south shore of Lake Superior, where a large party had come to trade. They inhabited the region around Lake Winnebago and on the river that bears their name, the Fox, on the watershed between Green Bay and the Wisconsin River. Earlier in the seventeenth cen-tury they may have occupied the upper Michigan peninsula, from which they were driven by their incessant wars with the Ojibwa to the north and east.

They can be found at war with and as allies of the Sioux on the upper Mississippi to the west, but they were inveterate foes of the Illinois to the south. Their closest allies were the Sauks (Sacs) and they had mixed relations with their other neighbours: Menominee, Winnebago, Mascouten, Kickapoo, with groups of whom they were frequently allied. In the seventeenth century they appear intermit-tently in the French records, often as spoilers and troublemakers, a characterization which likely reflects the French close partnership with the Ojibwa and the Illinois, Mesquakie enemies.

Unlike most other Algonquian-speaking nations of the Great Lakes area the Mesquakie were not proficient canoeists.[71] This seems not to have affected their ability to wage war successfully. Their loca-tion straddling access to one of the most productive source of pelts in Wisconsin, and the most convenient route to the upper Mississippi and the far west, stood in the way of French imperial and com-mercial ambitions. For the French, bringing the Mesquakie into a peaceful trade relationship with themselves and their neighbours was essential. For the Mesquakie, making peace with their ancient ene-mies and the French was something they were ultimately unwilling to do. Their reputation among their Amerindian neighbours, and the record of their behaviour, bespoke a fierce and defiant independence.

---

[71] R. David Edmunds and Joseph L. Peyser, *The Fox Wars: The Mesquakie Challenge to New France* (Norman and London: University of Oklahoma Press, 1993), pp. 8–9. This is the most recent and thorough study of the Mesquakie relations with the French and their neighbours.

Given that the Mesquakie enemies, the Ojibwa, Ottawa and Illinois played the major role in the wars against the Iroquois in the 1690s, it is not surprising that the Mesquakie kept aloof of the French and nourished peaceful relations with the Iroquois, especially the Seneca. Notwithstanding the Montreal peace of 1701, therefore, distrust of the Mesquakie lingered. Full scale war erupted in 1712 at Detroit.[72] Following the Montreal Peace the post commander there, Antoine Lamotte Cadillac, had invited all the Great Lakes Nations to establish villages at Detroit so that they could trade with the French. Several groups, including Ottawas, Potawatamis, Hurons, Ojibwa, Maskoutens, and Miamis. Mesquakies responded to the invitation. Bringing into close proximity groups who harboured resentments of past wrongs proved to be a dangerous policy. A murder, exchanged insults, and plots for revenge precipitated blows between Ottawas and Maskoutens, the latter seeking refuge in the palisade of their allies, the Mesquakies. When a large party of Illinois arrived, other opponents of the Mesquakies and Maskoutens were emboldened to slaughter their old foes. The post commander, Jacques-Charles Renaud Dubuisson, claimed he could not resist their demands for powder and shot, and ill-advisedly joined in the hostilities. In attempting to escape, an estimated 1,000 Mesquakie and Maskoutens, including women and children, were killed.

Thus began in earnest the "Fox Wars," which lasted 25 years and saw major French and Anishinabe expeditions against them in 1716, 1728, 1730 and 1735, the latter two attempts to exterminate them. Defiant and decimated, the Mesquakie effectively hampered French efforts to expand trade and exploration westward beyond them. They were nearly annihilated in 1731 when attempting a migration to settle with the Iroquois and finally found respite in making peace with the Sioux and resettling to the banks of the upper Mississippi River. One legacy of this non-canoeing people was to encourage the French to seek westward expansion to the north through the more hospitable waterways of the Ojibwa and Cree where the birchbark canoe was the proven transport of trade, alliance and empire.[73]

---

[72] For a succinct account of these events see Yves Zoltvany, *Philippe de Rigaud de Vaudreuil, Governor of New France 1703–1725* (Toronto, McClelland and Stewart, 1974), pp. 121–125.

[73] Dickason, *Canada's First Nations*, pp. 131–32.

The Ohio Valley

The Ohio valley was a different kind of frontier.[74] It had been a hunting and a war zone since the Iroquois wars of the seventeenth century.[75] Amerindians were active participants in the historical process during the French imperial era.[76] In the early part of the eighteenth century, they greatly assisted in undermining French imperial authority in the Great Lakes basin as well as in the Ohio country. The Ohio region had, for many years, remained the property of the Anishinabe and loosely linked to the Iroquois, acting as a buffer zone among the Thirteen colonies, the English and French imperial trading interests.

By the 1720's the French were buffered by the existance in the Ohio valley of the Five Nations, especially the Seneca. As well the Shawnees and Delaware were being pushed westward by the Pennsylvania and Virginian settlers, traders and land speculators who were steadily encroaching on their lands. These Nations kept their trading ties with the English in spite of being displaced. Protected by their Amerindian trading partners, English traders were now well-located to entice other Amerindian Nations, notably the western Huron on the Detroit River, the Potawatomi, the Ottawa, the Ouyatanons (Weas) and the Miami, to trade with them rather than with the French. The Huron Nation's loyalty to the French imperial Crown was of particular significance for the French because of the large village at Detroit where their territory produced pelts for trade and their warriors maintained hostilities with various southern Amerindian Nations allied to the English.[77]

A confrontation on Lake Ontario after 1720, nearly leading to armed conflict in 1727, led to the erection of a new fortified French post at Niagara, and an English one—Fort Ontario—at Oswego. This new situation placed constraints upon French choices of action against English penetration of the western trade. Here the disposition of the Iroquois Confederacy was of vital importance strategically. The Iroquois acted as a major barrier to the Ohio valley. When the

---

[74] This section is adopted from an unpublished paper, "Whose Frontier? Franco-Indian Relations on the Ohio Revisited, 1727–1747" presented at the conference "DIMENSIONI ATLANTICHE NELL'ETA DELL'ESPANSIONE EUROPA, at the Universitá di Genova, 19 October, 1992.

[75] Frese, "Canadian Canoe", 1999.

[76] Eccles, "Sovereignty Association", pp. 156–181.

[77] Standen, "'Personnes sans caractère'", op. cit.

Shawnees appeared increasingly on the Ohio in the late 1720's, French officials tried to entice them to the main trading post at Detroit or at least move to the Miami villages on the Maumee and Wabash rivers where they would reinforce the French buffer zone and "chemin de guerre." But this did not come about because the Shawnee had choices of where to trade and it was not in their interest to abandon their independent English trading partners located in Pennsylvania. For their part, the Miami and the Ouyatanons with kinship ties to the Iroquois and trade ties to the English also could not be relied on to do as the French wished. The reestablishment of Amerindian villages in the Ohio valley, trading regularly with the English, threatened the security which the French had maintained for their trade network in the Great Lakes area.

Later in the same decade, French officials found that they were powerless to prevent what they saw as a blood-feud which broke out among the Three Fires Confederacy of Ottawa, Potawatomi and Ojibwa on the one hand and a peace alliance between the Catawba and the Huron Nations on the other hand. The French had grave cause for alarm for the governor of New France—Charles de Beauharnois—to observe that "C'est une affaire bien délicate et qui demande un grande ménagement, . . . Les hurons étants alliez avec les cinq nations, Et les Outouais avec toutes celles des pays d'en haut." Over the next three years the French were powerless to change this situation, despite diplomacy which included increased gift-giving or trading opportunities. By the mid-eighteenth century the French empire in northeastern North America was being challenged by Amerindian traders and warriors in the Ohio valley.

The new reality for the French empire in the Ohio country on the eve of the Seven Years War was that both Anglo-American and Canadian traders were vying nose to nose along the waterway systems controlled by the Amerindian Nations and often in the same Amerindian villages. The French were clearly unable to organize an Amerindian coalition that was going to drive out the English traders. The buffer zone between French and English trade had been removed. French imperial policy which was characterized by containment within a system of trade outposts, was shattered by the maritime blockade of trade goods during the War of the Austrian Succession. Briefly in 1747, a coalition of Amerindian groups, including the Mohawks, joined in warring against French traders and western posts. The Anishinabe Nations had survived and remained independent and sovereign within their Territories. They changed their diplomatic and trade partners when it suited them and were not merely "subject tribes" as the French had hoped. In the end, it was the independent policies of the many Amerindian Nations of the Ohio valley which rendered French imperial ambitions impotent and ineffective by the mid-eighteenth century. And it contributed in no small way to the failure of the French to defend their empire in the Seven Years War.

The Seven Years War, 1755–1763

The canoe was modestly significant in the Seven Years War (1755–1763) and along the republican-monarchical borders during the War of the American Revolution. In this war the Amerindian Nations were fighting as active participants to protect their Territories, first and foremost, regardless of whether they were allied to Britain or the rebellious colonies. For the first time they faced large European armies and large vessels with cannon on the Great Lakes.

The primary role of the canoe in the Seven Years War came in the "Mi'kmaq War" in the Gulf of the St. Lawrence. As Olive Dickason has argued, this warfare was almost wholly at sea and not land-based. Mi'kmaq raiders guarded these inland coasts of the islands and peninsulas in their canoes and sloops while hounding and harassing the Royal Navy at the same time. But, in the end, let down by the ineptitude and weakness of the French Navy, especially after the French fortress at Louisbourg fell in 1758, the Mi'kmaq canoes were left to fight for their homeland alone against the English. Over the next few years the Mi'kmaq Nation had to enter into the treaty-making process with the English empire, for all of the Atlantic region, including Newfoundland between 1760 and 1763.[78]

Further to the west and south in the St. Lawrence valley and the Great Lakes regions, the Algonkian Nations, still very much allied with the French, assisted in defending their homelands from the forceful incursions of the British regular troops as well as the Iroquois forces under Sir William Johnson. The Anishinabe laid siege to and captured all the important English posts at Oswego (Fort Ontario)

---

[78] McNab, "Fragments", 1996. Sadly, and unfortunately, the solemn promises and terms of these treaties have remained outstanding to this day.

and at Fort William Henry in 1757 using forest warfare and the birchbark canoe. But the French could not keep their allies in the field to fight—no provisions, guns or gunpowder were forthcoming and starvation grew in the years that followed.

Outnumbered and outgunned by the Pennsylvanians, Virginians, the English and their old enemies, the Algonkian-speaking Nations without French help were no match for this wartime alliance. Forts William Henry, Duquesne, Detroit fell; the Anishinabe retreated, then came the forts at Niagara, Toronto and Fort Frontenac. Finally Quebec City (1759) and Montreal (1760) were laid siege to and sur-rendered in large part due to the presence of the Royal Navy; after 1763 New France was no more.[79]

The Seven Years War here was not won or lost by the Amerindian Nations using the birchbark canoe; the deciding factor in this European war, were the guns and the ships of the Royal Navy. The Anishinabe Nations who were allied with the French now had to enter into a new alliance system with the English empire. In this European war for northeastern North America, the birchbark canoe was becoming less militarily significant. The diplomatic invention of the Covenant Chain would, from the perspective of the Anishinabe Nations, some-how suffice, and new arrangements would follow in the Treaty of Montreal of 1760.

The Treaty of Montreal of 1760

For their part, the Anishinabe Nations who were independent and sovereign allies of the French Crown continued to occupy and use their Territories and to exercise local sovereignty and independence within them. This was reflected in the War itself by the Mi'kmaq Nation's actions in defence of its homeland. It was also observed by the English after the Capitulation of Louisbourg in 1758 and with it the fall of Prince Edward Island, then the fall of Quebec and Montreal during the next two years and was embedded in Article

---

[79] Schmalz, *Ojibwa*, pp. 50–62; Concerning the fall of Quebec at the Plains of Abraham, George Raudzens has written that "In the end ocean transport overcame canoe transport as well. The Maritime Evolution was stronger than the Military Revolution in the conquest of the Western Hemisphere.", "Military revolution or maritime evolution? Military superiorities or transportation advantages as main causes of European colonial conquests to 1788", *The Journal of Military History*, Vol. 63 (July 1999): 631–42.

XL of the Articles of Capitulation signed in Montreal in September 1760.[80] The English government guaranteed the rights of the Mi'kmaq Nation throughout the North Atlantic area.[81] And one year after the capitulation of New France, after the fall of Montreal and then Quebec, the English imperial government in the Atlantic region reaffirmed the Treaties of 1725 and 1752 with a "Burying of the Hatchet Ceremony" held at a public council at Governor Belcher's farm in Halifax. The Treaty of Halifax of 1761, was again in the form and the style and the substance of the Covenant Chain of Silver.[82]

Aboriginal oral traditions speak to the Treaty of Montreal that was entered into on September 6, 1760. This Treaty, which has been recorded in wampum belts, focuses on the waters of the territories of the Anishinabe Nations. Its purpose was to establish peace and friendship between the Anishinabe Nations and the English and French Empires after the defeat of France near the end of the Seven Years War. It was regarded by Aboriginal people as one of the founding documents in Canada's constitutional history in that it set out the relationship among the three founding Peoples to the new country of Canada.[83] In 1760 Anishinabe trade and the birchbark canoe were paramount.

The Anishinabe Nations, unlike the French Empire, were not in any way conquered in the Seven Years War. This was accepted as a fact by the English imperial government in the 1760 Articles of Capitulation and confirmed by the Peace of Paris and then the Royal

---

[80] Morantz, "Aboriginal land claims in Quebec", in *Aboriginal Land Claims*, p. 103.
[81] McNab, *Fragments of Time*, 1996.
[82] Provincial Archives of Nova Scotia, RG 1, Volume 165,162–165; Paul, *We Were Not the Savages*, pp. 149–154.
[83] Nin.Da.Waab.Jig. Files, Norman Miskokomon Paper, 1929. This oral tradition has been described in writing: "Then followed the French and English war which ended in 1759, and a short time later a treaty of peace was concluded at Montreal [the Treaty of Montreal of 1760]. This treaty provided for the French[-speaking] occupancy of [what became in 1867] the Province of Quebec, and the English occupancy of [what became in 1867] Ontario, reserving to the Three Tribes [the Ojibwa, Ottawa and the Potawatomi] a strip of ground, 66 ft. wide on each side of all rivers, 16 ft. wide on each side of all creeks and 99 feet wide along the shores of all lakes and around all lands entirely surrounded by water, also the use of all lands not fit for cultivation, and the right to hunt and sell timber in any forest, and to fish in any waters, also reserving to the Indians all stone, precious stones, and minerals. These strips of land were intended as a permanent inheritance to the Three Tribes, where they could camp and abide while fishing and trapping and cultivating the soil."

Proclamation in 1763 which is now an integral part of Canada's written Constitution reaffirming and recognizing Aboriginal title and rights. The Peace or Treaty of Paris of 1763 ended the French imperial influence, except for the two tiny islands of St. Pierre and Miquelon in the Gulf of the St. Lawrence. In addition, French rights to the fishery on the "French shore" in Newfoundland, confirmed by the Treaty of Utrecht in 1713, would continue for almost two hundred years. It was now certain Newfoundland would remain a colony of the English empire, at least until 1949, when it joined the Canadian Confederation.

The Anishinabe Resistance Movement of 1763

This resistance movement, which began in May of 1763 led by Pontiac, was fought by the Anishinabe Nations of northeastern North America against the British imperial government in the Great Lakes area to protect their traditional territories and cultures from "frauds and abuses."[84] The war began when the British commander in chief General Jeffrey Amherst ordered that the presents, extremely valuable commodities, given annually to the Amerindian Nations to maintain the diplomatic and military alliance system under the Covenant Chain, were no longer to be issued as of 1762. Much Amerindian discontent followed, intensified by a further edict to cut off all ammunition. The actual fighting broke out in the Spring of 1763.[85]

Two of the key battles fought in this war included a significant role for the canoe in Anishinabe victories against the English at Michilimackinac and also at the siege of Detroit. In June more than 400 warriors had come by birchbark canoe to Michilimackinac. There, using the ruse of a game of baggawataway (lacrosse), the warriors were able to capture this English fort and trading station killing seventy out of the ninety English troops and capturing the remainder. So successful was this victory that, using the speed of the canoe,

---

[84] Steele, *Warpaths*, pp. 246–247; Louis Chevrette, "Pontiac", *Dictionary of Canadian Biography*, Volume III, pp. 525–531.

[85] Steele, *Warpaths*, pp. 246–247. While some historians have named this resistance movement after him, Pontiac's role in it has been much exaggerated. Other leaders of the Western Confederacy had prominent roles as well such as Chief Wasson, Sekahos and Wabbicommicot, a Mississauga chief residing on the north shores of Lake Ontario (the Carrying Place, the modern-day Toronto area).

the word of this battle reached Detroit and then another English fort soon thereafter. Again using their canoes, a number of the warriors were able to come from the northern lakes to lay siege to Detroit later that same summer. Although the fort did not fall, the Anishinabe Nations initiated peace negotiations under the Covenant Chain of Silver and the resistance movement ended, successfully achieving its objectives. In this resistance movement the Anishinabe Nations were not conquered.[86] Even after the War, Sir William Johnson indicated that the English imperial government feared the military power of the Western Confederacy of Nations and wished to come to terms with them in a Treaty.[87]

The Royal Proclamation of 1763

The Royal Proclamation of 1763 was promulgated by King George III after the Seven Years War, partly in response to the Anishinabe resistance movement. The Royal Proclamation was an English imperial document, among other things, that established the administrative framework for the new English colonies in Quebec, and in the rest of North America. It also recognized and reaffirmed the "Indian territory." It established English imperial rules regarding the treaty-making process under the Covenant Chain as well as for Amerindian trade with non-Aboriginal people. This Proclamation also recognized the significance of the Amerindian trading system and, with it by extension, the canoe:

> And we do, by the Advice of our Privy Council, declare and enjoin, that the Trade with the said Indians shall be free and open to all our Subjects whatever, provided that every Person who may incline to Trade with the said Indians do take out a Licence for carrying on such Trade from the governor or Commander in Chief of any of our

---

[86] Steele, *Warpaths*, pp. 246–247. He reaches the following conclusion regarding Pontiac's resistance movement of 1763: "A diverse group of tribes, without the coherence of the successful Six Nations, Cherokee, or Creek confederations, had not been conquered, however, Amerindians had inflicted as many as two thousand casualties without any effective retaliation, a coup reminiscent of earlier massacres. The British army could not hope to conquer the Amerindians, given fiscal restraints and a peacetime army of only seventy-five hundred men. In the peace settlement, Amerindians appeared to recover the world they had lost; their presents were resumed, their lands were protected by the [Royal] proclamation of [1763]. . . ."

[87] Hamilton, *Sir William Johnson*, Vol. XI (13), pp. 134–135, 152, 155.

Colonies respectively where such Person shall reside, and also give Security to observe such Regulations as We shall at any Time think fit, by ourselves or by our Commissaries to be appointed for this Purpose, to direct and appoint for the Benefit of the said Trade . . .[88]

The Proclamation reaffirmed that the "Indian Territory" as well as the uses of that Territory by the First Nations and their citizens was to be their "absolute property." They retained control of their trading networks and their trade, of which the backbone remained the birchbark canoe.[89] These diplomatic initiatives came from the Amerindian Nations under the Covenant Chain of Silver—the Two Row Wampum symbolized by water and the canoe. It would be reaffirmed one year later in a grand council of Nations at Niagara in 1764. Since 1982 the Royal Proclamation has been a primary part of Canada's written Constitution.

The Twenty-Four Nations Wampum Belt and the Treaty of Niagara of 1764

The Treaty of Niagara is significant in that it reaffirmed the Covenant Chain of Silver with the Amerindian Nations of the Great Lakes. The English Empire and these Nations were now in an alliance that maintained the peace in northeastern North America. No longer at war they were traveling together in the same canoe in the historical process which has continued to this day, though not without disputes and long frayed and abused by the Anglo-Canadians. In July 1764 at the Treaty of Niagara, held at the "crooked place" on the Niagara River, the Amerindian Nations met with Johnson, the Northern Superintendent General of Indian Affairs, and other officials of the Crown. Johnson gave the Amerindian Nations, including the Western or the Lake(s) Confederacy, "the great Covenant Chain, 23 Rows broad & the year 1764 worked upon it." This action formally

---

[88] October 7, 1763, Royal Proclamation of 1763, *As Long as the Sun Shines and the Water Flows, A Reader in Canadian Native Studies*, ed. Ian A.L. Getty and Antoine S. Lussier, Vancouver: University of British Columbia Press, 1983, pp. 29–37.

[89] "Plan for the future management of Indian Affairs, referred to in the Thirty-Second Article of the Foregoing Instructions", *Constitutional Documents*, Sessional Papers, No. 18, pp. 614–619.

confirmed peace, through a Treaty, after Pontiac's resistance move-ment of 1763.[90]

Furthermore, Johnson made it clear that the major issues were trade as well as water, land under the water and its uses, and by extension, canoes. The next month, at the Treaty of Niagara, Johnson spoke (on July 31, 1764) at a "General Meeting with all the Western Indians in their Camp" and presented them with "... the great Covenant Chain [Belt], 23 Rows broad, & the Year 1764 worked upon it." An Ojibwa Chief stated he was "... of Opinion that it is best to keep the Belt of the Covenant Chain at Michilimackinac, as it is the Center, where all our People may see it. I exhort you to hold fast by it, to remember what has been said, and to abide by your Engagements." It will be recalled that Michilimackinac was an important northern trading post and military station located at a strategic isthmus on Mackinac Island and only could be reached by canoes.[91]

This latter Treaty is still known by the Amerindian Nations as the "Niagara Treaty Conference Twenty Four Nations Wampum Belt." The following are the First Nations' perspectives on the significance and the meaning of the Treaty:

> While the treaties are like stones marking a spot in time, the rela-tionship between the Nations is like two equals, respecting each of their differences but supporting each other for a common position on peace, order and justice for all. The brotherhood created by the Twenty Four Nations Belt represents a relationship of both sharing and respect. The sharing is reciprocal: as the First Nations shared land and the knowledge in the past, now that situation is reversed, the generosity of spirit and action is expected to continue. The respect is also reci-procal: respect for each other's rights, existence, laws and vision of the future.[92]

The 24 Amerindian Nations who were parties to the Niagara Treaty, reaffirming the Covenant Chain, were basically the "birchbark" Amerindian peoples who lived in the wide and long birch belt all centered in the St. Lawrence valley and Great Lakes waterway sys-tem. The birchbark canoe was central to their lives in both war and peace. (See Figure 8.4)

---

[90] Hamilton, *Sir William Johnson*, pp. 162–64.
[91] Hamilton, *Sir William Johnson*, pp. 221–222; 262–327.
[92] Nin.Da.Waab.Jig.Files, Treaty of Niagara of 1764.

The power of this oral tradition of the Niagara Treaty was also reaffirmed, emphasizing peace and friendship as well as the significance of trade and water, and with them the birchbark canoe, in the treaty-making process. Treaties embodying such provisions, were entered into at Detroit (1761, 1764–65),[93] Fort Ontario (Oswego, 1766),[94] Fort Stanwix (1786).[95] Johnson died in 1774, eight years after the Treaty of Lake Ontario was signed.[96] Things began to fall apart with the death of Sir William Johnson,[97] and by the 1820's the so-called second English Empire had embarked on an imperial strategy based on colonization rather than trade.[98]

The War of the American Revolution and the Treaty Making Process

The War of the American Revolution (1775–83) was fought between the United States and Great Britain.[99] In this War, canoes had a role to play in forest fighting, as they had previously, but this was primarily a "European civil war" and was largely fought where feasible using land forces and regular troops as well as small sailing vessels of the Royal Navy on the Great Lakes. The Amerindian Nations were not included as part of the Treaty negotiations or consulted about its terms. The new American republic proceeded to take their Territories and Reserves, by Treaty if possible, if not, then by military force.[100]

In the War of the American Revolution the Amerindian Nations, especially the Iroquois Confederacy, literally fought for their territo-

---

[93] Hamilton, *Sir William Johnson*, pp. 162–64, 765–767.

[94] NAC, RG 8, "C" Series, Microfilm Reel # C-2848, Vol. 248, pp. 1–3.

[95] Calloway, *American Revolution*, pp. 282–283.

[96] Gwyn, "Sir William Johnson", pp. 394–398.

[97] Ibid. See also RG 8, "C" Series, British Military and Naval Records, National Archives of Canada, Ottawa, Manuscripts Division, Microfilm Reel #C-2848, Vol. 248, pp. 251–257a.

[98] RG 8, "C" Series, British Military and Naval Records, National Archives of Canada, Ottawa, Manuscripts Division, Microfilm Reel #C-2848, Vol. 248, pp. 151–52; 155–156.

[99] Calloway, *Crown and Calumet*; *American Revolution in Indian Country*.

[100] Ibid. See also Reginald Horsman, *Matthew Elliott, British Indian Agent*, (Detroit: Wayne State University, 1964), pp. 113–114; RG 8, "C" Series, British Military and Naval Records, National Archives of Canada, Ottawa, Manuscripts Division, Microfilm Reel #C-2848, Vol. 248, pp. 251–257a.

ries. Their presence was first and foremost effective in the border (forest) warfare fought along the Great Lakes and connecting waterways. The Six Nations fared less well in that they had aligned themselves with the English empire and found themselves directly in the center of the conflict. After the battle of Wyoming in 1778, the American forces attempted to exterminate most of the Iroquois. By the end of the War a majority found themselves driven out of their territories in New York and Pennsylvania, and they moved as refugee Loyalists (1783–84) into what became Upper Canada in 1791 (created largely because of the arrival of Loyalists). Here they still remain on Reserve lands along the Grand and Shannon Rivers (in southwestern and eastern Ontario respectively). For their part, the Algonkian peoples of the Great Lakes, where they could, preferred and attempted to remain neutral. They fought in only one notable battle at Sandusky on Lake Erie and using the tried and true techniques of forest warfare and transported by birchbark canoes defeated the American forces. Outnumbered, with only about 400 Anishinabe, they faced 500 American mounted riflemen, emerging victorious with half of the American riflemen dead. They only lost some of their territories after this War due to encroaching expansionism of the American colonists.[101]

Although fighting ceased in 1781, the Treaty of Paris of 1783 ended the War of the American Revolution. Article II of that Treaty provided, in part, that the international boundary would be placed "through the middle of said Lake [Ontario] until it strikes the communication by water between that Lake and Lake Erie; thence along the middle of said communication into Lake Erie; through the middle of said Lake until it arrives at the water-communication between that Lake and Lake Huron;. . . ." The main diplomatic focus was on the waterways where the canoe was still a factor in transportation and communication.[102]

One of the Amerindian objectives intended to mitigate this "disaster" and enable them to survive into the twentieth century and beyond was to try to dovetail their situation with English imperial

---

[101] Schmalz, *Ojibwa*, pp. 97–101.
[102] James White, "Boundary disputes and treaties", in *Canada and its Provinces, A History of the Canadian People and their Institutions by One Hundred Associates*, Adam Shortt and Arthur G. Doughty (General Editors), Volume VIII (Toronto: Glasgow, Brook & Company, 1914), pp. 751–753.

strategies of trade, land and emigration policies and ultimately white colonization. This they tried to do by entering into a renewed treaty-making process which would safeguard their hunting territories, their waters and their economies built on the back of the birchbark canoe. For example, treaties were entered into in the 1780's and 1790's to lease or share certain areas with settlers while retaining Anishinabe sovereignty and water rights.[103] On May 19, 1790 the McKee Treaty was entered into at Detroit by the English Crown and the Bkejwanong First Nation. It is clear from the geographic description in it that the waters and the lands in Lake Erie, the Detroit River, Lake St. Clair, the St. Clair River and Lake Huron as well as the islands and the connecting waterways within the peninsula, were not included or referred to in that Treaty.[104] In addition, the Gun Shot Treaty of 1792 was one of the Treaties between the Western Confederacy, among other Amerindian Nations, and the English imperial government. It was entered into by Lieutenant Governor John Graves Simcoe, Sir John Johnson and the First Nations at the Bay of Quinte in 1792.[105] Specifically, it reaffirmed the Treaty entered into at Montreal in 1760.[106] The oral tradition asserts that the Gun Shot Treaty of 1792 was more than a sharing of the use of land:

> The Gov'r [Lieutenant Governor, Simcoe] stated although the Gov't wanted the land it was not intended that the fish and game rights be excluded or that they were to be deprived of their privileges of hunting, trapping and fishing as it was a source of their living and sustenance. These provisions were to hold good as long as the grass grows and water runs, and as long as the British Gov't is in existence. According to the ruling of the Gun Shot Treaty, the Indians to have first rights to all creeks, rivers and lakes, 16 feet on both sides of the said creek, 66 feet on both sides of all rivers and 99 feet around all lakes and island[s] on said lakes. This land mentioned is their inheritance where they can camp and abide while pursuing their occupa-

---

[103] Horsman, "Alexander McKee", *Dictionary of Canadian Biography*, Volume IV, 1771–1800 (Toronto: University of Toronto Press, 1979), pp. 499–500.

[104] Canada, *Indian Treaties*, Vol. 1, pp. 1–5.

[105] McNab, "'The promise that he gave to my grand father was very sweet': The Gun Shot Treaty of 1792 at the Bay of Quinte", Research Note, *The Canadian Journal of Native Studies*, 16(2), 1996, pp. 293–314.

[106] A copy of the Gun Shot Treaty of 1792 was deposited in the Provincial Archives of Ontario in a manuscript collection, A.E. Williams/United Indian Bands of Chippewas and Mississaugas Papers, F 4337, Microfilm Reels MS 2604–2607. The Gun Shot Treaty of 1792 is in F 4337-11-0-8.

tion of fishing and trapping and while occupying said land [,] no white men can order them off.[107]

Similarly Treaties respecting the centrality of the Amerindian trade, free trade and the necessity of border crossings along all the Great Lakes and the St. Lawrence River followed.[108]

The rights to the Aboriginal trade and free trade were synonymous, and these rights were intended by British imperial policy to protect the Aboriginal Nations, at a time when Britain was relinquishing its western posts (1796). They were also to be safeguarded in the Treaty-making process. The primary motivating factor was the real English fear that, if these rights were not reaffirmed, then there would be an "Indian war" in the Great Lakes which would have, so they thought, resulted in the loss of Upper Canada for the English imperial government. These Treaties are still at issue today and the subject of major litigious battles in Canada's courts.

The Jay Treaty of November 19, 1794

The Treaty of Amity, Commerce and Navigation of 1794 was named after the American negotiator of that Treaty, John Jay. Formerly the governor of the State of New York, John Jay was more than familiar with issues of First Nation Treaties, having negotiated some of them himself in his tenure as governor.[109] In 1794, Jay was Chief Justice for the United States government. Lord Grenville was the English negotiator. In this Treaty, made between the English and American governments, the English government gave up its posts in what became known as the American Midwest and, in doing so,

---

[107] Nin.Da.Waab.Jig. Files, Miskokomon Paper, "Treaties between the Whites and Indians, of Chippewa, Ottawa, and Pottawatomie Tribes" (1929).

[108] McNab, *Circles of Time* (1999) and "'Water is her lifeblood': The waters of Bkejwanong and the treaty-making process", in *Earth, Water, Air and Fire*, pp. 35–63. For example, in the Fall of 1794 Simcoe visited the Bkejwanong First Nation's Territory to make a Treaty, on behalf of the Crown, with their representatives. He met with the Walpole Island First Nation's representatives on October 10–13, 1794, regarding free trade. The Simcoe Treaty of 1794 at Brownstown was concluded while the negotiation of the Jay Treaty between the English government and the United States was being undertaken.

[109] NAC, RG 8, C Series, Volume 248, Microfilm Reel #C-2848, pp. 263–264.

abandoned its allies, the Amerindian Nations, including the Western Confederacy in July of 1796.[110]

On November 19, 1794, the English and the American governments signed the Jay Treaty. The English government did not notify or consult with the Amerindian Nations. The Treaty was ratified by the American and the English imperial governments and was proclaimed on February 29, 1796. The terms of the Jay Treaty included matters concerning amity or peace, privileges of settlers, commerce, survey and boundaries, indemnities, land tenures, private debts, navigation, trade and shipping, rules in time of war, extradition and ratification. Article III is entitled "Commerce and navigation; duties," addressing matters that specifically concerned the Amerindian Nations:

> It is agreed that it shall at all times be free to His Majesty's subjects, and to the citizens of the United States, and also to the Indians dwelling on either side of the boundary line, freely to pass and repass by land or inland navigation, into the respective territories and countries of the two parties, on the continent of America, (the country within the limits of the Hudson's Bay Company only excepted), and to navigate all the lakes, rivers and waters thereof, and freely to carry on trade and commerce with each other . . . No duty of entry shall ever be levied by either party on peltries brought by land or inland navigation into the said territories respectively, nor shall the Indians passing or repassing with their own proper goods and effects of whatever nature, pay for the same any impost or duty whatever.[111]

By the Jay Treaty the English imperial government also relinquished its trading posts and forts, including Detroit and Fort Ontario.[112]

"We Were Lashed Together Strongly": The St. Anne Island Treaty of 1796

The St. Anne Island Treaty was entered into by the English imperial government for military purposes-specifically to establish an Anishinabe buffer state against any future wars with the United States

---

[110] Calloway, *Crown and Calumet; The American Revolution in Indian Country.*

[111] Jay or Jay's Treaty, identified as "The treaty of amity, commerce and navigation, November 19, 1794".

[112] Nin.Da.Waab.Jig. Files, Norman Miskokomon, "Treaties between the Whites and Indians, of Chippewa, Ottawa, and Pottawatomie Tribes", 1929. "In 1818 Envoys representing England and the United States met the Three Tribes at

on the western frontier of the Great Lakes. From this perspective, Upper Canada was to be defended by First Nation warriors in canoes in conjunction with the Royal Navy on the Great Lakes.[113] In the summer of 1796 the situation of the First Nations was not diminished. Although the Americans "took possession of the forts at Detroit and Michilimackinac," Cleland wrote that this American presence was ". . . however, a very tenuous occupation at best." There was not then a great disruption, "much less a disaster," in the summer of 1796 created by the take-over of the posts by the Americans. In fact, the effect was to increase the economic and political power of the First Nations through "competitive gift-giving" as well as military power.[114]

The St. Anne Island Treaty of 1796 occurred at a Council Fire at which a Council Meeting was held, at the edge of the forest near the Ottawa village, on St. Anne Island on the northerly side of the Chenail Ecarte River [adjacent to, and across the river from present-day Wallaceburg] on August 30, 1796.[115] It could only be reached

---

Andarding or (Amherstburg) [the Treaty of Amherstburg of 1818] in conference on the subject of the protection of game for the Indian, at which time it was agreed that only those whites holding licenses would be permitted to hunt and fish and that the fees accruing should all be paid over to the Indians. Since 1822 when these first licenses were issued, there has been no distribution of the funds thus accrued and at this time (1929) the aggregate amount of the hunting and fishing licenses fees collected by the Provinces and by the several states should doubtless and does represent a very large amount of money, all of which belongs to the Indians as per the treaty.

In Jay's Treaty of 1794 between England and the United States, the right of all Indians to free passage across the border by land or water for all times was officially recognized by both nations. These rights were confirmed in an explanatory article the two Governments concluded at Philadelphia, May 4th, 1796.

The Indians of the Three Tribes feel that they possess a valid grievance and many claims against the Canadian Government and of the United States because of the complete failure of the latter to observe the obligations of these old treaties, and they cannot but recognize the difference in the treatment of the Oklahoma Indians by the United States Government and that accorded the Three Tribes on Walpole Island to whom treaty obligations are held as sacred and as inviolate as they should be by the Canadian or Dominion Government and the United States Government."

[113] E.A. Cruikshank (ed.), *The Correspondence of Lieutenant Governor John Graves Simcoe*, Vol. IV (Toronto: The Ontario Historical Society, 1932), p. 160.

[114] Charles E. Cleland, *Rites of Conquest, The History and Culture of Michigan's Native Americans* (Ann Arbor: University of Michigan Press, 1992), p. 159.

[115] At least four partial copies of the proceedings of this Council Meeting, from the Indian Department's perspective, have survived in the Peter Russell Papers (one copy) and in the records of the Department of Indian Affairs (two copies) and one

by canoes and according to the Bkejwanong oral tradition, the English
Crown's representation (Alexander McKee), "finding that our Fathers
were growing poor and wretched in the vicinity of the Long Knife
brought them up to the Island [St. Anne Island] on which you now
find us; he lept from his Canoe with a lighted Brand in his hand
and after having kindled the first Council Fire which had ever shone
upon it, he gave it to them forever." On August 30, 1796, McKee
addressed the "Chiefs Chippawa & Ottawa Nations":

> The change I allude to is the delivery of the Posts to the United States:
> these people have at last fulfilled the Treaty of [Paris] 1783 and the
> Justice of the King towards all the world, would not suffer him to
> withhold the rights of another, after a compliance with the terms stip-
> ulated in that Treaty: But he has notwithstanding taken the greatest
> care of the rights and independence of all the Indian Nations who by
> the last Treaty with America, are to be perfectly free and unmolested
> in their Trade and hunting grounds and to pass and repass freely and
> undisturbed to trade with whom they please.[116]

The solemn commitments of the Crown made at this Council Meeting
of August 30, 1796 constitute promises which were made by Alexander
McKee on behalf of the Crown. The Chenail Ecarte Reserve was
also discussed at this Council meeting and also was established as
an Indian Reserve.[117] It is clear from the oral tradition of the Walpole
Island First Nation that the St. Anne Island was a significant Treaty
with the English Crown for the matters discussed at the Council
meeting on August 30, 1796.[118] Once again it reaffirmed that diplomatic device of the Two Row Wampum and the pivotal symbol,
and the reality of the canoe which had been "lashed together strongly"
by the Anishinabe and the European Nations. This diplomatic practice
continued.[119] The Anishinabe trade would remain strong right into

---

copy in the Samuel Peters Jarvis Papers in the Metropolitan Reference Library in
Toronto, August 30, 1796, St. Anne Island Treaty, NAC, RG 10, Vol. 39, pp.
21652–21656. Another copy of the same document is in RG 10, Vol. 785, pp.
181477–181480.

[116] Samuel Peters Jarvis Papers, Metropolitan Toronto Public Library, Baldwin
Room, Toronto, S 125, Vol. B 56, pp. 29–36.

[117] September 2, 1796, "Return of Indians present at Treaty of Purchase", Chenail
Ecarte, E.A. Cruikshank (ed.), *The Peter Russell Papers*, Volume I, 1796–1797 (Toronto:
Published by the [Ontario Historical] Society, 1932), p. 37.

[118] NAC, Record Group 10, (RG 10), Indian Affairs Records, Vol. 58, pp.
59778–59781.

[119] Nin.Da.Waab,Jig., *Walpole Island, The Soul of Indian Territory*, Nin.Da.Waab,Jig.,
1987, Bkejwanong, Chapter 3, "Enaaknigewinke geeshoog Treaty Making 1790–1827",
pp. 17–26.

nineteenth and twentieth centuries.[120] Canoes were also paramount in this "golden age" of the fur trade in Canada's north country.

Canoes, Aboriginal Trade and Trading

The tradition of Amerindian trade and trading was primarily focused on the waterways flowing to the Atlantic and Arctic coasts, the St. Lawrence River valley, the Great Lakes and into the Ohio and Mississippi river valleys as well as to the Northwest. The canoe was the pre-eminent vehicle for transport and trade. In Canada land became a subject of trade largely through the Treaty-making process beginning in the late eighteenth century. It was only later when these Empires, with their military capabilities became overwhelming in terms of manpower, sea power and arms that the Amerindian trade became severely disrupted. Gradually, through the nineteenth century, the Amerindian trading networks either went underground or shifted northward and north westward.

In the late eighteenth century, in response to the Amerindian control of the trade and the presence of Montreal pedlars, the Hudson's Bay Company's traders set up secondary posts inland to attempt to effect more control over the fur trade. The first permanent inland post was established at Cumberland House on Pine Tree Island on the Saskatchewan River in 1783. Thereafter the Company did not succeed in controlling the trade, having less than 20% of its total. Even then, in the north and the west for much of the nineteenth century the role of canoes in this trade remained of considerable significance until the Second World War when bush planes proliferated and became a new means of travel and when limited road networks were built into Canada's vast northern region.

This trade, out of Montreal and into the Great Lakes, Laurentian Shield and the Ohio valley, was carried on by Amerindian and Metis in conjunction with many Scottish and Irish traders, like Peter Pond and John Askin, (1738–1815), Senior,[121] of Detroit, in the eighteenth

---

[120] Today, the citizens of Bkejwanong, on the southern most unceded Reserve in Canada still hunt muskrats and their pelts for food and trade them across the international border.

[121] David Farrell, "John Askin (Erskine)", *Dictionary of Canadian Biography*, Volume V, 1801–1820 (Toronto: University of Toronto Press, 1983), pp. 37–39.

and early nineteenth centuries. It spanned nearly all parts of the northeastern and much of mid-western North America, a vast geographical area. It lasted for more than four hundred years. Peter Pond has left us this description of the canoes and trade from 1774 when he arrived at Prairie du Chien for the annual rendezvous:

> . . . we saw a large collection from every part of the Mississippi who had arrived before us, even from Orleans eight hundred leagues below us. The Indian camp exceeded a mile and a half in length. Here was a sport of all sorts. The French were very numerous. There was not less than one hundred and thirty canoes which came from Mackinac, carrying sixty to eighty hundred weight apiece, all made of birchbark and white cedar for the ribs. These boats from Orleans and Illinois and other parts were numerous.[122]

Askin was one of the most prominent local traders at Detroit with extensive Anishinabe and European trading connections that stretched from Europe through the St. Lawrence to Montreal, Detroit and southerly deep into the Ohio and Mississippi valleys and north into the Canadian shield. The linkages between the trade and the military remained extremely close. The traders like Askin were the primary suppliers to the military establishments at the key points of the English empire in the St. Lawrence Valley and along the Great Lakes waterway system. Military posts like Mackinac, Niagara and Amherstburg (Fort Malden) and Detroit were not only the key places to guard the military frontier and safeguard the English colonies, they were also centers of trade. Although Askin used some larger sailing vessels on the Great Lakes, he also relied on large canoes with sails to carry freight.

Detroit had long been an important entrepot for Amerindian trade and then for the Indian trade which was between the Amerindian Nations and the European traders. It owed its location to the presence of the Amerindian Nations in the area of the Detroit River, Lake St. Clair and the connecting waterways. Anishinabe villages, located along the waterways, ringed Bkejwanong—the "place where the waters divide"—part of the Walpole Island First Nation Territory in the Lake St. Clair area. In the 1760's, for example, there were Amerindian villages—Wyandot, Ojibwa and Ottawa on the east side of the Detroit River—and a Potawatomi village on the west side.

---

[122] Frese, "The Canadian canoe", 1999; Cleland, *Rites*, p. 108.

All of these places were linked by waterways and the birchbark canoe.

The scope, extent and value of the Indian trade until the 1820's was extremely large. But the trade, although it included furs of all kinds, was not restricted to furs.[123] It included large quantities of foodstuffs, including corn and other vegetal products, among many other items.[124] Two-pronged this trade was mutual and an integral part of the local European economies.[125] It had been so for many years. And it would remain so well into the nineteenth century.

The trade and its infrastructure were also of strategic importance. In times of war, the trading as well as the Royal Navy's vessels and Amerindian canoes were commandeered for use in transporting the Amerindian warriors as well as English troops. In times of peace and war, the Amerindian Nations were an integral component in the defence of the English empire.

The Indian trade was big business linked as it was to large independent trading companies like the North West Company which was based in Montreal. While the relatively small traders may have found it difficult to make ends meet, this was not true for the McGillivrays,[126]

---

[123] *The John Askin Papers*, edited by Milo M. Quaife, 2 Volumes (Published by the Detroit Library Commission, 1928, 1931), pp. 1–6, 8–15, 46–47, 73–78.

[124] The articles traded were themselves wide-ranging and extensive. They included, at least in part, the following: 1. Indian corn; 2. food supplies, such as wheat, flour, tobacco, potatoes, Spanish beans, pumpkins, garden seeds; 3. wild rice; 4. fowl, especially wild ducks, and other wild game birds; 5. hay; 6. lye hominy [potash]; 7. Maple and black walnut sugar; 8. wood and wood products, timber for ships and ship-building, especially firewood, tree gum and bark, watap, which is a root of the spruce or fir tree used for making thread, string; 9. grease from animal fats; 10. lime; 11. sub-surface resources, including minerals such as gold, silver, copper, and other metals, flint and salt, or other minerals, oil from oil springs used for making and bartering liniments for medicinal purposes; 12. furs, including all kinds— deer, beaver, bear, raccoon, lynx, bob and wild cat, fox, otter, musquash [muskrat?], pichoux [red lynx]; 13. boats and canoes, for example, petiagers [a "petiager (variously spelled) was a boat made from a tree trunk, hollowed out, which was often provided with a plank bottom, the trunk being split in halves, each of which was made to serve as one side of the boat."]; 14. fish of all kinds, including: sturgeon, muskellunge, whitefish, pickerel, bass, perch, salmon, trout; 15. Wild berries and fruits of all kinds.

[125] In collaboration with Carol Whitfield, "Alexander Grant", *Dictionary of Canadian Biography*, Vol. V, 1801–1820 (Toronto: University of Toronto Press, 1983), pp. 363–367; *Askin Papers*, 365, pp. 75–78, 98–104.

[126] Sylvia Van Kirk and Jennifer S.H. Brown, "Duncan McGillivray", *Dictionary of Canadian Biography*, Vol. V, 1801–1802 (Toronto: University of Toronto Press, 1983), pp. 530–532; Jennifer S.H. Brown, *Strangers in Blood: Fur Trade Company Families in Indian country*, Vancouver: University of British Columbia Press, 1980; Sylvia Van Kirk, *"Many tender ties": Women in Fur Trade Society in Western Canada, 1670–1870* (Winnipeg, 1980).

McTavishes[127] and Frobishers[128] and Alexander Mackenzie[129] of Montreal. For instance, Askin wrote to Benjamin Frobisher in 1778:

> I will attempt writing to you by these Indians but cant say I will get through, having three Vessells to fit off now, your Canoes & my Public employment.
> St Cir [a North West Company guide] arrived last night. I have delivered him the Canoes, all your Corn, Sugar, Gum, Bark & Watap [spruce or fir root] now remaining here shall be delivered him to Day, all the rum comeing up in the Canoes he shall also have (I expect they will arrive to day).[130]

And these businesses continued to be aware of the impact of diplomacy on the trade. For example, Askin was aware of the long term consequences of the Jay Treaty on matters of free trade across the international boundary.[131]

Amerindian trade and trading also had a deeply political side; a side that was always present at Treaty negotiations between European Empires and the Amerindian Nations. All the parties arrived for these negotiations using canoes well into the nineteenth century.[132] This was later expanded to include the diplomatic and military relations between the English Empire and the American government in Washington. Trade could not be divorced from Amerindian Lands and Territories. In short, the First Nations had to remain, as Askin told his son, the "sole Masters of their Lands."[133] Aboriginal traders continued to be a significant part of the colonial economy until the mid-nineteenth century.[134] Thereafter, to protect themselves, Amerindian traders continued to attempt to control both the supply of the trading items as well as the credit system.[135]

---

[127] Fernand Ouellet, "Simon McTavish", *Dictionary of Canadian Biography*, Vol. V, 1801–1820 (Toronto: University of Toronto Press, 1983), pp. 560–567.

[128] Fernand Ouellet, "Benjamin Frobisher", *Dictionary of Canadian Biography*, Vol. IV, 1771–1800 (Toronto: University of Toronto Press, 1979), pp. 276–278.

[129] Barry M. Gough, *First Across the Continent: Sir Alexander Mackenzie* (Norman: U. of Oklahoma Press, 1997) and Barry M. Gough (ed.), *The Journal of Alexander Henry the Younger*, 2 Vols. (Toronto: The Champlain Society, 1988, 1992).

[130] *Askin Papers*, pp. 108–109.

[131] J.I. Cooper, "James McGill", *Dictionary of Canadian Biography*, Vol. V, 1801–1820 (Toronto: University of Toronto Press, 1983), pp. 527–530; *John Askin Papers*, pp. 505–509; Daniel J. Brock, "William Robertson", *Dictionary of Canadian Biography*, Vol. V, 1801–1820, pp. 718–719.

[132] Frese, "The Canadian Canoe", 1999.

[133] *Askin Papers*, Vol. 1, pp. 550–552.

[134] *Askin Papers*, Vol. 1, pp. 134–135; Cleland, *Rites*, pp. 158–159.

[135] *Askin Papers*, Vol. 1, pp. 153–154, 158–159, 165–166, 335–337.

The trade in Indian corn was particularly large and competitive. In one season, in 1799, one Anishinabe group alone had harvested 500 bushels of corn and traded them to the merchants at Detroit. The trade in maple sugar was also significant considering the fact there was no processed sugar manufactured locally and that was available cheaply. The Indian trade was so valuable that white settlers were complaining about it to their governments by the end of the eighteenth century. It was the Amerindian Nations which felt the effects. The Indian trade was a significant part of the economy of the Amerindian Nations which enhanced its diversity, creating richness and bounty.[136]

Even before the War of 1812 there was another threat to the Indian trade. Large American fur trading companies moved into the area to take advantage of it.[137] Nevertheless the Anishinabe trade remained strong well into the nineteenth century and beyond. It was greatly augmented by the increase in the trade of the commercial fishery on the Great Lakes early in the nineteenth century. The backbone of all this trade remained the birchbark canoe well into the nineteenth century. The American, Major Joseph Delafield, in his participation in the survey of the international Canadian-American boundary in the Great Lakes, noted about the trade at Manitoulin Island which was still considerable even in 1820:

> ... It is in the Autumn that the Indians come in to trade their articles and receive their presents. In some seasons they collect here 1,500 & 2,000 strong. Each Indian draws two days' rations besides his presents. They are principally Chippewas and Ottowas [Ottawa]. Formerly other Nations came here from the Mississippi, but they are now taken care of at more neighbouring Posts. In truth the American have brought the Indians within our Territories to trade more generally with us than they did a few years back.
> ... The Sault Ste. Marie is the great fishing ground. Fish have not been taken there yet this season. The Indians have a mode of taking white fish in the rapids of the Sault with what we call a scoop net. They take several at a time. The whites have not the skill. The white fish do not take the hook, are caught in gill nets and seines. The salmon trout & pike take the hook trowling [trolling]. The Indians take them all with the spear. ...

---

[136] *Askin Papers*, Vol. 2, pp. 206–207, 577–578.
[137] David A. Armour, "Alexander Henry", *Dictionary of Canadian Biography*, Vol. VI, 1821–1835 (Toronto: University of Toronto Press, 1987), pp. 316–319; Gough, *Alexander Mackenzie*; *Askin* Papers, Vol. 2, pp. 653–654.

> Shortly after my return, our old Indian messenger, who bro't [brought] the mail comes alongside in his canoe with a fine mess of fish, white fish and trout. He sold us a large white fish that weighed after it was cleaned 7 lb. 11 oz. (it would weigh 10 lbs. before cleaning) for 25 cents.[138]

All of this diplomacy, fishing, mail delivery was done by the birch-bark canoe in 1820.

The significance of the Anishinabe Nations and their presence on the waters of the Great Lakes in canoes was vividly captured by Anna Brownell [Jameson] Murphy, in her classic work *Winter Studies and Summer Rambles*. In July 1836 Jameson lyrically described the waters of Lake St. Clair, part of Bkejwanong: "The bateaux of the Canadians, or the canoes of the Indians, were perpetually seen glid-ing among these winding channels, or shooting across the river from side to side, as if playing at hide-and-seek-among the leafy recesses."[139] Later, on this same tour, she had an exhilarating ride in an Anishinabe birchbark canoe over the St. Mary's Rapids at Sault Ste. Marie.[140] (See Figure 8.5.)

By this time, however, the great Montreal-based fur trade to the far Northwest, even across the divide into the Athabasca country, had gone into severe decline. The era, after several years of extreme competition and violence bordering on corporate canoe warfare, of the Voyageurs (Metis, Mohawk, Ojibwa and French Canadian) ended with the merger in 1821. At this time the stronger North West Company was absorbed by the weaker, but better funded, Hudson's Bay Company. Most of the canoe brigades, supplemented by York boats in the lower reaches of the rivers, would henceforth travel down to and up from York Factory and Fort Churchill on the Bay. Nevertheless, the continuity continued and the birchbark canoe

---

[138] *The Unfortified Boundary, A Diary of the first survey of the Canadian Boundary Line from St. Regis to the Lake of the Woods by Major Joseph Delafield American Agent under Articles VI and VII of the Treaty of Ghent*, eds. Robert McElroy and Thomas Riggs, Privately printed in New York, 1943, pp. 319–320; Cleland, *Rites*, pp. 180–181. John Clarke, "The role of political position and family and economic linkage in land specula-tion in the Western District of Upper Canada, 1788–1815", *Canadian Geographer*, Vol. 19, 1975, pp. 18–34.

[139] Anna Jameson, *Winter Studies and Summer Rambles in Canada* (London: Saunders and Otley, Conduit Street, 1838; Coles Canadiana Collection, Toronto: Coles Publishing Company, 1970, 1972), Vol. 3, pp. 5–6.

[140] Calloway, *The American Revolution in Indian Country*, p. 15.

remained supreme as far as inland travel by both Amerindian and other Canadians in the north country.[141]

After more than four centuries, the pre-eminent place in the Amerindian trade was still held by the birchbark canoe. It still has a special place in the trade in recreation, a form of trade in the twentieth century. The canoe is shown prominently in historical sites, in heritage festivals and re-enactments, at fur trade gatherings and pow-wows in the late twentieth century as part of Amerindian cultures and traditions.[142] Its significance continued, and did not decline, and moreover became an issue in the treaty-making process and the determination of the international boundary in the decades that followed.

The War of 1812–14 and its Aftermath

During the War of 1812–14, along with the famous role played by Tecumseh, Anishinabe warriors, using birchbark canoes, defended the "Indian territory" against another American invasion, assisting in the defense of Upper Canada and thereby the maintenance of it as a colony within the British empire for their English allies. At first the Six Nations tried to remain neutral for the first few months of this War, causing much anxiety among the English military establishment. But soon they were heavily participating in the battle of Queenston Heights and later the battle of Chippewa (where ironically there were Iroquois fighting on the American side).[143] Further west, the Three Fires Confederacy once again rose to the occasion and inflicted early and overwhelming defeats on the Americans using the birchbark canoe as the most important tried and true methods of the speed of forest warfare.

During the summer of 1812, the Ojibwas and Ottawas captured Fort Michilimackinac through a canoe invasion, this was followed by victories in the south at Brownstown, Magauaga, which led to the capture of Detroit in August of that year. Indeed, Detroit fell largely

---

[141] Richard Pope, *Superior Illusions*, and Janet E. Clarke and Robert Stacey, *Frances Anne Hopkins, 1838–1919: Canadian Scenery*, Thunder Bay Art Gallery, 1990.

[142] Frese, "The Canadian canoe", 1999.

[143] Carl Benn, *The Iroquois in the War of 1812*, (Toronto: University of Toronto Press, 1998).

because the American commander, General Hull, both feared the
Indians and believed that he was surrounded by thousands of them.
John Baptist Askin (one of the Metis sons of John Askin, Senior,
then an interpreter in the Indian Department), summed up their
military significance using their canoes:

> ... without the Indians we never could keep this country, and that
> with them the Americans never will take the upper posts, for let them
> send forward as many men as they will, if we employ the ... Indians
> we can have equal number, which is more than is wanted, for in the
> woods where the Americans must pass one Indian is equal to three
> white men.[144]

They also fought successfully at battles at York (Toronto), Beaver
Dam, and Lundy's Lane (Niagara). In spite of the fact that the first
Canadian historian of the War of 1812–14 was an Aboriginal person—a Metis—Major John Richardson, Canadian historians have
failed until recently to give the Amerindian Nations their proper credit for both saving their homelands from the marauding Americans
forces and in safeguarding Upper Canada as part of the British
empire.

Fighting alone when the disgraced General Procter failed him, the
great Shawnee Chief Tecumseh was defeated at the Battle of the
Longwoods (on the banks of Thames River downstream from present-day London) in 1814.[145] His body was taken by his head soldier, Oshwawana (John Nahdee) to Bkejwanong. A monument in
his honour and to all Amerindians who fought in these—and other
wars—still stands overlooking the St. Clair river and the international
border between Canada and the United States which reminds all
visitors of the significant Amerindian role using the birchbark canoe
in this War. (See Figure 8.6.)

Yet the War of 1812–14, a "turntable in Canada's history,"[146]
changed fundamentally the military balance of power in northeastern North America. From the perspective of the English imperial
government, the Amerindian Nations were no longer required as
military allies. The "new" local Indian Department policy of "civilization" which began immediately after the War of 1812–14, became

---

[144] Schmalz, *Ojibwa*, p. 111.
[145] John Sugden, *Tecumseh, A Life* (New York: Henry Holt and Company, 1997),
pp. 355–367.
[146] Dickason, *Canada's First Nations*, pp. 131–32.

a primary factor in the removal attempted assimilation, centralization and "land loss treaties" of the nineteenth century. Simply put, after fighting, yet again, for the English imperial government in that War against the Americans, the Amerindian warriors received medals for their efforts while the white settlers ironically received gratis a considerable part of Amer-indian Territories.[147]

For a number of years after the War of 1812–14 the international boundary remained unsurveyed. The Treaty of Ghent, ratified in 1815, provided a process for the exact determination of the international boundary. After an arduous process in which canoes were used, the survey of the boundary through the Great Lakes was not approved until 1822. After the Treaty of Ghent was ratified in 1815, the Amerindian Nations gathered at Burlington Heights[148] for a Council Fire.[149] This Treaty guaranteed their freedom and independence and clearly included free trade as had always been the case. And this free trade was still being carried on by means of the birchbark canoe.[150] But the English did not keep their promises in these treaties.

In spite of the prominent role played in it by the Amerindian warriors, the War signaled a one hundred and fifty-year decline in the military significance of the "birchbark" Nations in what is now seen as southern Canada—the Great Lakes basin. Yet, the Amerindian Nations—largely thanks to their indomitable spiritual values, of which the canoe is symbolic—have survived and undergone a renaissance as we enter the twenty first century. In Canada's north and west, the canoe and the kayak have remained paramount.[151] The indomitable spirit of Tecumseh remains, like the birchbark canoe, to this day personifying the will of the Aboriginal Nations to resist and survive.

---

[147] Nin.Da.Waab.Jig., *Walpole Island*, pp. 17–26.

[148] This place of Council Fire is currently the site of Dundurn Castle in Hamilton, Ontario—formerly the home of Sir Allan Napier MacNab, a political opponent of John Sandfield Macdonald.

[149] NAC, RG 8, British Military Records, C Series, Vol. 258, Part 1, pp. 60–70a.

[150] NAC, Record Group (RG) 10, Vol. 628, pp. 68–73; Microfilm Reel #C-13, p. 396; McNab, "'What liars those people are': The St. Anne Island Speech of the Walpole Island First Nation given at the Chenail Ecarte River on August 3, 1815", in *Social Sciences and Humanities Aboriginal Research Exchange*, Vol. 1(1), Fall-Winter, 1993, pp. 10, 12–13, 15. Information on Chief Oshwawana, or John Nahdee, as well as a picture of him, can be found in Nin.Da.Waab.Jig., *Walpole Island*, pp. 25–29.

[151] See for one example the use by William Kennedy of the "tin kayak", modeled on his experience among the Inuit, while searching for Sir John Franklin in

Historical Retrospect on the Special Place of the Canoe

The Ojibwa artist from Manitoulin Island, Blake Debassige has observed that the birchbark canoe is a "technological wonder." Such canoes are constructed "out of fragile, natural materials," yet they could carry large loads and withstand surprisingly rough water." And, with "all the traveling that went on during their seasonal movements" during spring, summer and fall, "very few persons lost their lives." The canoe then was indispensable as a form of water transport and communication between Amerindian Nations and between them and the European empires for more than five hundred years of Canada's history.

The coming of European settlement did not reduce the need for the use of the canoe by either Aboriginal and non-Aboriginal peoples. Such a reduction would only come from the buildings of roads on the Indian trails in the nineteenth and twentieth centuries and especially after the Second World War in the northern regions. Even then, this change in the role of the canoe was only true in the south since more than 90% of non-Aboriginal Canadians live within one hundred miles of the border between Canada and the United States.

This can be seen in recent court decisions regarding harvesting Aboriginal and Treaty rights in this geographical area such as the Simon case. Interestingly enough, a high court in New Brunswick (1998), though recently overturned by an Appeal Court, substantiated the right of the Mi'kmaq people to cut timber by a prior right on all of their Treaty lands.[152] These cases, of course, have similar

---

1851–1852, in his *A Short Narrative of the Second Voyage of the Prince Albert in search of Sir John Franklin* (London: W.H. Dalton, Cockspur Street, 1853), pp. 36–37. Kennedy, Cree, Bear clan, was requested by Lady Franklin to command this expedition in search of her husband because of Kennedy's knowledge of the Arctic and canoe transportation and Aboriginal cultures. Kennedy's mother was Aggathas, in English "Mary Bear", a Cree woman from Pine Tree Island at Cumberland House in present-day northern Saskatchewan. Mary Bear was David McNab's great-great-great-great-grandmother on his mother's side of the Kennedy family. William Kennedy was his great-great-great grandfather. See his *Dreaming and Drawing: Autobiographical Fragments of Air and Fire*, with Lang for consideration 2000.

[152] The 1726 Treaty recognized and re-affirmed the Aboriginal rights to the natural resources on and under their Territories. This case unfortunately was overturned on appeal and will not be heard by the Supreme Court of Canada. But other legal cases of a similar nature are currently before the courts. Lumber leases may well continue to co-exist with Aboriginal and Treaty rights unless they are

overtones to recent court decisions in Australia and New Zealand, for example, the Mabo and Wik decision in Australia and the findings of the Waitangi Tribunal in New Zealand.

The economic displacement of Amerindians in the late nineteenth and twentieth centuries in northeastern North America parallels historically the decline of the use of the canoe which was replaced by the coming of other forms of land-based and then air transportation. Yet even then this transformation differed markedly from area to area. In the very south of what became Ontario, in the very heartland of English-speaking Canada, and in the St. John river valley, this process was characterized by its relative lack of violence as these areas saw the expansion of commercial agriculture. For a time, when they were allowed, and some Amerindian communities continue to do so, Amerindians engaged in this economic pursuit.

Further to the north and northwest, from that base on the St. Lawrence and from tiny European posts on James and Hudson Bay, and much later on the Red River, the process of economic displacement did not occur in border reaches until the late nineteenth century. And in the eastern Arctic it did not take place until well into the twentieth century. The canoe, the waterways, both along the inland bays and shores of the oceans and in the interior rivers and lakes—along with the Amerindian trade networks, continued to reign supreme.

In the far North, the significance of the "canoe" has continued down to the present. The skin kayak (in which one sits on the bottom and propels the canoe with a double-bladed paddle) is a part of the generic vessel called the canoe. Indeed, in the Arctic itself, the coastal kayak version of the canoe, the scientific invention of the Inuit, held sway. This canoe was used by the Inuit until the middle of the twentieth century. Could we also perhaps argue that the superior technology of the kayak was at least partly responsible for the emergence today of the Inuit-dominated Territory of Nunavut?[153]

---

superseded by another regime of land tenure which is agreed upon by indigenous peoples and governments. One might well expect and understand the nature of the uproar in 1998 from the private lumber interests and the provincial government in New Brunswick. The Saint John and other major rivers were important in the transition from the indigenous manufacture of canoes to canvas-covered ones used in the lumber trade and for recreation.

[153] *Canadian Geographic*, January–February 1999, Vol. 119 (1), Special Issue on Nunavut: "Nunavut, Up and Running", pp. 37–45, "Return of the Kayak", pp. 58–65.

If so, perhaps the importance of inshore coastal travel by great Arctic expeditions and the explosion in whale-hunting should be integrated into this story where it would share some significant place with the coastal kayak. The Inuit have maintained their autonomy to this day, even though the visitor Martin Frobisher had entered "his bay" as early as 1516. In April 1999 the creation of the autonomous Inuit Territory of Nunavut was one solid indication that resistance has continued unabated and that a new process of historical transformation of self-assertion and autonomy is indeed underway; one which encompasses the past, present and the future marking indeed circles of time.[154]

The canoe has continued to be renowned for its special place and uses in the expanding recreational travel in Canada's north country, covering, as it does, the vast extent of the landscape of Canada.[155] The birchbark canoe flows directly into the Peterborough canoe, the Fredericton-based Chestnut canoe and the Old Town canoes of eastern Maine. The wood-canvas canoe was used widely in the late nineteenth and twentieth centuries, for example in geological surveys and by the Royal Northwest Mounted Police in the North.[156]

For the Aboriginal people of Canada the canoe retains its spiritual character as a celestial craft of souls and a focal point for the four sacred directions. As the artist Michael Robinson has written, a person who "chooses to traverse a landscape by canoe is someone, who embraces the Spirit of our History as a mirror image of our future." It marks one's "moment in time" as well as one's "destination."[157] It helps us to discover whom we are—encompassing as it does the four natural elements of earth, water, air and fire. Metaphorically, in the end, the canoe is a vehicle which enables us to discover a true balance along the way on our inward journey from the natural realm to the world of the spirits. Truly the canoe retains its very special place in Canada's histories and its cultures.

---

[154] McNab, *Circles of Time*, 1999.

[155] Jamie Benidickson, *Idleness, Water, and a Canoe, Reflections on Paddling for Pleasure* (Toronto: University of Toronto Press, 1997).

[156] Hodgins and Margaret Hobbes, *Nastawgan, The Canadian North by Canoe & Snowshoe, A Collection of Historical Essays* (Toronto: Betelgeuse Books, 1985 (1987)), various articles.

[157] Wylie, *In the Wilds*, pp. 26–27.

INDEX

HISTORY
OF WARFARE

History of Warfare *presents the latest research on all aspects of military history. Publications in the series will examine technology, strategy, logistics, and economic and social developments related to warfare in Europe, Asia, and the Middle East from ancient times until the early nineteenth century. The series will accept monographs, collections of essays, conference proceedings, and translation of military texts.*

1. HOEVEN, M. VAN DER (ed.). *Exercise of Arms.* Warfare in the Netherlands, 1568-1648. 1997. ISBN 90 04 10727 4
2. RAUDZENS, G. (ed.). *Technology, Disease and Colonial Conquests, Sixteenth to Eighteenth Centuries.* Essays Reappraising the Guns and Germs Theories. 2001. ISBN 90 04 11745 8.
3. LENIHAN P. (ed.). *Conquest and Resistance.* War in Seventeenth-Century Ireland. 2001. ISBN 90 04 11743 1.
4. NICHOLSON, H. *Love, War and the Grail.* 2001. ISBN 90 04 12014 9

ISSN 1385–7827